T0133759

Fascia, Function, and Medical Applications

Fascia, Function, and Medical Applications

Edited by
David Lesondak
Angeli Maun Akey

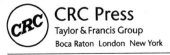

CRC Press
Taylor & Francis Group
Boca Raton London New York

CRC Press is an imprint of the
Taylor & Francis Group, an **informa** business

Cover Photo: Robert Strovers www.robertstrovers.com
Sculpture on cover: Michael Gard www.michaelgard.com

First edition published 2021
by CRC Press
6000 Broken Sound Parkway NW, Suite 300, Boca Raton, FL 33487-2742

and by CRC Press
2 Park Square, Milton Park, Abingdon, Oxon, OX14 4RN

© 2021 Taylor & Francis Group, LLC

CRC Press is an imprint of Taylor & Francis Group, LLC

Reasonable efforts have been made to publish reliable data and information, but the author and publisher cannot assume responsibility for the validity of all materials or the consequences of their use. The authors and publishers have attempted to trace the copyright holders of all material reproduced in this publication and apologize to copyright holders if permission to publish in this form has not been obtained. If any copyright material has not been acknowledged please write and let us know so we may rectify in any future reprint.

Except as permitted under U.S. Copyright Law, no part of this book may be reprinted, reproduced, transmitted, or utilized in any form by any electronic, mechanical, or other means, now known or hereafter invented, including photocopying, microfilming, and recording, or in any information storage or retrieval system, without written permission from the publishers.

For permission to photocopy or use material electronically from this work, access www.copyright.com or contact the Copyright Clearance Center, Inc. (CCC), 222 Rosewood Drive, Danvers, MA 01923, 978-750-8400. For works that are not available on CCC please contact mpkbookspermissions@tandf.co.uk

Trademark notice: Product or corporate names may be trademarks or registered trademarks, and are used only for identification and explanation without intent to infringe.

Library of Congress Cataloging-in-Publication Data

Names: Lesondak, David, editor. | Akey, Angeli Maun, editor.
Title: Fascia, function, and medical applications / edited by David
   Lesondak and Angeli Maun Akey.
Description: First edition. | Boca Raton : CRC Press, 2020. | Includes
   bibliographical references and index. | Summary: "Fascia, Function, and
   Medical Applications is essential reading for medical and allied health
   practitioners who want to bring scientific insights of the importance of
   fascia to human health into their clinical practices, providing the
   knowledge practitioners need to refer or add as an adjunct therapy to
   their department or rehabilitation team"-- Provided by publisher.
Identifiers: LCCN 2020013264 | ISBN 9780367531928 (paperback) | ISBN
   9780367196110 (hardback) | ISBN 9780429203350 (ebook)
Subjects: MESH: Fascia--anatomy & histology | Fascia--physiopathology
Classification: LCC QM563 | NLM WE 504 | DDC 612.7/5--dc23
LC record available at https://lccn.loc.gov/2020013264

ISBN: 9780367196110 (hbk)
ISBN: 9780367531928 (pbk)
ISBN: 9780429203350 (ebk)

Typeset in Times
by Lumina Datamatics Limited

Contents

SECTION I   Fascia

SECTION II   Function

SECTION III   Medical Applications: Interstitial Notes on Section 3
David Lesondak

Preface

Whenever something new appears on the medical horizon, it is wise to approach it with a healthy degree of cautious skepticism. It's endemic to human nature to hype the latest thing as the greatest thing, and this tendency is rife throughout both human history and the history of medicine. Conversely, it is also human nature to reject new information that might seem to threaten the status quo and thus, one's own view of how things work. This is the theory of "identity-protective cognition". It extends beyond individuals and can be more broadly applied to groups composed of diverse individuals who share a common set of values, experiences, or education. We tend to dismiss the evidence, or patterns of evidence, that challenge or threaten to upset the values and beliefs that predominate the group.

For the next 300 pages or so, I'm asking you to suspend those beliefs.

Fascia, that tough and gooey stuff that you were allowed to throw in the garbage during your first year of medical school, has a lot more to do with human health and proper functioning of the body than you were led to believe—if, indeed, you were led to believe anything about it at all.

When the first International Fascia Research Conference was held at Harvard Medical School in 2007, it was convened under the egalitarian ideal that researcher, physician, and clinician all have a place at the table. This same spirit infuses the Fascia Research Society, which evolved as a natural outgrowth of that first fascia congress (now approaching it's 6th iteration in 2021). So too, in this volume, you will hear from physicians, clinicians, therapists, surgeons, dissectors, and researchers. Often these individuals wear more than one hat. Such is professional life on the frontier. All are subject matter experts. It is our collective goal to present you with the most current evidence-based information, clinical impressions, and reasoned, relevant interpretations in the emerging field of fascia science and application.

There was a rather important paper published in 2018, entitled *Structure and Distribution of an Unrecognized Interstitium in Human Tissues.*[1] This paper demonstrated a fluid-filled "inner space" in the body, the boundaries of which are defined by collagen fibers. For the sake of absolute accuracy, let's quote the paper directly:

> We propose here a revision of the anatomical concepts of the submucosa, dermis, fascia, and vascular adventitia, suggesting that, rather than being densely-packed barrier-like walls of collagen, they are fluid-filled interstitial spaces. The presence of fluid has important implications for tissue function and pathology. Our data comparing rapidly-biopsied and frozen tissue with tissue fixed in a standard fashion suggest that the spaces we describe, supported and organized by a collagen lattice, are compressible and distensible and may thus serve as shock absorbers. All of the organs in which we have detected this structure are subject to cycles of compression and distension... The collagen bundles in the interstitial space are lined on only one side by cells, implying that the collagen matrix on the opposite side are in direct contact with interstitial fluid...

---

[1] Benais PC, Wells, RG, Sackey-Aboagye B, et al. 2018. Structure and distribution of an unrecognized interstitium in human tissues. *Sci Rep* 8(1); 4947.

In sum, while typical descriptions of the interstitium suggest spaces between cells, we describe macroscopically visible spaces within tissues—dynamically compressible and distensible sinuses through which interstitial fluid flows around the body. Our findings necessitate reconsideration of many of the normal functional activities of different organs and of disordered fluid dynamics in the setting of disease, including fibrosis and metastasis.

To those of us on the frontier this sounded like another, albeit an even more scientific, description of the tissue and system that we collectively refer to as *fascia*. Furthermore, it hypothesizes profound possibilities beyond making improvements to musculoskeletal disorders. It also points to the potential mechanisms through which broader changes, e.g., positive changes of autoimmune disorders, digestive function, etc. are possible. These sorts of physiological changes, and more, have all been observed by clinicians for decades.

This discovery was hyped in the media as "Science Discovers a New Organ". Of course, fascia is far from new. It's as old as we are. What is new is our understanding of the vital role fascia plays in human health and function, and our ability to study, observe, and draw conclusions based on our research and applications.

Welcome to the frontier!

David Lesondak
University of Pittsburgh Medical Center
Center for Integrative Medicine

Coeditor Preface

In the spring of 2018, I attended a whole-day continuing medical education (CME) workshop at the University of Florida. It was entitled *Fascial Approaches to Low Back Pain*. There, I was pleasantly surprised to meet a very funny, knowledgeable, and well-spoken man with a sonorous "radio voice". His name was David Lesondak, and he had just published a science-based book, *Fascia: What It Is and Why It Matters*. Over the course of the day, he shared his knowledge with us and also showed us ways to practically apply it. That day changed the trajectory of my clinical life.

Many of his slides were of anatomical dissections that presented the human body in ways I had never seen before. I clearly remember thinking that I must have been duped in the gross anatomy lab in medical school. No doubt the lab tech dissected out and "cleaned up" the white tissue, the fascia, in order for us medical students to learn origins and insertions of the muscles. Not to mention how, in retrospect, clearing out the fascia changed my perception in regard to the intricacies of the organs and the circulatory system. The fascia was just garbage in that paradigm of what I now know is "classical" anatomy. Now, thanks to David's class, I understand anatomy from a functional perspective and from that perspective, fascia is gold.

Despite my four board certifications, and 30 years of clinical experience, I had never heard any of this essential material until that fateful day when David Lesondak, one of the world-class educators on fascia, came to my hometown.

And then it took a very personal turn.

The week before I had been struggling with, and feeling incompetent to help, my then 17-year-old son, Derek. Derek is an elite athlete who at the time was a state finalist in discus and held a national record in power lifting. For the previous seven days, he had been complaining of intermittent, left-sided chest pain that was worse with respiration. His symptoms prompted two visits to the emergency room and two visits to the cardiologist. Pulmonary embolus (PE), acute myocardial ischemia, and supraventricular tachycardia were all ruled out. So, with a negative lower extremity ultrasound, normal computed tomography scan of the chest with contrast, echocardiogram, and labs, he was told he had "anxiety" and was sent home. I was very confused. Derek had never been the anxious type, and I felt sure it was PE because he was keeping his knee wrapped from a recent injury.

At the end of the morning CME workshop, David showed an *anatomy trains* arm dissection, and in that moment it all clicked into place. I knew Derek had a fascial injury to his right shoulder, his throwing arm, and due to the *biotensegrity* of the body, another brand-new concept, he was presenting with contralateral chest pain.

I figured that if anyone could help him, David could. At the lunch break I asked if he could treat my son. Being the kind and generous health care professional that he is, he said, "Sure, see if he can come in this afternoon".

After we finished our CME requirements, Derek became the extra credit teaching case for the whole class. David carefully examined my son's posture, checked range of motion of both shoulders, and noted asymmetric upper body relationships. He observed how rigidly Derek held his head with respect to the strain it was causing his cervical spine. Then he performed a series of slow, anatomically specific fascial manipulations with Derek. They were all based on the same principles we just learned for low back pain, just applied to his circumstances. It took about 30–40 minutes.

What I remembered most was that through manipulation on the right side of Derek's body, David elicited the same left-sided pleuritic chest pain of which Derek was complaining. In that moment, I knew that whatever was ailing Derek was musculoskeletal, or more precisely, *fascial* in origin. As a doctor, I was relieved and felt that no further work-up would be necessary. As a mom, I was even more relieved that his severe, intermittent chest pain was non-life-threatening!

David further instructed Derek with specific stretches, and how to become more aware of the motor patterns exacerbating his condition and how to correct for them. He followed through with his homework and simultaneously eliminated caffeine, added moist heat, slept more, and took anti-inflammatory and gut health supplements. Within a few weeks, his chest pain dissipated. As is often the case when multiple interventions are in play, it is hard to isolate which *one* intervention *fixed* the problem. In my professional opinion, however, I would say that the fascial intervention that started that day in class *was* the major component to changing Derek's trajectory of healing in a positive direction.

It sounds like a cliché, but when I think about that afternoon, I always come back to that line from *Amazing Grace*, "I was blind, but now I see", because that's exactly how I felt. I now saw clearly how fascia and its function was of critical clinical importance in understanding and approaching my patients. With this new way of "seeing" I realize that many of the pain syndromes I had seen in my 30-year career (including such diverse clinical settings as the emergency room, hospital, nursing home, internal medicine, and primary care) likely had a fascial component.

In most cases, when the presenting pain syndrome in my patients was deemed non-anatomic (in the classical sense), and the tests failed to show anything of significance, my patients would be labeled with *supratentorial pain* or given a psychiatric diagnosis. In hindsight, I now began to doubt the accuracy of those labels.

After that workshop, I changed. I became obsessed, I guess you could say, with learning everything I could about fascia, fascial syndromes, and all of the possibilities it could mean for human health and wellness. I was happy, even delirious, exploring this new territory I began to think of as "Fascia Land".

The information in this book will mean better care for your patients. Over the last two years, it has meant better care for mine. It is like having a new pair of glasses every time I walk into the exam room.

From my son, Derek, to the 40-year-old surgeon who has had three whiplash injuries from car accidents, to the 30-year-old woman who fell out of a tree at 5 years of age and landed on her left side and presented with chronic, right-sided, hemibody pain, to the 53-year-old woman who had not had coitus since a total abdominal hysterectomy, to the perimenopausal woman who had bilateral forearm aching pain with "pins and needles", to the 22-year-old man with aseptic necrosis of both of his proximal humerus bones due to recurrent steroid use for his autoimmune disease—their treatment plans have all been adjusted to incorporate the role of the fascia and with resultant excellent individual clinical benefits. With my old way of seeing, I could not have even conceived of their unique treatment plans, nor validated the relevancies of their prior experiences simply because *I did not know what I did not know.* Now, I do. Every patient I see, I now see differently.

In a new country, it helps to have a good guide. I remain eternally grateful to David for being my guide, mentor, and, well, my *Sherpa* in exploring Fascia Land. And now, dear reader, you too will benefit from his envisioning and overseeing the creation of this book you now hold in your hands.

Your patients will be grateful that you did.

Angeli Maun Akey, MD, FACP

Acknowledgments

A big thank you to all our authors for their time and devotion to this project.

Special thanks to Ingrid Kohlstadt for getting the ball rolling.

Gratitude also to Anita Boser, Emily Brown, Neilly Buckalew, Jeffery Burch, Melanie Burns, Gary Carter, Rachelle Clauson, Barry Craig, Caroline Cruz, Sarena Davis, Abby Denham, Brad Fullerton, Ginger Garner, Sue Hitzman, Leslie Hoy, Marye Lee, Reshma Mathew, Kayla Montero, Jasmine Nadayil, Laurie Nemetz, Coletta Perry, Noelle Perry, Rebecca Pratt, Hailey Schwab, Erin Sproul, Andrew Stevenson, Josh Summers, and Neil Thiese. You were all crucial to the successful completion of this project.

Extra special thanks to Heidi Patterson, MLIS, who was of great assistance and support to many of the contributors in this volume.

Editors

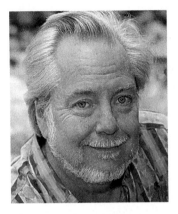

David Lesondak, BCSI, ATSI, FST, VMT, FFT is an Allied Health Member in the Department of Family and Community Medicine at the University of Pittsburgh Medical Center (UPMC). He is the author of the international bestseller, currently in nine languages, *Fascia: What It Is and Why It Matters* (Handspring). He also contributed to the second edition of *Metabolic Therapies in Orthopedics* (CRC Press).

He spent 10 years as "chief documentarian" of the Fascia Research Group at Ulm University, Germany, where he produced over 80 educational videos covering the full spectrum of fascia research. He provided similar services to the Fascia Research Congress in 2012 and directed and coproduced *Anatomy Trains Revealed*, a three-DVD, legacy media set, that takes Thomas Myers' myofascial meridians concept from the page into real-time exploration in the anatomy lab.

David's passion for the science of fascia as well as his excellent communication skills always shine through whether he's lecturing internationally, working through a translator, teaching a workshop, conducting a webinar or giving a podcast interview. Some of David's more notable appearances include the Fascia Research Congress, the Academic Consortium of Integrative Medicine and Health, University of Florida, University of Maryland, University of Arizona, Ulm University's Fascia Summer School program, the STTAR (Science, Technology, Training, Analytics, and Rehabilitation) Summit, the British Fascia Symposium, and the Australian Fascia Symposium as well as privately sponsored, hands-on workshops in the Netherlands, South Korea, and France.

Still, his greatest joy remains working one-on-one with patients at the UPMC Center for Integrative Medicine, where he is the resident Fascia Specialist, and Board Certified Structural Integrator. He focuses on helping individuals resolve chronic pain, improve physical performance (especially post-injury), and deal with pre- and post-surgical issues of all sorts.

David is also an avid songwriter who plays guitar and studies voice.

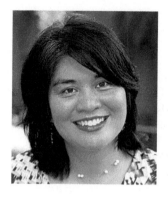

Dr. Angeli Maun Akey, MD, FACP, ABIHM, ABOIM, ABAARM, is board certified in internal medicine, integrative and holistic medicine, and anti-aging regenerative medicine, and has completed additional training in functional medicine. In clinical practice for over 30 years, she is the founding medical director of North Florida Integrative Medicine, Ageless Medical Solutions, and the Palm Beach Institute of Preventive Medicine. Her interests in other healing traditions have led her to teach at the Florida School of Acupuncture and Oriental Medicine. Currently she specializes in early-stage detection, delay, and reversal of chronic diseases.

Dr. Akey's undergraduate experience was at the University of Florida (UF), where she was accepted on five academic scholarships and a vocal performance music scholarship. She graduated Phi Beta Kappa and is a member of the UF Hall of Fame. Also of note is that she was the youngest person ever admitted to the University of Florida's College of Medicine in the Junior Honors Medical Program, where she was accepted to Alpha Omega Alpha and graduated with high honors. Dr. Akey did her internal medicine residency, served as a chief resident and taught as assistant clinical professor at Yale University.

She mentors medical students and pre-health care professionals in the Functional, Integrative, Regenerative, Restorative, Internal Medicine (FIRRIMup) model. An approach to navigating and solving complex medical problems, and promoting whole-person wellness, the FIRRIMup model is described in detail in Dr. Akey's book *Fine-Tune Your Hormone Symphony*. She is also the cofounder of an on-line teaching website, www.FIRRIMupDoctors.com, which teaches this model. A much sought-after speaker at home and abroad, she has taught and presented on the FIRRIMup model in Brazil, the Caribbean, Poland, Spain, Italy, France, and the United States. She lives with her family in her hometown of Gainesville, Florida, USA.

Contributors

Angeli Maun Akey, MD, FACP, ABIM,
ABAARM, ABIHM, ABOIM
University of Florida College of
Medicine
and
North Florida Integrative Medicine
Gainesville, Florida

Daniel Akins, LMT, BCSI
Private Practice
Portland, Oregon

Keith Baar, PhD
Department of Neurobiology,
Physiology & Behavior
and
Department of Physiology and
Membrane Biology
and
School of Medicine
University of California
Davis, California

Anita Boser, BCSI, CHP
Private Practice
Washington, DC
and
President, Ida P. Rolf Research
Foundation
Boulder, Colorado

Rachelle L. Clauson, BS, CMT, BCTMB
Private Practice
San Diego, California

James Earls, MSc
Born to Move
London, United Kingtom

Richard Finn, BA, PTS, CMTPT,
LMT, MCSTT
Private Practice
Pittsburgh, Pennsylvania

Chris Frederick, PT, ATSI
Stretch to Win Institute
Chandler, Arizona

Julie Hammond, ATSI
Anatomy Trains Australia &
New Zealand
Fermantle, Western Australia
and
Bodywork Education Australia
Perth, Western Australia

Nancy Keeney-Smith, LMT, MLD
Private Practice
Gainesville, Florida

David Lesondak, BCSI, ATSI, FST,
VMT, FFT
Department of Family and Community
Medicine
and
Center for Integrative Medicine
University of Pittsburgh Medical Center
(UPMC)
Pittsburgh, Pennsylvania

Jill Miller, C-IAYT, YA-ERYT
Tune Up Fitness Worldwide
Los Angeles, California

Thomas W. Myers, BCSI, ATSI
Anatomy Trains
Walpole, Maine

P. J. O'Clair, NASM-CPT
Praxis Performance & Wellness
Beverly, Massachusetts

Kathleen O'Neil-Smith, MD, ABIM
Treat Wellness
Newton, Massachusetts

Michael Polon, CAR
Private Practice
Denver, Colorado
and
Rolf Institute Faculty
Boulder, Colorado

Catherine Ryan, RMT
Private Practice
British Columbia, Canada

Dr. biol. hum. Robert Schleip,
Dipl. Psych.
University Institute of Health Sciences
(IUCS Barcelo)
Buenos Aires, Argentina
and
Conservative and Rehabilitative
Orthopaedics
Department of Sport and Health
Sciences
Technical University of Munich
Germany

Kirstin Schumaker, BA, BCSI, ATSI
Anatomy Trains Neurovascular Release
Certification Program
Private Practice
Portland, Oregon

John Sharkey, MSc
University of Chester
Chester, United Kingdom

Antonio Stecco, MD, PhD
Rusk Rehabilitation
New York University School of Medicine
New York, New York

Carla Stecco, MD
Human Anatomy and Movement
Science
University of Padua
Padua, Italy

Danielle Steffen
Biochemistry, Molecular, Cellular and
Developmental Biology
University of California
Davis, California

Jaap van der Wal, MD, PhD
Anatomy and Embryology (retired)
University of Maastricht
Maastricht, the Netherlands

Section I

Fascia

1 De Fabrica Humani Corporis—Fascia as the Fabric of the Body

Jaap van der Wal

CONTENTS

> Fascia is the fabric of the body; not the vestments covering the corpus, but the warp and weft of the material.

Stephen M. Levin, 2012

It was five centuries ago that Andreas Vesalius opened the eyes of the Western world to the way in which we, as modern people, still view ourselves and the world analytically and scientifically. His publication, *De Fabrica Humani Corporis*, represents nothing less than the birth of anatomy as a basic science, and as a basic attitude of modern medicine.

The word *fabrica* has several meanings: *factory* (building, construction); *fabric* (textile, weaving); and *structure* (organization, construction). There is little doubt that when choosing *Fabrica* for the title Vesalius did not think in terms of textiles or materials, but as the metaphor of the building.[1] He made that abundantly clear when he titled his atlas *About the Construction of the Human Body*. And thus, he ushered in the age of modern anatomy.

The anatomical mindset of today is still heavily influenced by the work of Vesalius (Figure 1.1). That mindset considers the human body to be something built from discrete parts and is sorely in need of an update. It is imperative that we come to embrace a new and more holistic view of the human organism in order to truly and fully understand the anatomy of fascia.

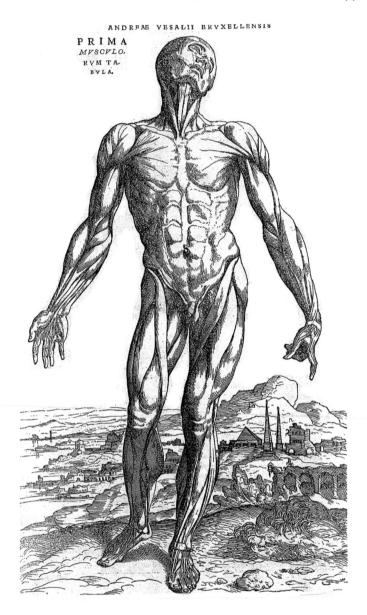

FIGURE 1.1   Classical muscle man/person engraving by Vesalius. (Courtesy of Wellcome Library.)

We must move beyond the mere building blocks concept to a deeper examination of the architecture—the structure—of the body. In so doing, we can examine, and come to fully appreciate the relationships between the so-called parts and elements of the body and their criticality. Such an updated view begins with a shift in thinking of *Fabrica* in the sense in which orthopedist Stephen Levin (a founding father of biotensegrity) meant when he described fascia as "the fabric of the body".[2]

WHAT IS IN A NAME?

Before moving on, let me be perfectly clear, this shift in thinking in no way diminishes the scientific genius of Vesalius.[3]

However, it is not surprising that the centuries of dissection research have shown the anatomical plates of Vesalius to be somewhat outdated. The paradigm that our bodies are made up of the organs and parts that the anatomists describe is still alive and kicking—as are the images of Vesalius burned on the retina of modern man and almost indelibly planted in our brains (Figure 1.1). For example, anyone who thinks of the musculoskeletal system sees the Vesalius muscle man/person. But in fact, this image is an artifact. The fundamental method of the anatomist is dissection—a process that disassembles the *whole* into *parts*.

This perhaps explains how the connective tissue, the fascia, has become the stepchild of medical anatomy. Even in the 2005 edition of *Gray's Anatomy*, fasciae are identified as "masses of connective tissue units large enough to be visible to the unaided eye". It continues: "In general collagen fibers in fascia tend to be interwoven and seldom show the compact, parallel orientation seen in tendons and aponeuroses".[4] It is the anatomist who has assigned parts to the connective tissue continuum that others call the fascial system.[5,6] In doing so, they create fasciae as anatomical structures related to body walls or regions (*fascia colli media*), organs (*fascia renalis*), or body parts (*fascia cruris or fascia lata*). Thus, the names of fasciae are almost always topographically related to either anatomical units or organs (*parts*). The names say nothing about the functionality—they are based solely on topographical anatomy.

The growing body of evidence supports the move away from thinking about fasciae as discrete anatomical elements and toward the definition of fascia as a system (a "whole").[5,7] Schleip puts it as follows: "Fascia is the dense irregular connective tissue that surrounds and connects every muscle, even the last myofibril, and every single organ of the body, forming continuity throughout the body".[8]

In his book *Fascia: What it is and Why it Matters*,[9] David Lesondak writes: "While I agree that embalmed cadaver fascia can appear as interesting as wet insulation, I do wonder if the very act of so very casually disregarding the connective tissue sets up an unconscious bias toward minimizing its importance". His rhetorical conclusion: "Does dissective exploration lead to dissective thinking?" Following this line of thought, is something such as the traditional "muscle person" merely then an artifact—something we made with our scalpels and our brains? Is it logically consistent to first divide the body into parts, tissues, and organs and then look for another tissue or organ that holds the body together as a whole? Or, in more philosophical terms, do Whole and Parts even belong to similar categories?

In functional anatomy the musculoskeletal *system* is still often thought of as a complex construct of separate elements (bones) connected by (hinged or non-hinged) joints that are moved by muscles that attach to the bones, innervated by a central nervous system. This construct can be questioned on both functional and physiological grounds. Moreover, would an anatomical concept such as the "musculoskeletal system" even survive a deeper reevaluation of the principles of anatomy?

ANATOMY AND ARCHITECTURE

Experiments in the 1990s at the University of Maastricht questioned the existence of ligaments in the elbow joint—at least in the way they are usually described as collagenous connective tissue structures that run from bone to bone.[10] A connective tissue-saving dissection was performed starting in the region of the elbow joint. The collagenous dense connective tissue that exists in this region as fasciae—inter- and intramuscular septa, aponeuroses, and tendons and so on—was made visible in its context and continuity in this dissection. Evidence showed that many of these connective tissue structures did not exist as discrete elements.[3,11,12]

As an example, the fascia antebrachii, like the fascia cruris, may be dissected as a separate anatomical structure, but such a discrete unit does not actually exist. In order to create it, one must break the continuity with hundreds of muscle fibers that attach proximally in the forearm, to this envelope of epimysium, or fascia. At that point, the epimysium is not an enveloping membrane at all, but an aponeurosis of regular, dense connective tissue along which the muscle fibers reach the humerus. The fascia is also continuous with intramuscular septa between the various forearm muscles. However, distally in the forearm, the fascia antebrachii is of a completely different nature. Here the fascia does function as a sort of enveloping sheath. The loose-meshed, fibrillary connective tissue beneath the fascia antebrachia creates a space between the underlying muscle and tendons where movement and gliding are possible.

Later in this chapter it will be argued a primary characteristic of fascia is that it may *connect* as well as *separate*. Fascia makes movement possible by creating spaces and fissures, for one example, between two skeletal elements. Fascia also creates relationships between adjacent muscles, and between muscle(s) and periosteum. These relationships both govern and influence the tensile forces of movement regionally and throughout the body as a whole.

It should be noted that connective tissue-saving dissections create a different type of artifact. Fascia dissected into individual "parts" can only be properly understood if the *relationship* between the connective tissue septa and layers and adjacent muscles is already known. It may come as no surprise that these relationships can only be seen and determined during the dissection procedure itself. In other words, one must know the architecture of the fascial system. Architecture is different from anatomy. Anatomy informs us *where*. Architecture tells us *how*.

How matters. Anatomical representation alone is insufficient. In anatomical atlases the muscle person is represented as a collection of discrete muscles. Likewise, a representation of the fascia person as a construct of layers, septa, aponeuroses, etc. existing as a separate model of isolated layers, could have the same shortcoming. Relationships between the two would be missing in such representations. The anatomy of "parts" must be supplemented with an architecture of force-controlled relationships between different anatomical elements.

This is now even inserting itself into *Gray's Anatomy*:

> From a morphological point of view, most anatomy books have described the skeletal muscles of the human body as being discrete activators with clear origins and insertions (van der Wal 2009). Recent analysis of published anatomical cadaveric studies

have challenged this assumption revealing that the active components of the locomotor system are directly linked by fibrous connective tissue.[4]

NOT *IN PARALLEL* BUT *IN SERIES*

The traditional approach of the anatomist has led to the idea that around a joint there exists a connective tissue construct called a capsule, as well as ligaments, that preserves the continuity between the skeletal elements. In this model the ligaments are passive collagenous connective tissue elements whose fibers are supposed to run from bone to bone, providing stability during movement only in certain positions of the joint. But is this anatomical model correct?

Anatomists think from outside to inside—from superficial to deep. On the outside (in the anatomical arrangement), above and parallel to those ligaments, the muscles function as joint-stabilizing units. This concerns the so-called shunt action of the muscle which, in contrast to the ligaments, maintains the continuity of the joint in a more dynamic manner. This would mean that the muscle is in continuous tone and can tension itself in all positions of the joint and thus dynamically transmit the tensile forces around it.

When connective tissue-saving dissection protocols are followed, it appears all too often that ligaments do not exist in objective, architectural reality but, rather, emerge as an artifact of the dissection process itself. This is explained by the example of the supinator muscle in Figure 1.2. Figure 1.2a shows the traditional anatomy: the joint capsule (blue) is reinforced by ligaments (yellow). In this example the latter are the collateral ligaments as well as the ligamentum annulare (considered as a kind of connective tissue ring), that would stabilize the head of the radius relative to the ulna. Once the ligaments are dissected away from the muscles and their connections severed; however, the shape of their respective layout forms a sort of *geometrical*

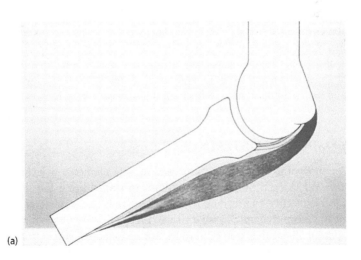

(a)

FIGURE 1.2 (a) Represents the capsule (blue) with ligaments (yellow) organized *in parallel* to the superficially situated muscle tissue. (*Continued*)

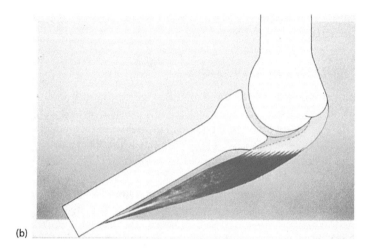

(b)

FIGURE 1.2 (Continued)   (b) Represents the capsule (blue) with periarticular connective tissue (yellow) organized *in series* with the muscle tissue.

parallelism. The muscles form a longer, outer layer in respect to the joint, and the ligaments form a shorter, inner layer. Thus, the muscles provide a dynamic positional control throughout the whole range of motion of the joint while constantly adapting and maintaining their tension or tonus in what is referred to as concentric and eccentric contraction, respectively. Meanwhile the inner ligament layer only passively controls joint stability, i.e., at the extremes of the range of motion when the ligaments are tightened.

Figure 1.2b shows the situation as it becomes visible with the connective tissue-saving dissection. The muscle fibers of the parallel and more superficially situated muscles (in this case the supinator muscle) appear to be organized in series with the periarticular connective tissue. The muscle fibers in this way attach to the epicondyle of the humerus via a system of epimysial and intermuscular layers of connective tissue. In the case of the supinator muscle, for example, the ligamentum annulare does not exist at all as an isolated structure but, rather, appears to run as a layer of connective tissue *in series* with the muscle fibers of the supinator muscle.

LET'S EXAMINE THE DIFFERENCES

Figure 1.2a shows the connective tissue and muscle elements working geometrically *in parallel* to each other when it comes to transmitting tensile forces and providing joint stability. In this model the connective tissue is relatively static compared with the more dynamic muscle tissue. Figure 1.2b represents a much more logical situation where the "outer" muscles are no longer in geometric parallelism to the "inner" (or deeper) connective tissue attachments across the joint. Rather, the muscles are now geometrically consecutive/serial or *in series* with the periarticular connective tissue. This allows them to form a morphological *dynament*, if you will, that functions by simultaneously providing a different mix of passive (periarticular connective tissues) and dynamic (muscle fibers) stiffness depending on the situational needs. A dynament can put the periarticular connective tissue under tension in all positions of the joint, functionally transmitting force *and* stabilizing the joint.

For years I have struggled with the idea that muscles are contractile organs. From physiology to embryology there are good arguments to help understand muscle tissue as a tissue that can both lengthen *and* shorten[13] and thereby view the muscle as a more dynamic form of connective tissue.[14] I propose designating the dynament as a new element in the construction of the Posture and Locomotion System (PLS)—not as a morphological, nor anatomical, nor (neuro) physiological unit, but as a hypothetical architectural unit. Here the notion PLS is preferred for reasons that will become clear—"system" instead of "apparatus" because the anatomical apparatus (consisting of bones, joint and ligaments, and muscles) is too narrow a concept. The nervous system should be incorporated in order to have a functioning PLS. Posture and locomotion because locomotion alone is not adequate. In humans, standing in equilibrium (posture) is typical and essential, keeping one's upright position is integral part of our bipedal locomotion. The notion "musculoskeletal system" will be shown in this text as a reductionistic concept.

The dynament consists of a zone of muscle tissue that is organized in series on both sides with connective tissue structures, or fascial units. These fascial units can manifest themselves as intermuscular septa, or muscle-covering epimysium, or intramuscular tendons (Figure 1.3a and b). In the example of elbow and forearm used here, the force-transmitting architecture is proximally organized *trans*-muscularly and distally *intra*-muscularly (in separate muscles). The architectural *How* relationships are here like warp and weft to the anatomical/topographical *Where* relationships.

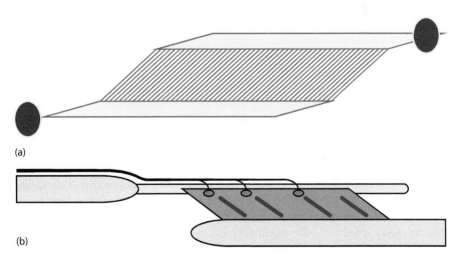

(a)

(b)

FIGURE 1.3 (a) Shows a schematic of a *dynament*, or dynamic ligament. (b) Shows that a *dynament* can be similar in organization to a unipennate muscle.

BIOTENSEGRITY—PULLING TOGETHER AND PUSHING APART

The tissue mix inside the dynament enables it to provide different proportions of passive and active stiffening/tensile force transfer, depending on the morphological priorities of a functional context related to posture and locomotion. It may therefore be seen as the force-transmitting, flexible cable element of what is now called a *biotensegrity* system. In the traditional biomechanical model of the musculoskeletal system (or PLS), the bones are joined by connective tissue structures, creating hinged/non-hinged joints that can be moved and positioned by active muscles.

In the classic architectural tensegrity model the rigid elements (struts) are suspended in a network of more-or-less flexible contiguous (sometimes continuous) cables. A biotensegrity system integrates both tension and compression—pulling together and pushing apart. The entire PLS can be considered a biotensegrity system, with the skeletal elements pushing outward (expansion) and the force-transmitting myofascial elements doing the inward pulling actions (compression). One could also characterize the tensional members as being responsible for the "togetherness" of the organism, whereas the compression members provide the "apartness" within the unity of the organism. In other words, a "sea of tension in which the rigid elements are suspended"[15] ensure the stability of the whole. The opposite, i.e., islands of compression in an ocean of tension, is also applicable. Biotensegrity systems are always about the relationship between the anatomical elements. A dynamic biotensegrity model is created if we replace "cables" with dynaments.

In the biotensegrity model, the relationships between the constituent elements can be constantly adjusted. On a gross anatomical level, in such a system, the tension and compression (pull and push) are transmitted by the dynaments and the skeletal elements respectively. This is how I think the ideal construction of a PLS is created. Then locomotion is not conceived as a movement of body parts but, rather, as a continuous positioning in space of the body as a whole—a lightning-fast change and adaptation of the spatial planning across the entire body.

The dynament is shown schematically in Figure 1.3a. The red striped zone is the central muscle tissue element/unit shown with yellow connective tissue structures on both sides (in series to the muscle tissue) and attached to the skeletal element (black circle). In terms of organization, the dynament resembles a unipennate muscle (Figure 1.3b). From this basic model all possible units can be conceived and represented where two skeletal elements are connected in such a way that, in each position of the joint, the relevant dynament can both give stability and transmit force (dynamic shunt operation). Figure 1.4a–e shows these options.

Whether the so-called locomotor apparatus (or PLS) is viewed as a biomechanical anatomical construct or as the architecture-based biotensegrity system also determines how the organization of proprioception is interpreted. It has been shown that the spatial organization of the morphological substrate of proprioception in the narrower sense (i.e., the mechanoreceptors in the muscle and connective tissue of the PLS) does not follow the anatomical relationships of bones, muscles, ligaments, and joints but, rather is organized around architectural, force-governing relationships.

(a)   (b)   (c)   (d)   (e)

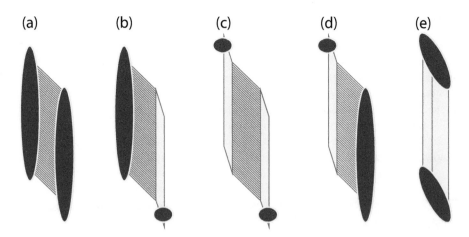

FIGURE 1.4   (a) Represents the extreme situation in which no separate connective tissue structures are needed, per se, and the muscle fibers adhere to the periosteum of both bones involved. (b) Represents an intermediate situation where muscle fibers adhere directly to the periosteum on one side and on the opposite side through a connective tissue structure (tendon, aponeurosis, septum, or fascial layer). (c) Represents the ideal template for a dynament: one connective tissue structure/layer (e.g., fascia, aponeurosis, septum, tendon) adheres to a proximal bone (higher in the graphic), and the other connective tissue structure/adheres to the distal bone (lower in the graphic). In between the two dense collagenous connective tissue structures there is an intermediate zone of muscle tissue (muscle fibers). (d) Represents the mirror intermediate situation of (b), where muscle fibers adhere to bone through a connective tissue structure, while on the opposite side, muscle fibers adhere directly to the periosteum. (e) represents the other extreme situation of a dynament, i.e., a dynament without intermediating muscle tissue between the connective tissue layers or structures. In this case, a dynament acts as a static tensile forces transmitting structure, in other words as a 'classical' ligament.

Perhaps in this respect the brain is not very interested in muscles and joints per se but, rather, in force transmission and movement relationships. In this context it also makes sense that all of the mechanoreceptors (muscle spindles, Golgi tendon receptors, etc.) are for detecting the variable tension or compression role that the same anatomical element of connective tissue can play, depending on the functional context. Perhaps the traditional dichotomy of joint receptors versus muscle receptors should be replaced by a "trans-anatomical" spatial arrangement in which the architecture of the muscle and connective tissue is instrumental for proprioception (instead of the anatomy of discrete anatomical elements of the muscle person).[3]

There are also researchers who argue that muscles and bones can also be considered specializations of fascia.[2,16] Would this mean that we have to distinguish a fascia in the narrower sense and a fascia in the broader sense? With the former being a complex of layers and structures that form a continuity with each other[8,17] and the latter being a kind of matrix–connective tissue–fluid continuum that forms the morphological substrate of our proprioceptive and interoceptive innerness?

ON THE ORIGIN OF FASCIA

We have seen that the traditional approach of dissecting discrete structures does not provide an appropriate basis for describing the functional architecture of the fascia in its continuity and connectivity. Perhaps we may find better answers to the question of "What is fascia and why does it matter?" by exploring where the fascia, the fascial system, and the connective tissue arises in embryonic development.

"Each being can only be understood from its becoming", is the way the German biologist Ernst Haeckel summarized the importance of the embryological science. Knowing how a certain organ or structure came about, simply tells more about what it is.[9] From the phenomenological stance, the functional meaning of forms is more important than their causal explanation. So, here the question of the origin of fascia will be: "Where does fascia come from? How is fascial body matrix shaped and what, if anything, does that tell us?"

In embryology the question "Where does it comes from?" usually leads to the so-called germ layers.[18] In human development these three germ layers appear in approximately the third week after conception.[19] In common embryology germ layers are regarded as *morphological organ-forming units* from which the various tissues and organs develop, resulting in a functioning organism. In most textbooks the three primary germ layers are referred to as ectoderm, mesoderm, and endoderm (some-times mentioned as ectoblast (or epiblast), mesoblast, and endoblast (or hypoblast).

Embryology textbooks usually summarize which germ layer gives rise to which organs and which tissue types. Nowadays it is no longer possible to trace every organ or tissue to a certain germ layer—almost every organ is at least a mixture of several germ layer derivatives. Despite these nuances, however, the germinal layers are still generally regarded as constituting elements of the body, supporting the idea that the body is built up from these three components. Like cells and organs, germ layers are considered building blocks. Under this model, we start as a fertilized egg that undergoes the process of cell multiplication and growth that forms the parts and the organs and the end result is the body.

In a phenomenological view on development, however, we do not start as a cell but, rather, as a zygote. A zygote is the first (unicellular) manifestation of the (human) body—not a cell but an organism that is constantly organizing itself into cells, and via those cells differentiating into organs and tissues. The embryo demonstrates this by the phenomenon of morphogenetic fields. In the developmental biology of the early twentieth century, a *morphogenetic field* is a group of cells able to respond to discrete, localized biochemical signals, leading to the development of specific morphological structures tissues. (This definition should not be confused with the extended view of this hypothesis as propagated by Sheldrake.)

Blechschmidt refers to them as kinetic metabolic fields—meaning that, within the embryo, new metabolic fields are constantly emerging in which the cells, con-trolled both by and in response to a changing environment, differentiate into new types of cells. In this view, the body is not the product of the parts but, rather, is a self-organizing, self-assembling organism, maintaining its unity throughout all those different fields and differentiations.[20] This is a lifelong process. The body is a performance in time.

THE MESODERM, OR MESO

From an embryological perspective, if one looks for the primeval fascia, one almost inevitably ends up with the mesoderm. The first appearance of the mesoderm is the mesenchyme. In the third week of human development, the bilaminar germinal disc (ectoderm and endoderm) is transformed by the process of gastrulation into a trilaminar disc. It is at this point that the mesoderm emerges. This tripartite or threefold organization is a biological necessity for the development of every animal or human body.

Applying the epitheton "-derm" to the name of all three components implies three more-or-less equivalent constituent elements of the human body. Histologically, however, this appears not to be the case. *Gray's Anatomy* underscores that it is not correct to consider the trilaminar disc as being constituted of three epithelial layers.[4] The ectoderm and endoderm clearly have the character of an epithelium. However, the mesoderm manifests itself as a connective tissue—the *mesenchyme*.[21] The German embryologist Erich Blechschmidt is emphatic that the primordial organization of a human body is already emerging at this point in embryonic development (Figure 1.5).[13]

In other words, this means we now deal with a body that can be described not as three equivalent elements but, rather, as two boundary layers and an intermediate "layer" of *inner tissue*. One could say the trilaminar disc is about an animal organization plan: the adult is characterized as existing in an anatomical and psychosomatic "inner space" between two body walls—broadly speaking, the outer parietal

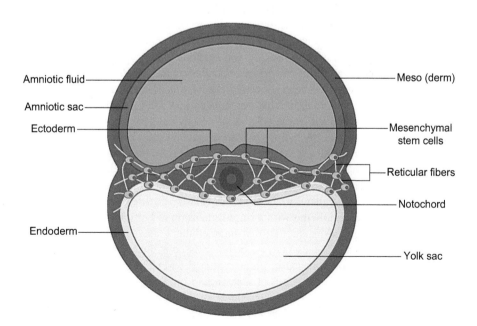

FIGURE 1.5   The human embryo. (Adapted from Lesondak, D., *Fascia: What It Is and Why It Matters*. Used with permission from Handspring Publishing, LTD.)

body wall from which the limbs and head develop; and the inner, visceral body wall from which the gut and its derivatives develop. Hence, the terms ectoderm and endoderm are accurate. They are the substrate of the skin, body walls, and boundaries. However, in this paradigm, the term meso*derm* no longer makes sense because mesenchyme is quite a different quality of tissue altogether: connective tissue. Here one can or should speak of "inner tissue" (in German: *Innegewebe*). Therefore, the term "meso" is applied here to emphasize that the trilaminar disc it is not a matter of three layers but, rather, of a three-part or triune body with an inner dimension of "meso" and with mesenchyme as the tissue of Innerness. Thus, we arrive at a completely different perspective that can also provide a new and special dimension to our understanding of fascia. In Blechschmidt's view, all cells are always kinetic or metabolically linked to each other through the transport of substances:

> There are cells that absorb nutrients from the environment or from neighboring cells and mutually attract each other through this physical absorption of substances. On the other hand, they also exert mutual rejection by producing and shedding metabolic by-products. This constant interaction between uptake and excretion, between attraction and repulsion is a condition for cells to organize themselves in relation to each other and thereby to bring about certain forms. "Limiting tissue" forms the boundary between fluid on the one hand and the inner tissue on the other. While the inner tissues are surrounded on all sides by boundary tissues and therefore permanently "on the inside"—that is: IN the body. Inner tissue can therefore also be described as undifferentiated connective tissue (mesenchyme).[21]

This model applied to the human body may give us a different view of the "inner" dimension. The organs that are usually described as viscera can therefore be considered as a body wall that limits us to the outside world and enables mainly metabolic and material interaction with that outer environment. The designation "inside" is therefore meant in this context literally and anatomically, it is an inside body wall. The "outside" body wall forms our parietal boundary to the world. This body wall also relates us to the outside world and allows a different kind of interaction with it: perception and action. One could argue that our "anatomical" (but also our psychological) interior is the space created by the original mesenchymal connective tissue, or meso. In this "inner", all organs, including the ectodermal and endodermal derivatives, plus those that can be understood as derivatives of the meso, are thus embedded. The mesenchyme, the original primal connective tissue, is the matrix tissue. It creates fasciae in broadest sense, forming the fabric of our body in which the organs are embroidered.[14]

Broadly speaking, it therefore is not three "blasts" or three "derms" but, rather, two limiting tissues (epithelia) with a third dimension in between them. While epithelia are characterized by the fact that intercellular space is virtually absent, the absolute characteristic of mesenchyme or inner tissue is the existence of interstitial space between the cells—the extracellular matrix (ECM). The ECM or *interstitium*[22] can be filled or formed by all kinds of substances from interstitial water, to cartilage substance, to calcified bone matrix and more. It always contains a third dimension, namely, *fibers* of all possible nature and quality. In this way, concepts such as fascia, connective tissue, matrix, and inner space are all congruent if not essentially the same. It is thus possible to conceive that meso and thus fascia represents the matrix, or *fabric* of our body organization.

MESENCHYME: CONNECTING AND SHAPING SPACE

In the previous quote from Blechschmidt, reference is made to intake and excretion, attraction and rejection as principles of interaction between cells. These principles of relationship can also be attributed to fascia, mesenchyme, and connective tissue. Mechanically, histologically, embryologically one can think of two different types of interactions in the mesenchyme, namely connecting and separating (or creating space). These two dimensions then have all kinds of histologic and physiologic appearances and display the principles of biotensegrity, namely pulling together and pushing apart.

If the cell component of the mesenchyme becomes dominant, then the cells, and thereby the mesenchyme, condense largely into cellular agglomerations. This is the case, for example, in fat or muscle tissue. The cells form a parenchyma embedded in a fibrous matrix. "… [remove] the parenchyma of muscle cells from the muscle tissue and you get a band or ligament".[2]

The opposite, shedding cells (in Blechschmidt's jargon), could then be recognized as the ability of the mesenchyme to create body cavities. Consider the pleural cavities or peritoneal cavity. Both of these membranes are often histologically described as mesothelium—an epithelium formed by mesenchyme (connective tissue). The essential difference is that the mesothelium defines and creates the interstitial space. Epithelium usually defines an outside wall or a lumen of a tube. Also, if the sliding movement is compromised, the mesothelial layers will tend to stick and adhere to each other. With a so-called body cavity such as the oral cavity, covered with epithelium, that tendency will not be as pronounced.

Perhaps, instead of thinking of these as cavities, we should think of them as "joint fissures"—places where two organs, or a body wall and organ, encounter each other but can still move against each other. One could rightly consider this the precept of creating a space that also makes movement possible.

Apply the concept of creating and connecting space to fascia in a broader context—namely, the *tensional network*[17] or system that is present everywhere in the body and that forms a network in which all organs and structures are both interwoven and embedded. This is the mature representation of our mesodermal innerness and primary mesenchymal framework of the body with regulatory roles on multiple functional levels.[6]

In a narrower sense, fascia is also the subcutaneous collection of anatomically recognizable connective tissue structures that connect, support, and enclose muscles, bones, nerves, blood vessels, and organs in the form of layers, membranes, laminae, and envelopes.[7,8]

Given these two characteristics of fascia, a picture emerges that meso (mesenchyme) can both densify, connect, and contract. It can also decentralize, stretch, and create space. These polar tendencies in the connective tissue can also be seen in the different qualities of interstitial substances as well as in different relationships between fibers, cells, and interstitium. Hence, most anatomy textbooks speak of fascia as a supportive *and* connective tissue.

Consequently, there are good arguments to consider body cavities and joint clefts as functions of fascia. The superficial fascia is a subcutaneous, loose connective tissue with a lot of interstitial space between the fibers. The functional principle here is focused on separating, creating space and enabling motion,[23] similar to tendon and muscle sheaths, and bursae. For intermuscular septa, the "classical" fasciae, such as epimysia, fascia lata, thoracolumbar fascia, etc. connect and guide tensile forces. In these cases, the appearance of the fascia is quite different. The fibers are denser with little room for interstitium or cells. This is the fascia we typically see in the PLS.[3,7,8]

It may also be the interstitial substance of mesenchyme that forms this mechanically connecting and separating dimension. Consider cartilage in this context. Cartilage types include the tough, chondrocyte-laden fibrous cartilage; elastin rich elastic cartilage (comprising much of your ear); and the collagen type II-rich, glasslike hyaline cartilage. Cartilage may provide relatively flexible structure and creates forms, like your ear. Cartilage can also serve motility by creating space, as is the case in the fissures of the synovial joints. It can also be seen in the formation of fissures in symphyses and in the intervertebral discs.

The interstitium is the third dimension of fascia and mesenchyme. It comprises a vast inner space that can be found everywhere between organs and tissue elements. It could be regarded as one continuous inter-anatomical body cavity along which chemical transport, communication, and organization are possible by means of various cellular substances.[22,24] From embryology we know that signaling proteins are organized and distributed via the mesenchyme. During human embryonic development the meso provides the metabolic conditions for the development of the ectodermal structures and plays a role in their differentiation.[21] Perhaps even epigenetic control molecules could be established via diffusion through the interstitial space.

BLOOD IS CONNECTIVE TISSUE

Mesenchyme is associated in the embryo with the formation of blood and blood vessels. Contrary to popular belief, blood is a tissue and not a fluid. Blood is categorized in many histology textbooks as supportive or connective tissue. The primary manifestation of blood is mesenchyme (via the formation of blood islands and blood strands) in which capillary vessels are formed. The capillaries transport "liquid tissue"—i.e., blood cells. The vast network of capillaries (estimates vary from 60 to 90,000 km) likewise creates what is typical of connective tissue—the blood connect the organs and create space between them in a dynamic, physiological way.

Blood vessels, often as neurovascular bundles, play a role in the shaping of the body. In the development of the embryo, strands of connective tissue surrounding a vascular structure may function as a restraining structure, providing resistance and biomechanical constraint to growth with flexure, or "flexion growth", if you will, as consequence. This may be observed in developing limbs or in the formation of pharyngeal arches.[13] The widespread presence of capillaries throughout the body also reinforces the idea of fascia in a broader sense as the matrix in which all organs are woven and embedded. Blood and fascia take the shape of the body, one might say, and literally create the web in which everything is both connected and separated.

FASCIA—THE "ORGAN OF INNERNESS"

All this is a logical consequence of the idea that fascia coincides with the meso or mesenchyme. Furthermore, I can't help but think that the concept of mesenchyme as inner tissue may lend credence to the very nonscientific concept, first espoused by Dr. Andrew Taylor Still, that fascia may constitute the space of the soul. He wrote: *"The soul of man, with all the streams of pure living water, seems to dwell in the fasciae of his body"*.[25]

While such speculations are far beyond the scope of this chapter, the goal here is to show that fascia in a broadest sense may be the literal representation of our inner being.

REFERENCES

1. Garrison, D.H. 2016. Why did Vesalius title his anatomical atlas "The Fabric of the Human Body"? In: *Transforming Vesalius*. Basel, S. Karger, A.G. (eds.). http://www.vesaliusfabrica.com/en/original-fabrica/inside-the-fabrica/the-name-fabrica.html
2. Levin, S.M. 2018. Bone is fascia. *Research Gate*. https://www.researchgate.net/publication/327142198_Bone_is_fascia
3. van der Wal, J.C. 2009. The architecture of the connective tissue in the musculoskeletal system—An often overlooked functional parameter as to proprioception in the locomotor apparatus. *International Journal of Therapeutic Massage and Bodywork (IJTMB)* 2(4): 9–23.
4. Standring, S. 2005. *Gray's Anatomy: The Anatomical Basis of Clinical Practice* 39rd/41st ed. Edinburgh: Elsevier Churchill Livingstone.
5. Adstrum, S. et al. 2017. Defining the fascial system. *Journal of Bodywork & Movement Therapies* 21(1): 173–177.
6. Stecco, C. 2015. *Functional Atlas of the Human Fascial System*. 1st ed. Warren I Hammer DC MS. London: Churchill Livingstone.
7. Stecco, C. 2016. A fascia and the fascial system. *Journal of Bodywork & Movement Therapies* 20: 139–140.
8. Schleip, R. et al. 2012. What is "fascia"? A review of different nomenclatures. *Journal of Bodywork & Movement Therapies* 16(4): 496–502.
9. Lesondak, D. 2017. *Fascia: What It Is and Why It Matters*. Edinburgh: Handspring Publishing Limited.
10. van Mameren, H. 1983. Reaction forces in a model of the human elbow joint. *Anat Anz* 152: 327–328.
11. van Mameren, H., Drukker J. 1984. A functional anatomical basis of injuries to the ligamentum and other soft tissues around the elbow joint: Transmission of tensile and compressive loads. *International Journal of Sports Medicine* 5: 88–92.
12. van der Wal, J.C. 1988. The organization of the substrate of proprioception in the elbow region of the rat [PhD thesis]. Maastricht, the Netherlands: Maastricht University, Faculty of Medicine.
13. Blechschmidt, E. 2004. *The Ontogenetic Basis of Human Anatomy*, 1st ed., edited and translated by Brian Freeman. Berkley, CA: North Atlantic Books.
14. Levin, S.M., Martin D.-C. 2012. Biotensegrity—The mechanics of fascia. In: *Fascia—The Tensional Network of the Human Body*, Section: 3.5 Biotensegrity, The mechanics of fascia. Schleip, R. et al. (eds.), 137–142. Edinburgh: Churchill Livingstone.
15. Myers, T.W. 2014. *Anatomy Trains: Myofascial Meridians for Manual and Movement Therapists*. Edinburgh: Churchill Livingstone.

16. Sharkey. J. 2019. Regarding: Update on fascial nomenclature—an additional proposal by John Sharkey. *Journal of Body Work and Movement Therapies* 23(1): 6–8.

17. Schleip, R. et al. (eds). 2012. *Fascia—The Tensional Network of the Human Body.* Edinburgh: Churchill Livingstone.

18. Sadler, T.W. 2019. *Langman's Medical Embryology*, 14th ed. Philadelphia: Wolters Kluwer.

19. Moore, K.L., Persaud, T.V.N. 2016. *The Developing Human—Clinically Oriented Embryology.* Philadelphia: W.B. Saunders Company.

20. Blechschmidt, E. 2011. *Die Frühentwicklung des Menschen—Eine Einführung.* München: Kiener Verlag.

21. Blechschmidt, E., Gasser, R. 2012. *Biokinetics and Biodynamics of Human Differentiation.* Berkley, CA: North Atlantic Books.

22. Theise, N.D. et al. 2018. Structure and distribution of an unrecognized interstitium in human tissue. *Science Reports.* March 27.

23. Guimberteau, J.C., Armstrong, C. 2015. *Architecture of Human Living Fascia: The Extracellular Matrix and Cells Revealed through Endoscopy.* Pencaitland, UK: Handspring Publishing.

24. Oschman, J. 2015. *Energy Medicine: The Scientific Basis.* London: Churchill Livingstone.

25. Lee, Paul R. 2005. *Interface. Mechanism of Spirit in Osteopathy.* Portland, OR: Stillness Press.

2 Fascial Anatomy

Carla Stecco

CONTENTS

INTRODUCTION

The vital role of the fascial system in maintaining and restoring proper function of the human body is being increasingly recognized by health care professionals. Knowledge of the fascial system's characteristics and functions is spreading from primary medical researchers to professionals in many health fields throughout the world. This includes doctors, therapists, and sports trainers who regularly treat soft tissue injuries and dysfunction. Understanding how the fascia works is even altering the way people are working out in the gym by changing the structure of their work-out regimen. Both superficial and deep fascia within the body can be treated with manual methods directly or indirectly and also with instrument-assisted modalities. Therapists in many areas are developing techniques to treat fascia and integrating it into their rehabilitation protocols. Surgeons are beginning to take connective tissue into account as an integral part of surgical procedures in order to promote wound healing, scar reduction, and tissue restoration. Now that fascial anatomy has been thoroughly researched, this knowledge must be integrated into our fundamental understanding of human anatomy.

Testut[1] and Chiarugi[2] wrote anatomy texts that included some analysis of fascia. However, the majority of anatomy researchers have considered fascia to be connective tissue that only filled the empty spaces of the body. So, in most contemporary anatomical studies, fascia is not new, but rather finally being understood as a functioning tissue and important to understanding the kinetic system.

Researchers are hampered by terminology that is not standardized.[3,4] In 1983, the International Anatomical Nomenclature Committee developed a classification system for all connective tissue structures. This nomenclature includes superficial and deep fascia. Under the superficial fascia is the deep fascia, or fascia profundus. The deep fascia is a denser and firmer type of tissue than the superficial fascia.

In 1998, the Federative Committee on Anatomical Terminology (FCAT)[5] proposed different terms. FCAT is still the highest authority for the nomenclature of anatomical terms. Their proposal was that the fascia should be described as "sheaths, sheets or other dissectible connective tissue aggregations". Different layers were also renamed.

In 2015 in Washington, DC, during the 4th Fascial Research Congress, many different opinions were expressed. Leading fascial researchers and clinicians presented and discussed the newest research in their areas of interest. Finally, a consensus definition of the fascia was reached:

> fascia is a sheath, a sheet or any number of other dissectible aggregations of connective tissue that forms beneath the skin to attach, enclose and separate muscles and internal organs.

A more functional definition was also defined for a general fascial system. Research groups are now making substantial progress toward the goal of creating new and useful fascial terminology. The new terminology will include both anatomical and functional aspects of the fascia[4] (Figure 2.1).

To understand the function and architecture of the fascial system, it is important to understand its composition. Fascia must be understood first and foremost as connective tissue (textus connectivus) (FCAT, 1998). Each fascial layer is distinct in

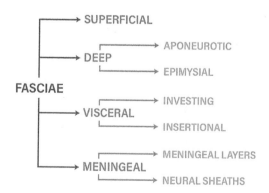

FIGURE 2.1   Classification of the human fasciae.

important ways from each other. Each layer has its own orientation and composition. For example, superficial fascia is loosely packed and irregular, whereas deep fascia is a well-organized fibrous layer.

SUPERFICIAL FASCIA

The superficial fascia (fascia superficialis) is a membranous layer of connective tissue formed by loosely packed interwoven collagen fibers mixed with abundant elastic fibers. Thicker in the trunk, it gradually becomes thinner in the limbs. The superficial fascia is connected to the skin by the *retinaculum cutis superficialis*, which presents vertical and thick collagen septa. It also connects with the deep fascia through the *retinaculum cutis profundus*, which presents loose oblique, very elastic collagen septa. The region between the skin and superficial fascia that includes the superficial retinacula cutis is called superficial adipose tissue (SAT), while the one between superficial fascia and deep fascia is called deep adipose tissue (DAT). Both impart the subcutis with specific mechanical proprieties.

The superficial fascia is homologous to the cutaneous muscle layer (panniculus carnosus) found in other mammals. Indeed, even in the human, muscle fibers can be found in the superficial fascia, particularly in the neck (referred to as the platysma muscle), in the face (the superficial muscular aponeurotic system, or SMAS), in the anal region (external anal sphincter), and in the scrotum (the dartos fascia). Functionally, the superficial fascia can participate in the integrity of the skin and provide support for subcutaneous structures. Furthermore, within the superficial fascia, many nerve fibers can be observed. On bony prominences and at some ligamentous folds, the superficial fascia adheres to the deep fascia. In some regions, the superficial fascia splits, forming special compartments, particularly around major subcutaneous veins and lymphatic vessels, with fibrous septa that extend out to attach to vessel walls. For example, the main superficial veins reside within the superficial fascia that splits into two sublayers to envelop these veins. The adventitia of these veins is connected with the superficial fascia by thin ligaments, ensuring their patency and preventing displacement of veins during movement.

THE DEEP FASCIA

The deep fascia can be divided into the aponeurotic and epimysial fascia according to orientation, composition, and architecture. Aponeurotic fasciae are formed by two to three layers of parallel bundles of collagen fibers. Each layer is separated from the adjacent one by a thin layer of loose connective tissue (Figure 2.2).

Aponeurotic fasciae envelope and connect whole groups of muscles. It covers the extremity muscles and includes both the thoracolumbar fascia (TLF) and the rectus abdominal sheath (RAS) in the torso. Epimysial fasciae covers and adheres to the whole muscle and can be used to refer to all the intramuscular connective tissue, which includes the epimysium, perimysium, and endomysium. Because it is so intertwined with the muscle tissue, it is not possible to separate the epymysial fascia from the muscle. It is in continuity, and the function of one is strongly dependent

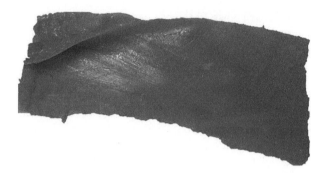

FIGURE 2.2   A sample of fascia lata in formaldehyde fixation. It is possible to see the different directions of the collagen fibers on the right side. On the left, two of the three layers are separated to show the interface.

on the other. In the extremities and in some parts of the trunk, such as the TLF and RAS, the aponeurotic fascia slides over the epimysium that covers the muscle and continues around the tendon (epitenon). Both epimysial fascia and epimysium proper transmit the force of the muscle to the surrounding areas thanks to myofascial expansions, but they have different thickness. Epimysial fascia is thicker, between 0.5 and 0.9 mm, whereas the epimysium is thinner, less than 0.1 mm. Both aponeurotic fasciae and epimysial fascia transmit the forces of muscle contraction. Closely associated with the epimysium is the perimysium, which covers the muscle fiber bundles and is in continuity with the endomysium located around every single muscle fiber.

Overall, the thickness of the deep fascia ranges from 0.5 to 1.8 mm.[4] Of particular importance is the scapula girdle and hip girdle, where the epimysial fascia and the aponeurotic fascia come together. The aponeurotic fascia can be represented as a long glove or sock that covers the superior and inferior limbs. The aponeurotic fascia splits at the inferior and lateral border of the gluteus maximus, merging the epimysial fascia over the muscle. In the anterior part of the aponeurotic fascia lata, the three layers of fascia split to include the three abdominal muscles, becoming, once again, epimysial fascia. A similar transformation occurs at the shoulder girdle. The epimysial fascia of the pectoralis major, deltoid, and latissimus dorsi merge into the brachial fascia to transmit force in the upper limbs.

This sophisticated anatomical arrangement allows the force of the trunk muscles to move different segments of the limbs. Smeulders et al.[6] proved that 37% of muscular attachments are connected to a fascial layer, not to the bone or tendon. Mechanical force transmission occurs when muscular tension is applied to fascia via myofascial expansions. These expansions work like a ship's sail, when it is pulled to one corner it gives the ship direction and force to move. In the human body, an example of this continuum is from the anterior part of the deltoid muscle toward the biceps brachii muscle. Fascia of biceps brachii forms the lacertus fibrosus (Figure 2.3), which covers the part of the forearm flexor attached to the aponeurotic deep fascia.

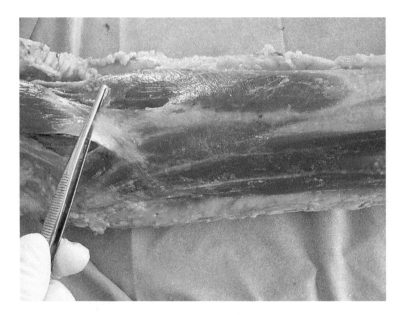

FIGURE 2.3   The lacertus fibrosis.

THE RETINACULA

As in the lacertus fibrosus, there are other areas of thickening in deep aponeurotic fascia like the retinacula. The term *retinaculum* is derived from Latin "retinere" (to restrain) or "rete" (a net). Retinaculum has been described as a structure that restrains an organ or tissue in place or as a network of collagen fiber bundles that form a cross pattern. Topographically, they are connective tissue bundles located near joints such as the knee, ankle, elbow, and wrist. They resemble ligaments, but composition and function differ. Ligaments bond two bones together and have a resistant structure, with fibers that are arranged along a more uniform line of traction, acting as a support structure for joints. Retinacula are actually reinforcements of the deep fascia attaching to capsules (bones), muscles, and tendons, fusing with the superficial fascia.

Similar to aponeuroses, retinacula consist of collagen fibers arranged in layers with each layer oriented in a different direction. A retinaculum is a network or grid of collagen fibers arranged according to multiple lines of traction that, at the same time, slide independently from one another. Smooth sliding of retinacula layers is extremely important for proper proprioception and pain reduction.

From a classical point of view, retinacula are described as a passive type of tissue. The most commonly known retinacula are in the wrist and ankle areas. Since the time of Vesalius (1543),[7] retinacula have been designated as pulley systems for tendons, or lately, as a load–shear system. If retinacula were just a tendon holder, why does it have such a complex structure? The complexity of its architecture reveals a functionally complex action. A reinvestigation of anatomy demonstrates that retinacula are not only passive stabilizers or pulley systems.

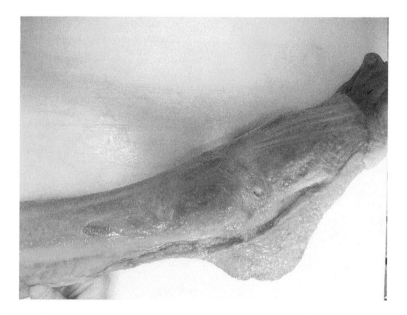

FIGURE 2.4   The ankle retinaculum.

Contrary to classical understanding, retinacula should be seen as a specialized proprioceptive organ that perceives joint movement (Figure 2.4).

Retinacula are a three-layered structure containing layers of collagen fibers that are able to glide independently from one other within the ground substance. Another interesting fact about retinaculum anatomy is its innervation. Retinacula are the most highly innervated fascial tissue, rich in free nerve endings and Ruffini and Pacinian corpuscles. Obviously, this structure is much more than a passive stabilizer.

Based on our studies, retinacula act as a specialized fascial reinforcement for local proprioception of joints. Retinacula have connections to muscle and bone, which makes them able to sense both bone movement and muscular contraction. While retinacula do have a connective tissue system, allowing them to have a stabilizing role, their complex multilayered structure and rich innervation better supports the idea of a proprioceptive-like organ than just a passive stabilizing system.[8]

1. The superior retinacula of the extensor muscles of the foot are situated at the inferior third of the leg where tendons do not require retinacula support as they might under the inferior retinaculum.
2. If the only role of the inferior retinaculum of the foot were that of a restraint, then all of its fibers would be inserted onto bone, instead of many of its fibers continuing with the posterior fascia.
3. Around the knee, the patellar retinaculum and the popliteal retinaculum do not maintain any tendons close to the bone.
4. In the wrist, the transverse carpal ligament restrains the flexor tendons, while the flexor retinaculum is effectively independent and slides over the ligament.

The retinaculum of the ankle is a structure that researchers have attempted to define in various ways (Figure 2.4). C. Stecco[8] studied 27 dissected ankles. In this study, magnetic resonance imaging scans were performed *in vivo* to 7 healthy subjects: 17 with sprained ankles and 3 with limb amputation. The study demonstrated the retinaculum of the ankle is a reinforcement of the deep fascia. This may explain why so many authors define this structure in different ways. The retinaculum of the ankle is a dynamic structure, and stress makes it stronger and thicker. Thus, after an ankle sprain it is crucial to restore its function. In addition, examination should ascertain what other structures might be involved via the leg (crural) fascia extending toward the limbs and pelvis (fascia lata).

THE VISCERAL FASCIA

The Terminologia Anatomica[9] defines the visceral fasciae as "a generic term for the fascia which lies immediately outside the visceral layer of the serosae together with that which immediately surrounds the viscera". In a general sense it is a structural component that refers to the connective tissue covering the organs, muscles, and the pelvic side wall. Historically, ligaments have been defined as a condensation of this fascia. On dissection "fascia" appears white and it is often assumed that this is a purely collagenous layer. Biopsies of ligaments, "fascial" layers of the vagina, and the attachments between organs all show the same results: collagen, elastin, smooth muscle, blood vessels and nerves; albeit in different proportions. There are also well-defined fascial connections with different viscera. The rectovesical fascia, for example, is a membranous layer that connects the prostate, the urinary bladder, and the rectum and covers the seminal vessels. It has been demonstrated that fasciae support the interconnections between the viscera, providing not only a proper isolation but, at the same time, guarantee the appropriate motility of the organs. Additionally, the visceral fascia connects various organs with the muscles of the trunk. They are capable of force transmission and, in particular, of regulating possible imbalances that could interfere with the normal motility and mobility of the organs. As a result, sometimes organs from different systems can reflect different dysfunctions at the same time.

Accordingly, in the normal healthy state, the visceral fasciae are relaxed and can stretch and move without restriction, but physical trauma, scarring, infection, or inflammation can alter their pliability. They may become tight, producing pain or restriction of motion of the organs.

CONNECTIVE TISSUE

The basic composition of connective tissue contains three components: cells, fibers, and ground substance.

CELLS

Cells provide the metabolic properties of biological tissue. Fibroblasts produce collagen fiber types I and III, while other intercellular materials [such as glycosaminoglycans (GAGs)] are produced by fasciacytes, hyaluronan-secreting cells.[10] Adipocytes (adipose or fat cells) are found in the connective tissue. The adipose cells can be divided into white (unilocular cells) and brown fat cells (multilocular cells). Overall, fat cells store energy and they are extremely important for insulation,[11] as interstitial fillers, and for facilitation of gliding.

FIBERS (COLLAGEN, ELASTIC)

The fibers provide the mechanical properties of the connective tissue. The fibers have the power to transfer force generated by muscle cells, and they seem to get stronger and thicker when tensional stress is applied.[12,13] There are two types of fibers in connective tissue: collagen fibers and elastic fibers. Collagen is the main structural protein in the connective tissue. The name *collagen* comes from the Greek κόλλα (*kólla*), meaning "glue", and the suffix -γέν, -*gen*, denoting "producing". A collagen fiber's lifespan varies depending on its collagen types. To describe the length of the life of a collagen fiber, researchers use the term "turnover time" to indicate a biogeochemical cycle. It is a measure of how long it takes to fill or empty a particular nutrient reservoir. The human collagen turnover time has been estimated from 300 to 500 days. In animal studies, the rate differs. For instance, rat collagen fibers turnover time varies even more: intestine 20 days, liver 30 days, muscles 50 days, tendon 110 days.[14] The metabolism of the rat is much faster than the human (estimated seven to ten times), therefore those findings are not comparable to human subjects.[15]

There are many types of collagen, and almost 90% of the collagen of the muscles can be found in the perimysium.[16,17] Although there are parallel collagen fibers in the deep fascia, there are other layers that have different fiber orientation. This allows force transmission to occur in a variety of multidirectional planes.[18,19] Also, mechanical load and tension increase collagen synthesis and make it more resistant to load stress.

Elastic Fibers

Elastin fibers are thinner than collagen fibers and they create a three-dimensional network around collagen fibers. Elastin is a protein that gives collagen the ability to tolerate stretch and distension. Elastic fibers and collagen fibers are not parallel. They lie across one another and/or spiral around one another so that they form a three-dimensional interacting superstructure, which gives final strength and elasticity to the whole tissue matrix.[4,20]

GROUND SUBSTANCE

Ground substance provides viscosity and plasticity to the tissues. The ground substance is composed of water and GAGs (glycosaminoglycans). Ground substance itself is a gel-like material including extrafibrillar matrix, but no collagen or elastin fibers. In other words, the collagen and elastin fibers create the previously mentioned three-dimensional network, and the ground substance surrounds and fills the empty spaces. GAGs are long-chained polysaccharides attached to a core protein of the proteoglycan. Several different groups of GAGs have been identified. The most common are: hyaluronan, chondroitin-sulfate, dermatan sulfate, and heparan sulfate (Figure 2.5). Extra cellular proteins stabilize the aggregates of proteoglycans and

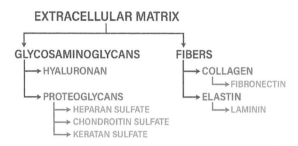

FIGURE 2.5   The composition of connective tissue.

together form a "bottle-brush-like" structure. GAGs have a negative charge and this attracts water, forming a hydrated gel. This gel is responsible for turgidity and visco-elasticity as well as for controlling the diffusion of various metabolites.[4,12]

Hyaluronan (HA) is the most common GAG in the loose connective tissue. It is not a typical GAG because it has no sulfate group and it has a very long and rigid construction. HA provides moisture for the skin and creates the ability of muscles, tendons, and fascia to move against one another. HA also participates in the wound healing process.

Primarily, HA acts as a lubricant, protecting normal tissue viscosity and allowing the fascial layers to glide upon one another. It exists in all connective tissue from the periosteum to the skin. In the musculoskeletal system, HA is ubiquitous, especially between the layers of the aponeurotic fascia, between the deep fascia and muscles, in the loose connective tissue surrounding muscle bundles, and within the intra-muscular fascial layers. HA also serves an important function in both perivascular and perineural areas. In the perivascular areas, especially around veins, and in the perineural areas around nerves, the normal properties of HA are necessary to allow adequate gliding on these structures. This relationship is similar to the relationship between deep fascia and muscles. Without adequate gliding, there is the potential for nerve entrapment and vascular inhibition.

INNERVATION OF THE FASCIA

Fascial architecture of the nerve is similar to the fascial architecture of the muscle. The nerve trunk is surrounded by epineurium, and the fascicles are surrounded by perineurium. Collagen fibers surround and are attached to the capsules of corpuscles and free nerve endings. The main sensory receptors in the musculoskeletal system are the proprioceptors, usually referred to as mechanoreceptors. Tissue function determines the amount of receptors in different parts of the body. The type of mechanical force transmission that is necessary in different parts of our body determines the number of mechanoreceptors that will be available. Mechanoreceptors are integrated into the fascial system. Many studies demonstrate the importance of mechanoreceptors in the fascial layers, especially highly innervated are the superficial layers of the deep fascia.[12,21–23]

Free nerve endings and Ruffini and Pacinian corpuscles are present within the fascial layers. The amount of free nerve endings, which can also sense temperature, mechanical stimuli, and nociception, may be up to seven times more numerous than other mechanoreceptors. This furthers the importance of fascia as a sensory system.

Ruffini corpuscles, or endings, and Merkel discs are slow adapting touch receptors. They are responsive only to prolonged stimuli. Merkel discs are abundant in the fingertips, hands, lips, and external genitals. Ruffini endings lie deep in the dermis, ligaments, tendons, and fasciae. Ruffini corpuscles are most sensitive to stretch resulting from muscle movement, particularly movement in the limbs or digits. Meissner corpuscles are rapidly adapting touch receptors that react at the onset of a stimulus. They also are located in hairless skin. Pacinian corpuscles react to pressure against a broad area as opposed to a localized touch area. They are rapidly adapting receptors and are located in the dermis and subcutaneous tissue, tendons, and joints. Ruffini and Pacinian corpuscles are also present in deep fascia and retinacula.[7]

Together with the retinacula, the superficial and intermediate layers of the deep fascia are the most highly innervated.[22] The superficial tissues are rich in free nerve endings. These nerve endings are aligned perpendicularly to the collagen fibers, so stretching the muscle and fascia stimulates these receptors easily. Free nerve endings act as sensory receptors. In addition to pressure, they react to temperature, tickle, itch, and some touch sensations. A percentage of free nerve endings transmit pain.

Some studies show that pain from the fascia can be even more aggravating than pain from the muscles. People use different words to describe pain. Fascial pain is usually described as a stabbing, irritating, stinging, or beating sensation, whereas muscle pain is described as a more dull and aching type of pain.[24] This indicates that different anatomical locations can produce different sensory feedback. A skillful therapist can make use of this during a diagnostic examinations.

MUSCLE SPINDLES

Another important neural element in connection with the fascial system are the muscle spindles. They are located in the periphery of the muscle in direct connection with the muscle connective tissue. Muscle spindles are part of the perimysium.[25] And are composed of intrafusal fibers and noncontractile connective tissue. The intrafusal fibers provide tension to the spindle in order to maintain tautness and are therefore sensitive to stretch across a wide range of muscle. Motor unit contraction can be activated via efferent gamma impulses resulting from the stretch reflex mechanism (gamma loop).

Another important function of muscle spindles is the pre-activation of the motor units. When a muscle contracts, two motor nerves from the central nervous system are involved: the alpha motor neuron, which is responsible for the muscle contraction, and the gamma motor neuron, whose main responsibility is to activate (in this case stretch) the spindle cell. It is hypothesized that activation of the intrafusal fibers will contract the capsule of the muscle spindle that will stretch the adjoining perimysium and epimysium. Deformation of the spindle cell capsule stimulates the annulospiral (flower spray) endings of the Ia fibers and type II fibers, all of which generate input to the spinal cord. If no peripheral or central inhibition occurs, activation of the alpha motor neuron will take place. This activation will generate the contraction of the extrafusal fiber of the motor units, creating what is called a gamma loop, essentially a feedback loop that regulates muscle tension.

The gamma loop is just one function of the spindle. Muscle spindles also have excitation and inhibition generating properties. They can activate motor units that are suddenly necessary or deactivate ones that are no longer required. This function of creating quick adjustments is called *indirect enhancement.*

Indirect enhancement means that muscle spindles can add impulses coming down from central neural pathways and thereby increase potential for full activation via the alpha pathway. Quick adjustment means that the spindle can reduce the alpha motor neuron output and reduce the number of motor units activated, if necessary. In this way, muscle spindles are working like light dimmers, controlling how much light you have in the room, and potentially throughout the house.

Tension of the perimysium can affect the function of the muscle spindle. Abnormal tension can create dysfunction in the force generation system through the fascial layers. Because spindles are adhered to intramuscular fascia, fascial dysfunctions can alter the normal function of the spindles. Tensional changes in the fascial system can alter spindle's ability to react, and because of that, it may lead to motor control dysfunction.

SUMMARY POINTS

1. The pivotal role of the fascial system in maintaining and restoring proper function of the human body is being increasingly recognized.
2. Now that fascial anatomy has been more thoroughly researched, this knowledge must be integrated into our fundamental understanding of human anatomy. For example, surgeons are beginning to take connective tissue into account as an integral part of surgical procedures in order to promote wound healing, scar reduction, and tissue restoration.
3. Researchers are hampered somewhat by terminology that is not standardized. Research groups are now making substantial progress toward the goal of creating new and useful terminology that will include both anatomical and functional aspects of the fascia.
4. The basic composition of connective tissue contains three components: cells, fibers, and ground substance.
5. Fascia is highly innervated, particularly with proprioceptive nerves, making it a complex sensory system as well as a tissue.

REFERENCES

1. Testut L, Doin O. 1895. *Traité d'anatomie humaine*, in French, 3th ed., rev., corr. et augm.
2. Chiarugi G, Bucciante L. (eds.). 1975. *Apparecchio muscolare*. Istituzioni di anatomia dell'Uomo, Vallardi Soc Ed Lib, Milano.
3. Schleip R, Jäger H, Klingler W. What is "fascia"? A review of different nomenclatures. *J Bodyw Mov Ther.* 2012;16(4):496–502.
4. Stecco A, Busoni F, Stecco C, Mattioli-Belmonte M, Soldani P, Condino S, Ermolao A, Zaccaria M Gesi M. Comparative ultrasonographic evaluation of the Achilles paratenon in symptomatic and asymptomatic subjects: An imaging study. *Surg Radiol Anat.* 2015;37(3):281–285.

5. Federative Committee on Anatomical Terminology (FCAT). 1998. Stuttgart: Georg Thieme Verlag. ISBN-10: 3-13-114361-4. ISBN-13: 978-3-13-114361-7. 300 pp.

6. Smeulders MJ, Kreulen M, Hage JJ, Huijing PA, van der Horst CM. Spastic muscle properties are affected by length changes of adjacent structures. *Muscle Nerve.* 2005;32(2):208–215. PubMed PMID: 15937875.

7. Vesalius A. 1543. *De humani corporis fabrica* libri septem. Basel: Johannes Oporinus.

8. Stecco C, Macchi V, Porzionato A, Morra A, Parenti A, Stecco A, Delmas V, De Caro R. The ankle retinacula: Morphological evidence of the proprioceptive role of the fascial system. *Cells Tissues Organs.* 2010;192(3):200–210.

9. *Terminologia Anatomica* (TA) is the international standard on human anatomic terminology. It was developed by the Federative Committee on Anatomical Terminology (FCAT) and the International Federation of Associations of Anatomists (IFAA) and was released in 1998.

10. Stecco C, Fede C, Macchi V, Porzionato A, Petrelli L, Biz C, Stern R, De Caro R. The fasciacytes: A new cell devoted to fascial gliding regulation. *Clin Anat.* 2018;31(5):667–676.

11. Drake R, Wayne Vogl A, Mitchell ADM, 2015. *Gray's Anatomy for Students*, 3rd ed. Philadelphia, PA: Churchill Livingstone.

12. Schleip R, Muller D. Training principles for fascial connective tissue: Scientific foundation and suggested practical application. *J Bodyw Mov Ther.* 2013;17(1):103–115.

13. Magnusson SP, Langberg H, Kjaer M. The pathogenesis of tendinopathy: Balancing the response to loading. *Nat Rev Rheumatol.* 2010;6:262–268.

14. Gerber G. Studies on the metabolism of tissue proteins. 1. Turnover of collagen labeled with proline UC-14 in young rats. *J Biol Chem.* 1960;235:2653–2656.

15. Carano A, Siciliani G. Effects of continuous and intermittent forces on human fibroblasts in vitro. *Eur J Orthod.* 1996;18(1):19–26. PubMed PMID: 8746174.

16. Müller WEG. The origin of metazoan complexity: Porifera as integrated animals. *Integr Computational Biol.* 2003;43(1):3–10.

17. McCormick RJ. The flexibility of the collagen compartment of muscle. *Meat Sci.* 1994;36(1–2):79–91. doi:10.1016/0309-1740(94)90035-3. Elsevier.

18. Purslow P. Muscle fascia and force transmission. *J Bodyw Mov Ther.* 2010;4:411–417.

19. Benetazzo L, Bizzego A, De Caro R, Frigo G, Guidolin D, Stecco C. 3D reconstruction of the crural and thoracolumbar fasciae. *Surg Radiol Anat.* 2011;10:855–862.

20. Kannus P. Structure of the tendon connective tissue. *Scand. J. Med. Sci. Sports.* 2000;10(6):312–320.

21. Stecco C, Gagey O, Belloni A, Pozzuoli A, et al. Anatomy of the deep fascia of the upper limb. Second part: Study of innervation. *Morphologie.* 2007;91(292):38–43. PubMed PMID: 17574469.

22. Schilder A, Magerl W, Klein T, Treede RD. Assessment of pain quality reveals distinct differences between nociceptive innervation of low back fascia and muscle in humans. *Pain Rep.* 2018;3(3):e662.

23. Tesarz J, Hoheisel U, Wiedenhöfer B, Mense S. Sensory innervation of the thoracolumbar fascia in rats and humans. *Neuroscience.* 2011;194:302–308.

24. Schilder A, Hoheisel U, Magerl W, Benrath J, Klein T, Treede RD. Deep tissue and back pain: Stimulation of the thoracolumbar fascia with hypertonic saline. *Schmerz.* 2014;28(1):90–92.

25. Boyd-Clark LC, Briggs CA, Galea MP. Muscle spindle distribution, morphology, and density in longus colli and multifidus muscles of the cervical spine. *Spine* (Phila Pa 1976). 2002;27(7):694–701.

3 The Fascial Net Plastination Project

Rachelle L. Clauson

CONTENTS

OVERVIEW

In January 2018, the Fascia Research Society, Somatics Academy, the Plastinarium, and Body Worlds (Figure 3.1) collaborated to form the Fascial Net Plastination Project (FNPP). This international effort of over 50 scientific advisors, academic supervisors, and volunteer dissectors is headquartered at the Plastinarium laboratories in Guben, Germany. The goal of this three-year project is to create the first three-dimensional, full-body plastinate that highlights fascia and the fascial system. The resulting specimen will first be displayed at the Sixth International Fascia Research Congress in Montreal, Canada, in 2021, after which it will become part of the Body Worlds permanent collection. Some of the early proof-of-concept plastinates were first shown at the Fifth International Research Congress in Berlin, Germany, November 2018 in *Fascia in a NEW LIGHT: The Exhibition*.[1] Six of the specimens from that collection are now a part of the Body Worlds permanent exhibits in Berlin and Heidelberg (Figure 3.2).

In this chapter we will discuss how the fascial system as a body-wide network is lacking representation in mainstream anatomy education, the emergence of fascia in the

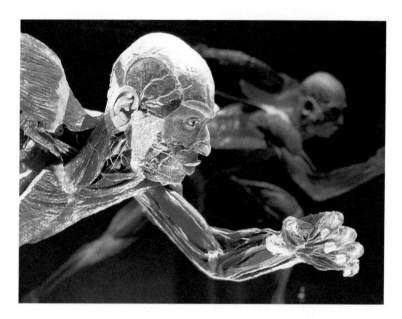

FIGURE 3.1 Full-body plastinate from the Body Worlds permanent collection. Body Worlds. Berlin, Germany. (Courtesy of Rachelle L. Clauson. Reproduced with permission from the Fascial Net Plastination Project, www.fasciaresearchsociety.org/plastination.)

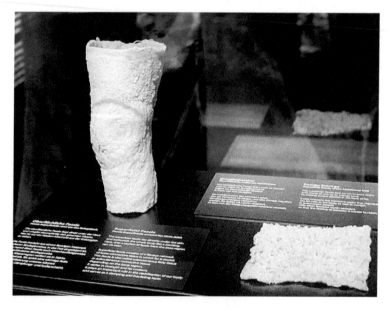

FIGURE 3.2 Plastinated superficial fascia of the knee and abdomen. Body Worlds. Berlin, Germany. (Courtesy of Robert Schleip. Reproduced with permission from the Fascial Net Plastination Project, www.fasciaresearchsociety.org/plastination.)

world of science, and the process of how the fascial system is being brought into the realm of three-dimensional illustration through the art and science of anatomical plastination.

FASCIA TERMINOLOGY AND ILLUSTRATION: MISSING CONNECTIONS

The heart of anatomical study through dissection is the act of separating the body and naming the parts. This method proves useful and effective for systems made of countable structures such as the bones, muscles, organs, nerves, and vessels. A problem arises when applying the method to fascia, however, the very nature of which is *connection*. Soft connective tissues interpenetrates the entire human form, and complete separations exist only when created by either pulling things apart or cutting with a scalpel (Figure 3.3). This state of connectivity makes terminology and illustration very challenging.

A wide variety of perspectives on soft connective tissue exists across disciplines that has contributed to a lack of consensus on the definition of fascia for some time. The Fascia Research Group in Ulm, Germany, suggests that "no area of anatomical science is characterized by such divergent terminology, as is the case in fascia-related connective tissues".[2] Highly respected references such as the *Terminologia Anatomica*[3] and *Gray's Anatomy*[4] define fascia quite differently, each including and excluding different tissues, making it difficult to find a common language to study and discuss fascia, let alone illustrate it.

Illustrations can fragment fascia into seemingly isolated structures omitting many important connections and relationships, never fully appreciating it as a whole-body network. In education we are quite reliant on dissection images and drawings to show

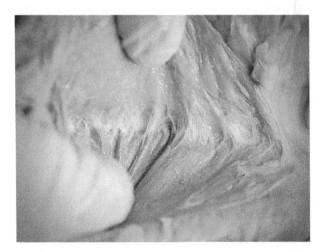

FIGURE 3.3   Superficial fascia being separated from the deep fascia of the abdomen. (Courtesy of Thomas Stephan. Reproduced with permission from the Fascial Net Plastination Project, www.fasciaresearchsociety.org/plastination.)

fascia, along with whatever divisions their creators chose, due to the limitations of modern imaging techniques for capturing fascia in detail such as with X-ray, basic ultrasound, or magnetic resonance imaging. Three-dimensional anatomical digital imaging technology and virtual/augmented reality may have the potential to illustrate fascia the most completely, but currently most systems represent limited fascial structures and appear to have not yet attempted to represent fascia as a continuous, body-wide network.

Images of fascial continuities *can* be found in some higher level anatomy texts related to the specific disciplines of medicine or osteopathy, and some exist in older atlases such as those of Jean-Baptiste Marc Bourgery;[5] however, current basic anatomy education is rather devoid of fascia as a complete system and lacks the images that would illustrate it as such.

THE EMERGENCE OF FASCIA RESEARCH

In the past two decades there has been a remarkable groundswell of new research on fascia. This surge can largely be credited to two major factors: the development of new assessment technologies and the changing perspective of fascia as one large, networking organ.[2]

A rising demand for more complete explanations for how fascia is impacted by exercise, manipulation, injury, and recovery methods are continuing to push forward this emerging field of research.[6] Fascial behavior research requires the ability to precisely measure changes in fascial tissues *in vivo*. Until recently, measurement devices lacked the precision required for meaningful research. High-resolution ultrasound,[7] bioelectric impedance,[8] and myometry[9] are among the promising technologies surfacing that aid in measuring living fascia.

Aware of the lack of consensus on fascia nomenclature and the growing desire to study fascia as a body-wide network inclusive of structures involved in force transmission and proprioception, the Fascia Research Society has proposed two definitions of fascia: one defines "a fascia" with a narrower morphological and histological focus, and another defines "the fascial system" with a broader focus on the functional aspects of the larger fascia net.[10] This second, more inclusive definition continues to spark new thoughts of how we might illustrate the fascial network. As interest in fascia grows, so too does the demand for more complete fascia illustrations and images.

Modern pioneers of fascia research are creating new images, building on the work of their predecessors. In 2015, after 10 years of research, orthopedic surgeon and professor of anatomy, Dr. Carla Stecco, published *The Functional Atlas of the Human Fascial System*.[11] This ground-breaking atlas of fascia as a body-wide system serves as a milestone in the field, featuring over 300 photographs of unpreserved fascial dissections. In March 2018, Dr. Hanno Steinke, using Thiel-fixed cadavers, published *the Atlas of Human Fascial Topography*[12] in cooperation with the award-winning German photographer Anna Rowedder.

Other pioneers of note include hand surgeon Dr. Jean-Claude Guimberteau with his book *Architecture of Human Living Fascia*[13] and video series[14] that document the sliding functions and behaviors of fascia at 50× magnification in living human patients. Dr. Gil Hedley's video series, *Integral Anatomy*,[15] approaches the dissections in full-body layers, and Tom Myers' *Anatomy Trains Revealed: Dissecting the*

Myofascial Meridians[16] highlights his proposed maps, or "trains", which illustrate lines of force transmission through the fascial system. These all are huge steps forward in fascial anatomy education, but showing the body-wide ubiquity of the fascial system remains an unexhausted frontier.

A BRIEF HISTORY OF PLASTINATION

Plastination is a method of permanently preserving anatomical specimens by infusing the tissue with silicone rubber. As developed by Dr. Gunther von Hagens in 1977 at the University of Heidelberg's Institute of Anatomy, the idea of plastination struck in a moment when von Hagans was observing a kidney specimen in a polymer block, which was a commonly used method of preservation at the time. It occurred to him that the process was backwards: the polymer should be in the kidney, not the other way around.[17] Later that year, he filed a patent for the plastination process, and the method continued to evolve.

In the first 20 years, only small specimens were plastinated for medical study. Full-body specimens did not become possible until the early 1990s. The Institute for Plastination was founded in Heidelberg in 1993, with the first Body Worlds exhibit following in 1995. Since then Body Worlds has travelled to over 90 cities, with more than 44 million visitors worldwide.[18] In 2006, Gubener Plastinate GmbH was founded in Guben, Brandenburg, Germany, with laboratories for the plastination process and a permanent public exhibition space under one roof: the Plastinarium (Figure 3.4).

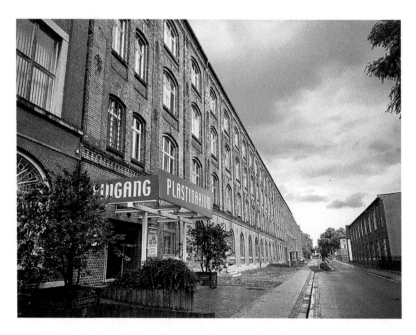

FIGURE 3.4   Plastinarium. Guben, Germany. (Courtesy of Lauri Nemetz. Reproduced with permission from the Fascial Net Plastination Project, www.fasciaresearchsociety.org/plastination.)

THE PLASTINATION PROCESS

Modern plastination at the Plastinarium begins with formalin-preserved cadavers and consists of five distinct stages: dissection, dehydration and defatting, vacuum-forced impregnation, positioning, and curing.

DISSECTION

The dissection phase for a full-body plastinate can take up to six months, depending on the complexity of the anatomy being revealed. Gentle pulling, prying, and cleaning of surfaces is a fiber-by-fiber process requiring precise dissection skills and tremendous patience.

DEHYDRATION AND DEFATTING

Once the dissection is completed, the specimen goes through a series of low- and high-temperature acetone baths for dehydration and defatting, respectively. Dehydration involves a series of low-temperature acetone baths that slowly replace the tissue's water content with acetone. Technicians continually transfer the specimen to fresh acetone, measuring the released water each time. The tissue is considered dehydrated once the water in the bath is less than 1%. Next, the lipids are dissolved in high-temperature acetone baths, which completes this stage.

VACUUM-FORCED IMPREGNATION

Once dehydration and defatting is complete, the specimen is ready to be infused with a plastic polymer. This step requires the specimen to be submersed in liquid polymer under vacuum pressure, which draws out the acetone, causing it to bubble up to the surface. The silicone rubber impregnates the specimen down to the cellular level.

POSITIONING

The series of acetone and silicone baths take approximately six months for a full-body specimen; after which the specimen is removed from the liquid polymer, drained, and prepared for positioning into its final shape. Positioning is a meticulous process that can take many months for full-body plastinates and requires the use of metal rods, cables, wires, blocks, mesh, and hundreds (sometimes thousands) of pins, to hold the malleable tissues in place. Every nerve and vessel are accounted for with great precision. The positioner must possess an extremely elevated knowledge of anatomy in order be able to maintain anatomical accuracy, as well as an esthetic sensibility required to bring the form "to life". When the final shape has been achieved, the specimen is ready for the final stage, curing.

CURING

There are two processes for curing, one for three-dimensional specimens and one for sheet plastinates. Once positioned, three-dimensional specimens are placed into an airtight container filled with gas that chemically transforms the liquid plastic polymer into a firm, rubber consistency. Sliced specimens are placed between sheets of glass, heat cured, and infused with epoxy resin to create sheet plastinates 1–5 mm in thickness. Once the curing is completed, the plastinates are prepared for final display.

THE FASCIAL NET PLASTINATION PROJECT

In the fall of 2017, the director of the Fascia Research Group at Ulm University and co-founder/Vice President of the Fascia Research Society (FRS), Robert Schleip, approached Rurik von Hagens, Managing Director of von Hagens Plastination, and Dr. Vladimir Chereminskiy, Director of Anatomy and Plastination of von Hagens Plastination, with a proposal. In this proposal the Fascia Research Society would provide three teams over the course of one year to produce three full-body fascial plastinates. The first would be a seamless, singular specimen of the fascia superficialis, or superficial fascia. The second would highlight the fascia profunda, or deep fascia. The third would illustrate the deep fascial structures of the "core body". The concept was to provide a sequential view of the fascial system from superficial to deep, enabling the observer to view distinctions in types of fascia, their relationships, and continuities throughout the body.

There were reasonable objections to such an ambitious proposal. First, fascial tissue had never been the focus of a plastinate to this scale, largely for reasons of practicality. In the typical plastination preparation as outlined above, much of the fascia is cleaned away from the specimen because it obstructs the view of the structures within and beneath it. The remaining lipids are dissolved through the series of high-temperature acetone baths. Fascia could potentially create problems in this "defatting" process given that the superficial fascia is mostly composed of fat, and deep fascia left in place could risk trapping some lipids in the body, causing the curing process to fail. Second, the original deadline was too short. In order to have the plastinates in time for the Fifth International Fascia Research Congress in Berlin, Germany, they would need to be completed by November 2018, which was barely enough time to complete the plastination and positioning process, let alone enough time to first create proof-of-concept specimens. It was decided the project would be better served by a three-year timeline.

The revised proposal began with the first critical step of producing several fascia-only specimens to answer the primary question of whether plastinating large amounts of fascia would meet both the necessary functional and aesthetic qualities, or if they would just look like shriveled up pieces of off-white plastic resistant to curing. One cadaver and two upper limbs and three lower limbs were provided for this task. A dissection plan was created by project Drs. Schleip, Chereminskiy, and Professor Carla Stecco, assisted by clinical anatomist John Sharkey. In addition, expert anatomical advice from Dr. Jaap van der Wal and Gil Hedley, PhD, was obtained via video conferencing. The subsequent plan included the following specimens:

1. Superficial fascia of the knee region
2. Superficial fascia of the elbow region
3. Superficial fascia of the abdomen

4. Deep fascia of the thigh, the fascia lata
5. Five-centimeter axial cross sections of the thigh, deep fascia and septa
6. Five-centimeter axial cross sections of the leg, deep fascia and septa
7. Thoracolumbar fascia
8. Fibroserous pericardium with respiratory diaphragm.

In January 2018, an international team of 16 volunteer dissectors from the FRS assembled at the Plastinarium lab, producing a collection of clean dissections over four days, from which ten were chosen to proceed through the plastination process.

SUPERFICIAL FASCIA

Despite the obstacles it posed to the defatting process, it was important to include superficial fascia in the project design as a recognized tissue in the fascial *system*.[19] Resembling bubble wrap, superficial fascia is primarily composed of two parts: the collagen-rich scaffolding that forms the structure of the spaces, and the adipose cells that fill them. This architecture makes no easy exit route for the fat to escape. The thick sheets of tissue were easily dissected away from the form, but the question of how to remove the fat imbedded within the thousands of tiny pockets remained to be answered.

Two different approaches were employed to test the defatting process on the superficial fascia of the abdomen, which was divided into two pieces, a left and a right half. The first approach was applied to the left half, using solely the high-temperature acetone baths to dissolve the lipids, or fats, which is one of the standard steps in the plastination process. The second approach was applied to the right half, pretreating the specimen with a pressing tool covered in metal pins creating dozens of small holes, and then massaging and squeezing the fat lobules free. Hot water and dish soap were also used to aid in the squeezing process. Six months later, after the dehydration, defatting, and vacuum-forced impregnation steps were complete, the results showed surprisingly very little difference between the two specimens. Some destruction of the honeycomb-like structure was only slightly visible on the pretreated half. This damage was caused by all the extra hole-poking and squeezing, making it the less desired result in the end. The untreated specimen defatted well from the high-temperature acetone bath alone, which meant larger portions of superficial fascia would likely also plastinate well with no additional preparation and successfully create a whole-body plastinate with large amounts of superficial fascia left in place.

Superficial fascia specimens of the elbow and knee regions also turned out well and were stitched back together to form their original cylindrical shape. It was a surprise to see that blood vessels could be clearly observed when the specimens were held up to light, which were otherwise masked by the specimen's relative opacity (Figure 3.5). This discovery was part of the inspiration of the exhibit title later that year: *Fascia in a NEW LIGHT: The Exhibition.*

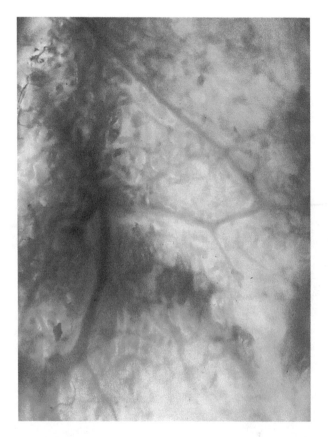

FIGURE 3.5   Plastinated superficial fascia of the knee with backlighting. (Courtesy of Stefan Westerback. Reproduced with permission from the Fascial Net Plastination Project, www.fasciaresearchsociety.org/plastination.)

DEEP AND VISCERAL FASCIA

The deep and visceral fascia specimens, though requiring little additional preparation in terms of defatting, were much more challenging to dissect. Removing the heart from its fibroserous pericardium with the respiratory diaphragm still attached was arguably the most complex. The pericardium is harnessed to the sternum anteriorly, the vertebral column posteriorly, the lungs and vessels laterally, the thoracic outlet superiorly, and the diaphragm inferiorly. The specimen creation began by first separating the respiratory diaphragm from the vertebral column, rib cage, and endoabdominal fascia and from the ligaments of the liver, stomach, spleen, and strong vascular network inferiorly. Next, the respiratory apparatus was removed from the sides and top of the heart, preserving only the aortic arch and the superior vena cava. Last, the heart was removed from the pericardial sac. In order to create an exit for the heart, several 2-inch incisions were made in the central tendon of the diaphragm where the pericardium and respiratory diaphragm come together as one structure. After carefully prying the heart from the pericardium, it was then ungloved inferiorly, leaving behind the empty pericardial sac still attached to the respiratory diaphragm.

The pericardium with attached diaphragm plastinated successfully (Figure 3.6). Again, shining light through the specimen revealed details that were otherwise obscured in the mostly opaque plastinate. Distinct muscle fibers of the diaphragm radiating outward around the central tendon and delicate vessels of the pericardium shone in bold relief.

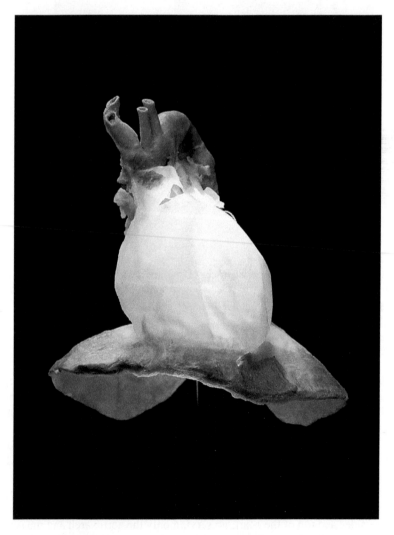

FIGURE 3.6 Plastinated pericardium and respiratory diaphragm. (Courtesy of Stefan Westerback. Reproduced with permission from the Fascial Net Plastination Project, www.fasciaresearchsociety.org/plastination.)

The fascia lata was less complex, but not without obstacles of cleanly removing all the muscle fibers embedded within it and preserving the septa that connect it to the femur. It was deemed important to show the fascia lata as a complete cylindrical structure, emphasizing the fact that the iliotibial band is a thickening of the entire structure and not a separate strip as it is so often shown in traditional anatomical illustrations. This was achieved in two specimens. The first was a 5-cm axial cross section of the thigh. The muscles were removed one fiber at time leaving only the fascia lata, septa, neurovascular bundles, and bone. This same approach was also taken in the lower leg with the fascia cruris, which is a continuation of the same fascial plane as the fascia lata (Figure 3.7). With the second specimen, the attempt was made to spare the entire fascia lata, from the iliac crest to just superior of the knee. In order to open the compartments to remove the muscle tissue and femur, a long incision was made following the path of the sartorius muscle. The gluteus medius, vastus medialis, and vastus lateralis were removed from the fascia lata. The gluteus maximus and tensor fascia lata are imbedded within and fully continuous with the

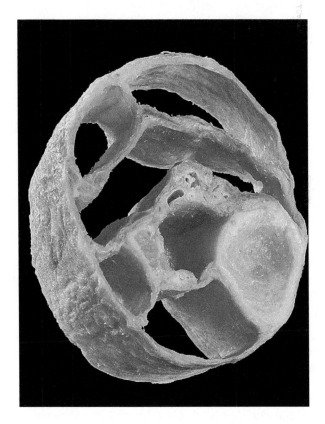

FIGURE 3.7 Plastinated deep fascia 5-cm cross section of the leg. The fascia cruris and muscular septa are visible as well as the tibia, fibula, and neurovascular bundle. (Courtesy of Plastinarium. Reproduced with permission from the Fascial Net Plastination Project, www. fasciaresearchsociety.org/plastination.)

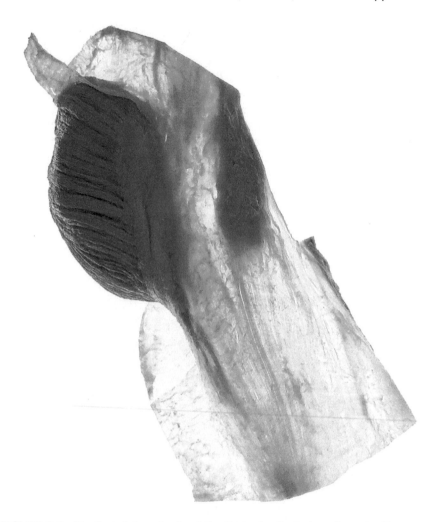

FIGURE 3.8 Plastinated deep fascia of the thigh, the fascia lata, from the iliac crest to above the knee with backlighting. The gluteus maximus and tensor fascia lata remain intact. (Courtesy of Rachelle L. Clauson. Reproduced with permission from the Fascial Net Plastination Project, www.fasciaresearchsociety.org/plastination.)

fascia lata; for this reason, they were included in the specimen. The attempt was made to preserve the fascial septa that divide the thigh into three muscular compartments. Like its other fascial counterparts, the fascia lata also revealed more than anticipated with lighting (Figure 3.8). Beyond just showing thickening of the iliotibial band, illumination showed clearly delineated fiber directions, revealing the force transmission-driven loading pattern of this fascial structure created over many years of use and development[20] (Figure 3.9).

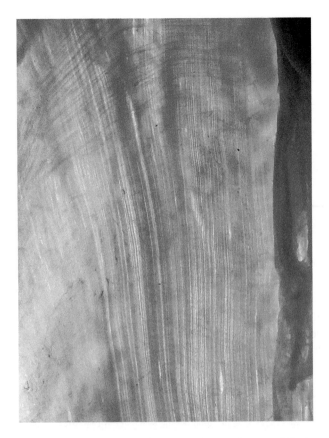

FIGURE 3.9 Plastinated fascia of the thigh, the fascia lata, close up of the deep surface with backlighting showing the dense collagen organization at the iliotibial tract region. (Courtesy of Stefan Westerback. Reproduced with permission from the Fascial Net Plastination Project, www.fasciaresearchsociety.org/plastination.)

FASCIA IN A NEW LIGHT: THE EXHIBITION

By mid-July, a total of ten fascia plastinates were completed from the dissection week in January 2018. A showing of the specimens debuted in *Fascia in a NEW LIGHT: The Exhibition*, at the Fifth International Fascia Research Congress in Berlin in November 2018. The exhibit was co-created by FNPP members Rachelle Clauson and Gary Carter with the support of Dr. Vladimir Chereminskiy, Alexander Crasemann, on-site FNPP team members, and the Plastinarium (who generously provided the exhibit's construction elements and eight additional plastinates from the Plastinarium collection). FNPP member Lauri Nemetz and phone app creator Eric Feinstein facilitated the creation of an audiovisual guide for the exhibit via the Otocast app for both iOS and Android platforms. The entire exhibit can still be

FIGURE 3.10   The audiovisual guide for *Fascia in a NEW LIGHT: the Exhibition* is available in English, German, and Portuguese on the Otocast app. There is no fee for the app or the guide.

viewed in English, German, and Portuguese after downloading the Otocast app and searching the term "fascia". There is no charge associated with the Otocast app[21] (Figure 3.10).

NEXT STEPS

After successful proof-of-concept specimens and a strong positive response at the Berlin congress, the project is advancing to the next phase: creating the first whole-body, fascial-focused plastinate set to debut at the Sixth International Fascia Research Congress in Montreal, Canada, fall of 2021. Though challenges still remain for creating a full-body specimen, the Fascial Net Plastination Project is optimistic they will achieve their objective to present fascia as a body-wide network, highlighting fascial continuities and relationships in three dimensions. If successful, they will bring us closer to understanding the body as a whole, through the art and science of anatomical plastination.

REFERENCES

1. Fascia Research Society. 2019. Plastinatination Project. Accessed December 17, 2019. https://fasciaresearchsociety.org/plastination
2. Schleip, R., H. Jager, and W. Klingler. 2012. What is "fascia"? A review of different nomenclatures. *Journal of Bodywork & Movement Therapies* 16: 496–502.
3. Federative Committee on Anatomical Terminology. 1998. *Terminologia Anatomica*. New York: Thieme.
4. Standring, S. (Ed.). 2016. *Gray's Anatomy—The Anatomical Basis of Clinical Practice*, 41st ed. Edinburgh: Churchill Livingstone.
5. Bourgery, J.M. 1831–1854. *Atlas of Human Anatomy and Surgery/Traite complet de l'anatomie de l'homme*, Vols. 1–8. Paris: Delaunay.

6. Chaitow, L., T.W. Findley, and R. Schleip. 2012. *Fascia Research III—Basic Science and Implications for Conventional and Complimentary Health Care.* Munich: Keiner Press.

7. Tozzi, P., D. Bongiorno, and C. Vitturini. 2011. Fascial release effects patients with non-specific cervical or lumbar pain. *Journal of Bodywork and Movement Therapies* 15 (4): 405–416.

8. Kim, C.T., T.W. Findley, and S.R. Reisman. 1997. Bioelectrical impedance changes in regional extracellular fluid alterations. *Electromyography and Clinical Neurophysiology* 37 (5): 297–304.

9. Gavronski, G., A. Veraksits, E. Vasar, and J. Maaroos. 2007. Evaluation of viscoelastic parameters of the skeletal muscles in junior triathletes. *Physiological Measurement* 28 (6): 625–637.

10. Stecco, C., and R. Schleip. 2016. A fascia and the fascial system. *Journal of Bodywork and Movement Therapies* 20 (1): 139–140.

11. Stecco, C. 2015. *Functional Atlas of the Human Fascial System.* Edinburgh: Churchill Livingstone.

12. Steinke, H. 2018. *Atlas of Human Fascial Topography.* Leipziger: Leipziger University.

13. Guimberteau, J.C. 2015. *Architecture of Human Living Fasica.* Edinburgh: Handspring Publishing.

14. Guimberteau, J.C. 2009–2019. *Strolling Under the Skin.* Bordeaux, France: Endovivo Productions. www.endovivo.com.

15. Hedley, G. 2005–2009. *The Integral Anatomy Series.* Vols. 1–4. New York: DVD.

16. Lesondak, D. 2009. *Anatomy Trains Revealed: Dissecting the Myofascial Meridians.* DVD, performed by T. Myers. Pittsburgh, PA: Singing Cowboy Productions.

17. Whalley, A. 2014. *Pushing the Limits.* Heidelberg: Arts & Sciences.

18. Korperwelten. 2019. FAQ. Accessed November 21, 2019. https://bodyworlds.com/about/faq/.

19. Adstrum, S., G. Hedley, R. Schleip, C. Stecco, and C.A. Yucesoy. 2017. Defining the fascial system. *Journal of Bodywork & Movement Therapies* 21 (1): 173–177.

20. Blechschmidt, E., and R.F. Gasser. 2012. *Biokinetics and Biodynamics of Human Differentiation: Principles and Applications.* Berkeley: North Atlantic Books.

21. Otocast. 2019. Otocast. Accessed December 17, 2019. www.Otocast.com

4 Physiology of the Fascia

Antonio Stecco

CONTENTS

FASCIA AND BIOMECHANICS

Recent studies have expanded the understanding of the role of fascia in fundamental functions such as force transmission and nerve proprioception. Superficial fascia, superficial and deep adipose tissue, deep fascia, and myofascial expansions, all form the network necessary for the manifestation of these functions. Deep fascia is responsible for both force transmission and proprioception. Loose connective tissue works as a gliding and shearing system between the fascial layers and other connective tissue so that both proper sliding and more rigid stability can be achieved.[1]

The two types of deep fascia, aponeurotic and epimysial, have a different ability to transmit muscle force. Aponeurotic fascia slides over the epimysium and transmits force at distance. Epimysial fascia is also capable of force transmission over shorter distances, at the local level. Also, epimysial fascia is tightly adherent to the underlying muscles, giving it the ability to transmit the full force of the muscle in multiple directions. Many authors report similar findings of fascia as a force transmitter.[2,3] The concept of force transmission through synergistic muscles groups and myofascial tissue connectivity is further supported by the study by Cruz-Montecinos et al.[4]

Aponeurotic deep fascia consists of sublayers with in-between loose connective tissue. When a force is transmitted to an area, aponeurotic fascia adapts to the tension and transmits the force, not only to the nearest contiguous area of the muscle but also to muscles that are distal and proximal.[3] For instance, the thoracolumbar fascia (TLF) permits the gluteus maximus and latissimus dorsi to contract simultaneously, owing to its fascial layers allowing connection between the two halves of the body. Vleeming et al.[5] showed the transfer of forces occurring through this layer from the biceps femoris to the sacrotuberous ligament to the erector spinae to the TLF to the contralateral latissimus dorsi. Because of this connection the gluteus maximus muscle is appropriately positioned between the TLF and the fascia lata (the deep fascia of the thigh) to coordinate muscular forces relating to both the lower extremity and torso. Jan Wilke et al.[6] studied the continuity of the iliotibial tract to the crural fascia (the deep fascia of the leg), and the strong connections between them was present in every examined subject.

Tension is one of the most important features relating to collagen orientation. Tension lines occur in patterns consistent with the orientation of the collagen fibers. There is a contradiction with classical anatomy where force transmission is demonstrated only as longitudinal vectors from tendon to tendon, from the origin of the muscle to the insertion of the muscle. While 70% of force transmission is directed (in series) through tendons, new information shows that 30% of muscle force is transmitted through the connective tissue in parallel, as non-spanning fibers that never reach the tendon.[2,3] To reiterate, 30% of muscle force is transmitted by the connective tissue, myofascial expansion and deep fascia. The endomysium's collagen fibers are not longitudinal, they exist in multidirectional form, giving us indications of multidirectional tensions.

The term *myofascial expansion* indicates each fascial connection that originates from a skeletal muscle, or from its tendon, inserting into the aponeurotic fascia.[7] Myofascial expansions have also been described or proposed by other authors from Chiarugi[8] to Standring et al.[9] Similar descriptions are found in Da Vinci's famous writings over 500 years ago where he described deltoid muscle anatomy "which part insert to bone and which are inserted to other muscles". Myofascial expansions (MFEs) refer to all the anatomical connections from muscle to deep fascia. MFEs are not just muscle–fascia links, but all links between muscles. For example, these links are often found where the tendon inserts into the bone. The tendons arise from their insertions to fascial sheets that cover the surrounding areas. Therefore, it is no longer correct to define muscle attachments by way of singular origins and insertions.

Perhaps the most "famous" MFE is the lacertus fibrosus, which arises from the biceps brachii muscles' insertional tendon to cover the flexor muscles of the wrist (or the antebrachial fascia, the deep fascia of the forearm). When looking carefully, other expansions can be found similar to the lacertus fibrosus. The brachialis and biceps are not exceptions; almost all muscles have similar expansions. For example, the quadriceps inserts into the tibial tuberosity but also expands to the anterior retinaculum of the knee. The quadriceps expands to the lateral side of knee to the iliotibial tract (or IT band) and medially to the pes anserinus. The gluteus maximus has numerous expansions, some proximal, attaching to the iliac crest and sacrum and then into the trunk via the TLF. Distally, the gluteus maximus inserts into the femur (tuberosity of glutei), with most of its fibers traveling to the deep fascia of the thigh (fascia lata), and into the iliotibial tract that inserts laterally below the knee.

FASCIA AS ENERGY STORAGE

Most of the studies about the elasticity of the deep fascia are described at the aponeurotic type of fascial layer. Collagen fibrils cannot be completely taut, at least some elasticity must be present to permit movement. Tendons, for instance, have the potential to be stretched around 3%–4%.[10] The Achilles tendon has an estimated 4% elasticity.

Elastic properties are exhibited in two ways: during active contraction of the muscle and passively, when mechanical loading is applied. Tendons, ligaments, and deep fascia contain different percentages of elastin (primarily responsible for elastic capacity) and other elements that determine the tissue's overall elasticity. In addition to elasticity, other factors contribute to the capacity for movement. There is tissue shearing between contiguous tissues, and the different levels of elastic potential in these tissues. The loose connective tissue provides a gliding interface between layers of dense connective tissue that allows structures to move relative to one another. The lubricant capacity of the loose connective tissue between fascial layers allows the deep aponeurotic fascia to adapt to different tensions, thus allowing changes in the direction of the collagen fibers in the different layers. This elastic adaptability is important for energy storage and fascial recoil.

All soft tissue is elastic to some degree. This elasticity allows movement and affects how efficiently tissues produce movement, absorb stress, and tolerate strain. All soft tissue, including collagen, has at least some ability to store mechanical energy. Stored energy is used to produce the next movement. This system permits the energy saving and movement efficiency known as hysteresis. Hysteresis is the energy storage between loading the tissue and its return to the original shape and size. The quantity of energy storage and reuse is determined principally by the shape, or architecture, of the tissue in question.

FASCIA AND PROPRIOCEPTION

Recent research has claimed that the deep fascia is richly innervated and can play an active role in proprioception.[11] The epimysial fasciae is rich in free nerve endings. These type IV mechanoreceptors are immersed in a fibrous stroma and sensitive to the traction of the muscles due to the tendinous expansions into the fascia. Superficial fascia is innervated with free nerve endings and Ruffini and Pacinian corpuscles. There is a difference in the density of innervation of fascia in relation to their location.

For example, both the tendinous expansions of the pectoralis major and the lacertus fibrosus in the forearm are less innervated than the brachial and the antebrachial fascia, probably because they have a function of mechanical transmission rather than proprioception. Samples taken from the flexor retinaculum, however, are much better innervated. So rather than just functioning primarily as a transmitter of mechanical load, the flexor retinaculum has other functions, such as acting like a pulley for the flexor tendons and as an extrinsic ligament for the carpus and, most importantly, it contains a thickening of fascia, giving it a fundamental role in motor perception as well as signaling variations dealing with joint volume. The Pacini corpuscles, as compared with the Ruffini corpuscles, are relatively few in this region. Comparing the few studies that report a quantitative analysis of these encapsulated receptors of the upper limb, we see that the fascia is relatively rich with these elements.[13]

The mechanoreceptors within the fascia carry out different functions, and they are activated in different situations. Pacini corpuscles only perceive rapid variations in their state of compression/relaxation, whereas Ruffini corpuscles respond to more continuous stimuli. It is probable that when the fascia is stretched, the compression exerted by the surrounding collagenic fascicles activates the Pacini corpuscles. Quite differently, the Ruffini corpuscles are activated by traction on the capsule by the surrounding collagenic fibers.

FASCIA AND MUSCLE SPINDLE

Muscle spindles are localized in the periphery of the muscle. The capsule that encloses the muscle spindle is part of the perimysium, giving the muscle spindle the ability to perceive the level of tension of all the connective tissue of the muscle (endomysium, perimysium, and epimysium) and of the surrounding fascia. If the fascia is altered, the spindle cells may not function normally, depriving the central nervous system (CNS) of necessary information about muscle coordination and position. Spindle cells are stretched during muscle contraction or passive stretch. It is therefore probable that if the spindle cells are embedded in thickened, densified fascia, its ability to be stretched would be affected and normal spindle cell feedback to the CNS would be altered.

Siegfried Mense, MD, one of the world's leading experts on muscle pain and neurophysiology was questioned about fascial alteration having an adverse effect on spindle cells and answered, *"Structural disorders of the fascia can surely distort the information sent by the spindles to the CNS and thus can interfere with a proper coordinated movement"* and *"the primary spindle afferents (1a fibers) are so sensitive that even slight distortions of the perimysium will change their discharge frequency"*.

By understanding the important role of the muscle spindle in pre-activation, we can see how an alteration of the ability of the muscle spindle to be activated can change the amount of muscle fibers recruited for a specific task. This can explain the weakness or fatigue that many subjects present, even in the absence of pain or muscle atrophy, when they perform specific movements. It was also shown that a decrease in fascial stiffness can increase active movement[12] in spastic patients and increase the muscle recruitment of the masseter and temporalis muscle[13] in subjects suffering with temporomandibular joint disorders.

HORMONAL STIMULATION

Nallasamy et al.[14] have demonstrated that progesterone and estrogen play distinct and complementary roles in regulating synthesis, processing, assembly, and structural reorganization of both collagen and elastic fibers in the cervix during pregnancy and in regulating the mechanical tissue function. It was found that fascia becomes stiffer with low hormone levels, equal to the menopause period of a woman. By increased collagen deposition, especially cross-linking collagen I, the extracellular matrix (ECM) stiffens, disrupting the normal tissue morphogenesis. In menopause, the collagen III and the fibrillin content decrease, consequently decreasing the elastic properties of fascial tissue.

When hormone levels rise, such as during pregnancy, the fascial tissue becomes more elastic. After administration of β-estradiol, the collagen I level goes down, whereas collagen III and fibrillin levels increase. This change in the ECM composition permits the adaptation of the tissue during the pregnancy processes, such as during the ovulatory period of a woman, in which we observe the same trend of ECM changes. When adding the hormone relaxin-1 to the culture, these evident and rapid changes are smoothed, confirming the antifibrotic function of relaxin-1 by the ability to reduce matrix synthesis. It is hypothesized that women with hormonal dysfunctions may have myofascial pain by the dysregulation of ECM production, causing stiffness, fibrosis, and inflammatory activities that create a sensitization of fascial nociceptors.[15] This may explain why oral administration of estrogen can help to resolve myofascial pain in women.[16]

LOOSE CONNECTIVE TISSUE

Throughout the body, the loose connective tissue cushions and separates different structures from each other. The chief component of the loose connective tissue is hyaluronan (HA), which has the role of providing a substance for the smooth gliding between surfaces such as the fascial layers or different muscle fibers surrounded by epimysium.[17] This suggests that the layer of HA between the fascia and the muscle bundles functions as a lubricant, and its widespread presence in the perimysium and endomysium could provide planes of potential movement.

In addition to the histolocalization of HA between fascia and muscle, the studies by Piehl-Aulin et al.[18] show that perivascular and perineural connective tissue stain positive for HA. In those studies, quantitative measures of HA were measured and the effect of exercise examined. The retention of HA after exercise, combined with endomysial location, supports the concept that HA not only lubricates but also facilitates movements between muscle fibers. Changes of HA function can occur with changing concentrations and aggregation properties in response to van der Waals and hydrophobic forces. In increasing concentrations, HA chains begin to entangle, conferring distinctive hydrodynamic properties on HA solutions, with a dramatic increase in viscosity.[19]

The hydrodynamics of HA solutions may provide the viscoelasticity needed for skeletal muscle movement. Interchain interactions are reversible, with disaggregation occurring with an increase in temperature and by alkalinization. We have observed, in a number of samples, fibroblast-like cells aligned on the inferior surface of fascia. We term these cells *fasciacytes* and suggest these are a new class of cells.[1] Fasciacytes may be related to other fibroblast-like cells in the body but have a more specialized function of HA synthesis and secretion. As ascertained by surface marker studies, fasciacytes are of the monocyte/macrophage lineage. Whereas the myofibroblast, another cell that actively secretes HA and other ECM components,[17] is not of monocyte/macrophage origin.

Temperature, chemical elements, and pressure can modulate the physical–chemical properties of HA. When HA assumes a more dense conformation, its viscosity increases, compromising the behavior of the deep fascia and underlying muscle. There is much evidence that proper activation of the mechanoreceptors is strongly dependent on the viscoelasticity of the surrounding tissue.[20] Tissue viscoelasticity shapes the dynamic response of the mechanoreceptors. This could be the origin of the common phenomenon of myofascial pain.

PATHOPHYSIOLOGY OF FASCIA

A series of studies address the possible involvement of the deep fascia in myofascial pain. Variations in deep fascia thickness occurs in subjects with chronic low back pain[21] or with chronic neck pain.[7] The ingrowth of nociceptive fibers and immuno-reactions to substance P have been found in the loose connective tissue of the deep fascia (retinaculum) of patients with patella–femoral alignment problems,[22] whereas a loss of nerve fibers in the TLF has been reported in patients with chronic lum-balgia.[23] Innervation of the TLF, by both A and C fiber nociceptors, has been sug-gested by the long-lasting sensitization of the deep fascia in response to mechanical pressure and chemical stimulation.[24,25] Interestingly, the same authors demonstrate that the sensitized free nerve fiber endings within muscle fascia are stimulated more effectively when the fascia is "pre-stretched" by muscle contraction.

Given that free nerve endings and the proprioceptive corpuscles are completely embedded inside the fascia, it is possible that the viscoelasticity of fascia can modify activation of the proprioceptors within the fascia. If the deep fascia is either over-stretched or it becomes too viscous, it is probable that the nerves inside the fascia will be activated in a negative way.

The concept of gliding within the fascial system is critical for normal function. When HA assumes a more packed conformation, in other words when the loose connective tissue inside the fascia alters its density, the behavior of the entire deep fascia and the underlying muscle would be compromised. There is evidence that if the loose connective tissue within the fascia has increased viscosity, the receptors will not be activated properly. Densified HA also alters the distribution of the lines of force within the fascia. In this environment, pain and stiffness may be created with stretching even within the normal physiological range.

Langevin et al.[21] have shown that TLF shear strain was ~20% lower in human subjects with chronic low back pain. This reduction of shear plane motion may be due to intrinsic connective tissue alterations. If the tensional system is impaired, fascial dysfunction might create excessive local compression under prolonged stress, generating tissue damage. Schilder et al.[25] demonstrated that fascia is the most pain-sensitive deep tissue in the low back and can cause widespread referred pain. Fascia, as a complex network, can also interfere with the physiology of the nerve by altering the gliding movement of its surrounding fascial layers: the epineu-rium and perineurium.

HA turnover time is about 2–4 days, whereas the other glycosaminoglycans (GAGs) have a lifetime of 7–10 days. Therefore, it is important for patients to keep moving. Inactivity and static activities, like sitting in front of the computer for hours every day, create isometric contractions that are risk factors for a change in the quantity and quality of the ground substance. This change in viscoelasticity is defined as densification.[15] Prime reasons for fascial densification are trauma, surgery, overuse, or misuse. These conditions allow HA chains to aggregate, increasing the viscosity of the loose connective tissue, with resulting stiffness and irritation of free nerve endings and mechanoreceptors. When HA chains entangle, it prevents the normal gliding between fascia and muscles, changing the normal biomechanics of human body.

Particular attention should be placed in the interaction between HA, lactic acid and alterations of pH in fascial tissues. Different authors[26,27] document that the pH inside muscle can decrease until pH 6.6 is reached. This level represents the point of exhaustion during heavy sport activities. This value is far lower than the mean pH value found in the blood stream, which ranges from 7.4 to 7.2. At pH 6.6, the viscosity of HA present in the endomysium and perimysium of muscle can increase considerably. This is demonstrated by the experiment of Gatej et al.[28] He documents that at pH 6.6, the complex viscosity of the HA approaches 4.5 Pa s. (this is the measure of the dynamic fluid viscosity: N s m^{-2}) instead of the typical 3.8 (the normal value at pH 7.4).

This increase in viscosity can explain the typical stiffness experienced by athletes after prolonged intense activity (marathons, endurance games, etc.). We postulate that lactic acid is not the only component that creates such stiffness, but it is also the substance that catalyzes the reaction. The fascia assumes a fundamental role here, with two of its components: dense connective tissue (collagen fibers type I and III) and loose connective tissue (adipose cells, GAGs, and HA). The alteration of pH stimulates the reaction that increases HA viscosity. The dense connective tissue spreads the stiffness throughout the surrounding areas, driving even further the sensation of muscle stiffness.

The stiffness can be reversed soon thereafter, thanks to the degradation of the lactic acid in muscle. For this reason, stiffness disappears quite soon with rest in athletes, with a full restoration of range of motion and cessation of symptoms. We postulate that this same mechanism can underlie alterations that do not permit full restoration nor relief of symptoms. We further speculate that specific areas may not be restored to complete normal viscosity, so a high viscosity profile is maintained. From a clinical point of view, such areas can be defined as undergoing densification and constitute potential myofascial pain syndrome (MPS).

Heating modalities and deep friction manipulation can locally increase the temperature of muscles and their associated fascial tissue. The three-dimensional superstructure of HA chains by inter- and intra-molecular water bridges (van der Waals and hydrophobic forces) break down progressively when the temperature is increased to over 40°C. There is a change in viscosity of HA solutions at precisely that temperature.[29] This decrease in viscosity is able to restore normal gliding and normalizes the activation of the mechanoreceptors in that area. It is reasonable to assume that the quantity of HA in that area will not be altered by increases in temperature but that its behavior and structure will be. For this reason, it is postulated that with rest, the aggregative properties of HA can be regenerated soon thereafter. This hypothesis can also explain short-lasting effects that simply increase temperature.

Noble[30] has defined a self-resolving inflammatory reaction cascade where, under conditions of stress, HA becomes depolymerized and lower molecular mass polymers are generated. These HA fragmentation reactions result in smaller polymers that in a size-dependent manner are highly angiogenic, inflammatory, and immunogenic.[30,31] HA fragments promote inflammation, angiogenesis, and immune reactions by driving endothelial cell proliferation and migration, by stimulating production of inflammatory cytokines, and by promoting macrophage chemotaxis. Mary Cowman et al.[32] hypothesize that manual manipulation of the subcutis, with deep compression and friction, is able to catalyze this reaction. Stern et al.[33] demonstrated that as soon as fragments of 1,000 Da in size are generated, particular inflammatory reactions are catalyzed. However, the smallest HA fragments, 4 Da in size, have no inflammatory effect but, rather, do the exact opposite. They decrease the effect of the other larger HA fragments by stopping the full reaction.

We hypothesize a correlation between this reaction and the soreness referred to by patients in the days following manipulation treatments. Even if soreness will be present, patients can appreciate the improvements of quality of life following this short period of an inflammatory reaction that will be even better at its resolution in 48–72 h. We consider this self-resolving inflammatory reaction the actual mechanism that restores the correct quantity and quality of loose connective tissue in MPS in critical areas [trigger points (TrPs), areas of high viscosity, densified areas, etc.] where the clinician has worked. In other words, the real efficacy of the manipulation of deep tissue has a twofold affect: to restore the gliding and to catalyze this specific self-resolving inflammatory reaction.

FASCIA IMAGING

Different investigators and clinicians have used ultrasonography or magnetic resonance imaging (MRI) scans (Figure 4.1) to compare the thickness of fascia in different area of the body between healthy and symptomatic subjects.

All of these authors are in agreement that the thickening of the fascia is a well-established criterion for the diagnosis of MPS.[7,21,34] The variation in thickness of the fascia correlates with the increase in quantity of loose connective tissue (black layers) and not with the dense connective tissue (white layers) (Figure 4.2).

MPS is characterized by the presence of TrPs, which are hard, palpable, localized nodules located within taut bands of skeletal muscle[35,36] and characterized as an elliptical hypoechoic (darker) region in ultrasound.[37,38] Authors describe TrPs as larger blobs with a lower echo intensity[39,40] and therefore a relatively hypoechoic signal whose size was similar to the one detected clinically by palpation.

Given that myofascial pain is present in more than 85% of the population at the least once in a lifetime, it is critical to determine whether stiffness is related to dense connective tissue or to "fluid"-like densification areas.[41] In fact, it was shown that visually apparent hypoechoic regions associated with palpable myofascial TrPs were significantly different from those of healthy controls.[42]

In densification-like areas, high-molecular-weight and semi-flexible chains of HA are key factors leading to the high viscosity due to mutual macromolecular crowding.[32] It is becoming commonplace to use dynamic ultrasonography methods in order to visualize the gliding between different structures and to collect data regarding the movement of one structure in comparison to others. In elastography images, the densification seems to be visible in the deep fascia. In particular, myofascial pain seems to be associated with not only reduction of gliding between fascial sublayers but also changes in the elasticity of the deep fascia. Elastography imaging seems to be a useful tool to help clinicians in diagnosing myofascial pain owing to its ability to quantify the tissue stiffness (Figure 4.3).

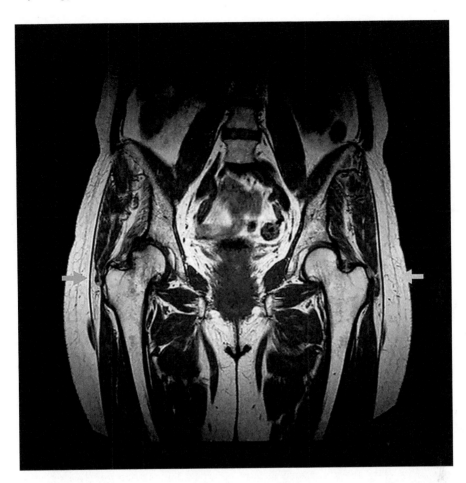

FIGURE 4.1 Magnetic resonance imaging scan of the pelvic region. Orange arrow indicates the superficial fascia. Blue arrow indicates the deep fascia.

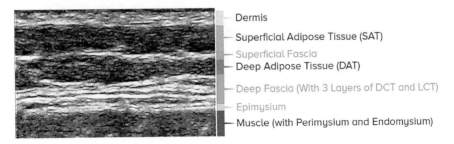

FIGURE 4.2 Ultrasonography of the subcutis. DCT: dense connective tissue; LCT: loose connective tissue.

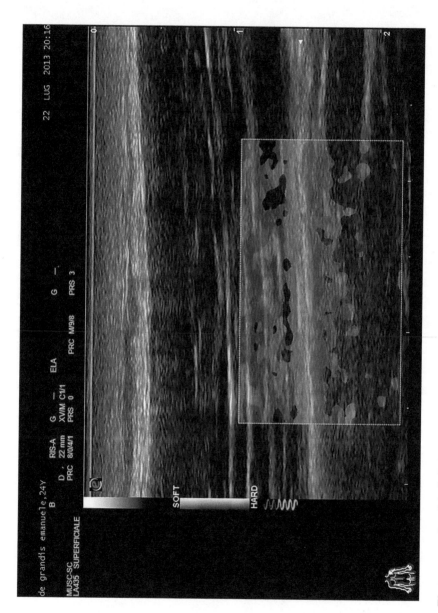

FIGURE 4.3 Elastosonography of the inferior border of the trapezius fascia. Green = soft tissue; red = hard tissue.

Also very promising is the new T1ρ MRI imaging that is sensitive to the chemical exchange of large macromolecules such as HA with protons in bulk water, making it a useful tool to quantify GAG content in muscles before and after treatment.[43]

SUMMARY

1. Superficial fascia, superficial and deep adipose tissue, deep fascia, and myofascial expansions form a body-wide network necessary for the manifestation of the fundamental functions of fascia, such as force transmission and proprioception.

2. Tension is one of the most important features relating to collagen orientation. There is a contradiction with classical anatomy where force transmission is demonstrated only from the origin of the muscle to the insertion of the muscle. While 70% of force transmission is directed this way, in series through tendons, new information shows that 30% of muscle force is transmitted through the connective tissue in parallel.

3. If fascia is altered (thickened, densified, or damaged) muscle spindle cells may not function normally, depriving the CNS of necessary information for muscle fiber recruitment.

4. The hydrodynamics of HA provide the viscoelasticity needed for skeletal muscle movement. Aggregations of HA occur with both injury and immobility, which can further restrict and disorganize movement. This situation is reversible, with disaggregation of HA occurring with an increase in temperature and by alkalinization.

5. We have observed fibroblast-like cells aligned on the inferior surface of fascia in a number of samples. We term these cells fasciacytes, a new class of cells with a specialized function of HA synthesis and secretion. These cells are of the monocyte/macrophage lineage.

6. The myofibroblast is not of monocyte/macrophage origin but is actually a modified fibroblast. The myofibroblast is active in wound repair and associated with scarring and contractures.

7. HA fragments promote inflammation, angiogenesis, and immune reactions by driving endothelial cell proliferation and migration, by stimulating production of inflammatory cytokines, and by promoting macrophage chemotaxis.

8. The concept of gliding within the fascial system is crucial for normal function. When HA assumes a more packed conformation, or in other words when the loose connective tissue inside the fascia alters its viscosity, the behavior of the entire deep fascia and the underlying muscle would be compromised.

9. Imaging techniques have validated the existence of alteration of the loose connective tissue.

REFERENCES

1. Stecco C, Fede C, Macchi V, Porzionato A, Petrelli L, Biz C, Stern R, De Caro R. The fasciacytes: A new cell devoted to fascial gliding regulation. *Clin Anat.* 2018;31(5):667–676.
2. Patel TJ, Lieber RL. Force transmission in skeletal muscle: From actomyosin to external tendons. *Exerc Sport Sci Rev.* 1997;25:321–363. Review. PubMed PMID: 9213097.
3. Huijing PA, Baan GC. Myofascial force transmission via extramuscular pathways occurs between antagonistic muscles. *Cells Tissues Organs.* 2008;188(4):400–414.
4. Cruz-Montecinos C, González Blanche A, López Sánchez D, Cerda M, Sanzana-Cuche R, Cuesta-Vargas A. In vivo relationship between pelvis motion and deep fascia displacement of the medial gastrocnemius: Anatomical and functional implications. *J Anat.* 2015;227(5):665–672.
5. Vleeming A, Pool-Goudzwaard AL, Stoeckart R, van Wingerden JP, Snijders CJ. The posterior layer of the thoracolumbar fascia. Its function in load transfer from spine to legs. *Spine* (Phila Pa 1976). 1995;20(7):753–758. PubMed PMID: 7701385.
6. Wilke J, Engeroff T, Nürnberger F, Vogt L, Banzer W. Anatomical study of the morphological continuity between iliotibial tract and the fibularis longus fascia. *Surg Radiol Anat.* 2016;38(3):349–352.
7. Stecco A, Meneghini A, Stern R, Stecco C, Imamura M. Ultrasonography in myofascial neck pain: Randomized clinical trial for diagnosis and follow-up. *Surg Radiol Anat.* 2014;36(3):243–253.
8. Chiarugi G, Bucciante L. 1975. *Istituzioni di Anatomia dell'uomo*, 11th ed. Vallardi-Piccin, Padova.
9. Standring, S. 2008. *Gray's Anatomy: The Anatomical Basis of Clinical Practice*, 40th ed. London: Churchill Livingstone Elsevier.
10. Ker RF. The design of soft collagenous load-bearing tissues. *J Exp Biol.* 1999;202(Pt 23):3315–3324. Review. PubMed PMID: 10562514.
11. Stecco C, Gagey O, Belloni A, Pozzuoli A, Porzionato A, Macchi V, Aldegheri R, De Caro R, Delmas V. Anatomy of the deep fascia of the upper limb. Second part: Study of innervation. *Morphologie.* 2007;91(292):38–43. PubMed PMID: 17574469.
12. Raghavan P, Lu Y, Mirchandani M, Stecco A. Human recombinant hyaluronidase injections for upper limb muscle stiffness in individuals with cerebral injury: A case series. *EBioMedicine.* 2016;9:306–313.
13. Sekito F et al. Myofascial pain of the jaw muscles: Comparison of conventional odonatological intervention and fascial manipulation method. *Sleep Med.* 2019 (under revision).
14. Nallasamy S, Yoshida K, Akins M, Myers K, Iozzo R, Mahendroo M. Steroid hormones are key modulators of tissue mechanical function via regulation of collagen and elastic fibers. *Endocrinology.* 2017;158(4):950–962.
15. Pavan PG, Stecco A, Stern R, Stecco C. Painful connections: Densification versus fibrosis of fascia. *Curr Pain Headache Rep.* 2014;18(8):441.
16. Sarajari S, Oblinger MM. Estrogen effects on pain sensitivity and neuropeptide expression in rat sensory neurons. *Exp Neurol.* 2010;224(1):163–169.
17. McCombe D, Brown T, Slavin J, Morrison WA. The histochemical structure of the deep fascia and its structural response to surgery. *J Hand Surg Br.* 2001;26:89–97.
18. Piehl-Aulin K, Laurent C, Engström-Laurent A, Hellström S, Henriksson J. Hyaluronan in human skeletal muscle of lower extremity: Concentration, distribution, and effect of exercise. *J Appl Physiol.* 1991;71:2493–2498.
19. Tanaka S, Ito T. Histochemical demonstration of adrenergic fibers in the fascia periosteum and retinaculum. *Clin Orthop Relat Res.* 1977;126:276–281.

20. Song Z, Banks RW, Bewick GS. Modelling the mechanoreceptor's dynamic behaviour. *J Anat.* 2015;227(2):243–254.
21. Langevin HM, Fox JR, Koptiuch C, Badger GJ, Greenan-Naumann AC, Bouffard NA, Konofagou EE, Lee WN, Triano JJ, Henry SM. Reduced thoracolumbar fascia shear strain in human chronic low back pain. *BMC Musculoskelet Disord.* 2011;12:203.
22. Sanchis-Alfonso V, Roselló-Sastre E. Immunohistochemical analysis for neural markers of the lateral retinaculum in patients with isolated symptomatic patellofemoral malalignment. A neuroanatomic basis for anterior knee pain in the active young patient. *Am J Sports Med.* 2000;28(5):725–731. PubMed PMID: 11032232.
23. Bednar DA, Orr FW, Simon GT. Observations on the pathomorphology of the thoracolumbar fascia in chronic mechanical back pain. A microscopic study. *Spine* (Phila Pa 1976). 1995;20(10):1161–1164. PubMed PMID: 7638659.
24. Deising S, Weinkauf B, Blunk J, Obreja O, Schmelz M, Rukwied R. NGF-evoked sensitization of muscle fascia nociceptors in humans. *Pain.* 2012;153(8):1673–1679.
25. Schilder A, Hoheisel U, Magerl W, Benrath J, Klein T, Treede RD. Deep tissue and back pain: Stimulation of the thoracolumbar fascia with hypertonic saline. *Schmerz.* 2014;28(1):90–92.
26. Nielsen JJ et al. Effects of high-intensity intermittent training on potassium kinetics and performance in human skeletal muscle. *J Physiol.* 2004;554:857–870.
27. Juel C, Klarskov C, Nielsen JJ, Krustrup P, Mohr M, Bangsbo J. Effect of high-intensity intermittent training on lactate and H+ release from human skeletal muscle. *Am J Physiol Endocrinol Metab.* 2004;286:E245–E251.
28. Gatej I, Popa M, Rinaudo M. Role of the pH on hyaluronan behavior in aqueous solution. *Biomacromolecules.* 2005;6:61–67.
29. Juel C, Bangsbo J, Graham T, Saltin B. Lactate and potassium fluxes from human skeletal muscle during and after intense, dynamic, knee extensor exercise. *Acta Physiol Scand.* 1990;140:147–159.
30. Noble PW. Hyaluronan and its catabolic products in tissue injury and repair. *Matrix Biol.* 2002;21:2529.
31. Horton MR, Olman MA, Noble P. Hyaluronan fragments induce plasminogen activator inhibitor-1 and inhibit urokinase activity in mouse alveolar macrophages: A potential mechanism for impaired fibrinolytic activity in acute lung injury. *Chest.* 1999;116:17S.
32. Cowman MK, Schmidt TA, Raghavan P, Stecco A. Viscoelastic properties of hyaluronan in physiological conditions. *F1000Res.* 2015;4:622.
33. Stern R, Asari R, Sugahara KN. Size-specific fragments of hyaluronan: An information-rich system. *Eur J Cell Biol.* 2006;85:699–715.
34. Stecco A, Busoni F, Stecco C, Mattioli-Belmonte M, Soldani P, Condino S, Ermolao A, Zaccaria M, Gesi M. Comparative ultrasonographic evaluation of the Achilles paratenon in symptomatic and asymptomatic subjects: An imaging study. *Surg Radiol Anat.* 2015;37(3):281–285.
35. Gerwin RD. Classification, epidemiology and natural history of myofascial pain syndrome. *Curr Pain Headache Rep.* 2001;5:412–420.
36. Shah JP et al. Biochemicals associated with pain and inflammation are elevated in sites near to and remote from active myofascial trigger points. *Arch Phys Med Rehabil.* 2008;89:16–23.
37. Sikdar S et al. Novel applications of ultrasound technology to visualize and characterize myofascial trigger points and surrounding soft tissue. *Arch Phys Med Rehabil.* 2009;90:1829–1838.
38. Adigozali H et al. Reliability of assessment of upper trapezius morphology, its mechanical properties and blood flow in female patients with myofascial pain syndrome using ultrasonography. *J Bodyw Mov Ther.* 2017;21:35–40.

39. Kumbhare DA, Elzibak AH, Noseworthy MD. Assessment of myofascial trigger points using ultrasound. *Am J Phys Med Rehabil.* 2016;95:72–80.

40. Sikdar S et al. Assessment of myofascial trigger points (MTrPs): A new application of ultrasound imaging and vibration sonoelastography. *Conf Proc IEEE Eng Med Biol Soc.* 2008;2008:5585–5588.

41. Fleckenstein J et al. Discrepancy between prevalence and perceived effectiveness of treatment methods in myofascial pain syndrome: Results of a cross-sectional, nationwide survey. *BMC Musculoskelet Disord.* 2010;11:article 32.

42. Ballyns JJ et al. Objective sonographic measures for characterizing myofascial trigger points associated with cervical pain. *J Ultrasound Med.* 2011;30:1331–1340.

43. Menon RG, Raghavan P, Ravinder R. Quantifying muscle glycosaminoglycan levels in patients with post-stroke muscle stiffness using T1ρ MRI. *Regatte Sci Rep.* 2019;9:14513. Published online October 10, 2019.

5 Innervation of Fascia

Robert Schleip

CONTENTS

QUANTITY OF INNERVATION

Fascial tissues are richly innervated (Figure 5.1).[1–3] A recent calculation by Grunwald[4] estimated the total number of fascial nerve endings in an average human body at 100 million. This estimation related to the total mass of dense fibrous connective tissues, which based on the standard data set of Tanaka et al.[5] was estimated at 5 kg for an average male body. However, if one includes the loose connective tissues, as is done in the current nomenclature recommendations relating to "the fascial system",[6] then the total mass of fibrous collagenous connective tissues, based on the same data set by Tanaka et al.[5] increases to 12.5 kg. Taking this into account, the total quantity of nerve endings in the fascial net can then be estimated to be approximately 2. 5 times larger than the 100 million endings suggested by Grunwald, which arrives at the impressive number of 250 million nerve endings in the fascial net. Compared with an estimated quantity of 200 million nerve endings in the skin[4] or with the estimated 120 million to 130 million endings for vision in our eyes, this improved calculation of approximated 250 nerve endings, which are embedded in fascial tissues of some sorts in the human body, suggests that the body-wide fascial network may possibly constitute our richest sensory organ. However, this assumes that the innervation density in the loose connective tissues is not significantly lower than in the dense fibrous tissues, used in the original calculation from Grunwald.[4] As will be

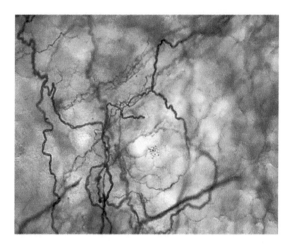

FIGURE 5.1 Demonstration of the rich presence of nerves in a fascia specimen. Immunostaining of a piece of rat lumbar fascia with a pan-neuronal marker (PGP 9.5) reveals the rich network of visible fibers. Image length: approx. 0.5 mm. (Courtesy reproduced with permission from Hoheisel et al., *Neuroscience*, 300, 351–359, 2015.)

examined in the following paragraph, there is some histological evidence to support this assumption. However, the above quantification is only a rough estimation, based on the best data available at this time, and future investigations may improve that estimation in an augmented or attenuated direction.

LOCAL DIFFERENCES IN INNERVATION

There are several indications that the distribution of intrafascial nerve endings is not uniform throughout the body. First, the histological investigations from Tesarz et al.[2] from Heidelberg University, Germany, have shown that in human, as well as rat, lumbar fascia, the density of sensory neurons tends to be significantly higher in the superficial tissue layers between the dermis and fascia profunda when compared with the respective density within the deeper tissue layer, called the lumbodorsal fascia, just underneath these superficial layers.[2] A similar tendency for an augmented innervation density of superficial layers of the human lumbar fasciae was also reported by Benetazo et al.[7]

The second recent insight regarding areas of increased density of sensory nerves in the fascial net comes from Stecco et al.[1] at Padua University in Italy. Their histological examinations of upper and lower limb fasciae in human cadavers revealed severe differences in the density of proprioceptive nerve endings, such as Golgi, Ruffini, and Pacinian corpuscles. Their data indicated that fascial tissues, which clearly serve an important force-transmitting function (such as the lacertus fibrosus on the upper forearm as an extension of the biceps femoris), hardly contain any proprioceptive endings. On the other hand, these investigators observed that some fascial structures seem to have very little role in force transmission, as witnessed when dissecting them away, as is the case of the retinaculae around the ankle and wrist regions. Interestingly, these more obliquely running fascial bands seem to be located at specific approximations to major joints and they contain a very high density of proprioceptive nerve endings. The investigators even suggested that the prime function of these fascial bands may not be their biomechanical but their sensorial function in providing detailed proprioceptive to the central nervous system. If this finding is verified for other body regions as well, it might offer important recommendations for surgical interventions, particularly in situations in which several access options exist for entering a specific internal location.

DIFFERENT NERVE ENDINGS TYPES AND THEIR ASSUMED FUNCTION

Fascia contains different types of nerve endings (Figure 5.2). The vast majority can be characterized as sensory nerve endings. Among these, the free nerve endings are the most numerous. These endings are associated with either C-fibers (also called type III) or with Aδ (type IV) fibers.[3,8] A large number of these are sensitive to mechanical stimulation, whereas the majority can be described as "polymodal receptors", meaning that they are sensitive for different types of stimulation, including nociception. Studies by Tesarz et al.[2] clearly demonstrated the presence of nociceptive endings in fascial tissues. These findings have been supported by provocation tests with injection of hypertonic saline into human lumbar fascia,[9] which indicated that the stimulated interstitial neurons are particularly responsive to repeated mechanical or biochemical irritation. Whether some of the free nerve endings may be able to serve proprioceptive function is a matter of debate.[10–12]

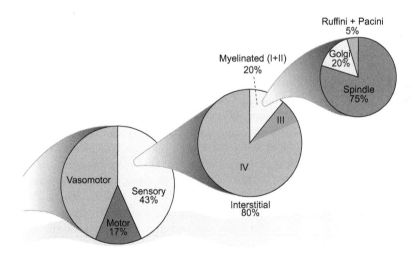

FIGURE 5.2 Composition of neurons in musculoskeletal tissues. The quantities of respective axons were derived from detailed analysis of the combined nerve supplying the lateral gastrocnemius and soleus muscle of a cat. Although a small portion of the interstitial neurons may terminate inside bone, the remaining neurons can all be considered to terminate in fascial connective tissues of some kind, including endo-, peri-, and epimysium. Interstitial neurons include group III (C) fibers as well as group IV (Aδ) fibers, both of which terminate in free nerve endings. Vasomotor neurons are sympathetic, a majority of which regulates the local blood flow. (Image: © fascialnet.com.)

Some of the free nerve endings are sympathetic, a majority of which seems to serve a vasomotor function. However, a significant portion of them seems to serve other unknown functions given that they terminate in areas not associated with blood vessels. Neuhuber et al.[13] suggest that they might serve a trophic function.

Fascia is also innervated by mechanosensory neurons with thick myelin sheets.[1] They are assumed to serve proprioceptive functions. These include Pacinian, Ruffini, and Golgi nerve endings, as well as muscle spindles. The Pacinian corpuscles are rapidly adapting receptors and are, therefore, suspected to mediate rapid joint motion. Ruffini endings, on the other hand, are slow-adaptive mechanosensors, which are particularly sensitive to differences in shear loading. They seem to be involved in perceiving directional differences in tensional loading between different adjacent tissue layers. While the Golgi receptors were previously considered to exist in tendinous tissues only, their presence in other fascial tissues has been securely confirmed by several independent studies.[1,14] Stimulation of Golgi receptors tends to trigger a relaxation response (autogenic inhibition) in skeletal muscle fibers that are directly linked with the respectively tensioned collagen fibers. Golgi receptors can, therefore, contribute to the proprioceptive sense of force and heaviness of muscles. Muscle spindles inform the central nervous system about the changing status of muscle tone, movement, and joint position. These spindles are embedded in the perimysium of the muscle. Changes in stiffness and other viscoelastic properties of the perimysial connective tissue may, therefore, corroborate spindle sensitivity.[15]

SEGMENTAL INNERVATION ZONES

The term "fasciotome" was introduced by Tesarz[2] in relation to hypothesized existence of segmental innervation zones in the fascia profunda of the human lumbar region. He postulated that these fascial tissues might contain a regional innervation by specific medial and lateral branches of dorsal neurons, with correspondences similar to the lumbar musculature underneath. The term has subsequently been taken over by others[16,17] and used hypothetically for other fascial regions as well.[17]

A recent review by Stecco et al.[17] suggests that the term "fasciotomes" should be used for dense layers of fascia profunda, while the innervation of superficial fasciae (or subcutaneous loose connective tissues) should be considered to be organized in the same "dermatomes" as the overlying skin. According to this concept, the term "dermatome" represents the portion of tissue composed of cutis and subcutaneous loose connective tissue, supplied by all the cutaneous branches of an individual spinal nerve. In contrast the term "fasciotome" then includes the portion of deep fascia supplied by the same nerve root. The dermatome is considered to be important for exteroception, whereas the "fasciatome" is important for proprioception. If pathologically altered, the dermatome tends to express clearly localized pain while the "fasciatomes" tend to express as irradiating pain according to the organization of the fascial anatomy.[17]

However, there are indications that the primary innervation of fascial regions might not be exclusive, and that additional secondary innervation from other spinal nerves might exist, as was suggested by a study of rat crural fasciae.[8] If verified, this could mean that the regional precision of fasciotomes might be partly similar to the dermatomes, whose specialization tends to be less precise and less uniform than had been generally assumed.[18]

INNERVATION OF VISCERAL CONNECTIVE TISSUES

According to Stecco et al.[19] visceral fascia can be divided into two large groups. On one hand, "investing fasciae", which are closely related to individual organs, give shape to the individual organs and support the respective parenchyma. Investing fasciae are usually quite thin and elastic and are well innervated. On the other hand, the "insertional fasciae" consist of fibrous sheets that form the compartments for the organs and also connect these organs with the musculoskeletal system. Insertional fasciae are relatively thick, are less densely innervated, and also contain larger myelinated neurons, which are rarely found among the investing fasciae. In particular, those myelinated neurons were found in insertional fasciae of the liver, heart, and the visceral fascia of the abdomen. The authors suggest that their findings are congruent with the innervation pattern reported by Standring[20] that fasciae close to organs have only autonomic innervation, whereas the visceral fasciae of the abdomen and thorax also contain a sensitive innervation from the somatic nervous system.

INTEROCEPTIVE FUNCTION

INTEROCEPTION AND THE INSULAR CORTEX

Free nerve endings in fascial tissues are sometimes associated with an interoceptive function. Their stimulation then provides the brain with information about the condition of the body in its constant search for physiological homeostasis. A large quantity of interoceptive free nerve endings are located in visceral connective tissues and constitute an important part of what is frequently referred to as the enteric brain. However, other interoceptive interstitial neurons are located within musculoskeletal connective tissues, such as the endomysium or perimysium. Interoceptive signaling is associated with feelings like warmth, hunger, thirst, nausea, muscular effort, soreness, and heaviness or lightness as well as a sense of belonging or alienation regarding specific body regions, etc.[21] The upstream neural pathway from interoceptive nerve endings does not follow the usual afferent pathways toward the somatosensory cortex of the brain. Instead, they project to the insular cortex inside the forebrain. In this cortical area, sensations related to internal somatic sensations are associated with emotional preferences and affective attitudes. As described by Damasio,[22] patients with disturbed functioning of the insula may still have full biomechanical functioning and achieve high IQ levels in respective tests; however, they usually tend to be socially dysfunctional and are unable to make reasonable decisions in complex situations.

Several health-related conditions, such as low back pain, scoliosis, or complex regional pain syndrome, are associated with a diminished proprioceptive acuity. In contrast to these, several other conditions are apparently more clearly related to dysfunctional interoceptive processing. These latter conditions include irritable bowel syndrome, anorexia, anxiety, depression, and alexithymia (inability in recognizing and expressing one's own emotional states) (Table 5.1).

TABLE 5.1

Associations of Proprio- and Interoceptive Dysfunctions with Specific Pathologies

Proprioceptive Impairment	Interoceptive Dysregulation
Chronic low back pain	Eating disorders
	Irritable bowel syndrome
Complex regional pain syndrome (CRGP)	Posttraumatic stress disorder
Whiplash	Depression
	Panic disorder
	Generalized anxiety disorder
Attention deficit hyperactivity disorder (ADHD)	Substance use disorders
Systemic hypermobility	Autism spectrum disorders
	Depersonalization/derealization disorder
Scoliosis	Somatic symptom disorders
	Functional disorders
Other myofascial pain syndromes	Chronic fatigue syndrome

INNERVATION OF EPI-/PERINEURIUM

Most peripheral nerves are enveloped in a three-layer fascial model. Their axons are surrounded by endoneurium, which offers only little mechanical support. Groups of endoneurium-covered axons are then enveloped by a think but dense perineurium, which offers strength in tension, and also maintains the so-called blood–nerve barrier. Finally, the perineurium is again covered by the epineurium, a thick and areolar layer of connective tissue that is highly vascularized and acts as a cushion for the whole nerve bundle. All three fascial layers of the nerve are innervated and contain a thin plexus of potential nociceptors that is likely responsible for some cases of nerve trunk pain. Experiments with rats have shown that inflammation tends to change respective neural axons by making them sensitive to mechanical stimuli.[23] Such nerve trunk pain may then appear either as local tenderness of a nerve, or a "doorbell" type of response, where local spot palpation may evoke symptoms in a more distal region.

FASCIAL ENTRAPMENT NEUROPATHIES

The term "nerve entrapment" is generally used to describe the entrapment or compression of a peripheral nerve as it passes through a musculoskeletal structure such as a fascial opening, a fibro-osseous tunnel or below a dense overlying fascial retinaculum. Only very few of these are attributed to muscles. Among these are cubital tunnel syndrome and piriformis syndrome, which are attributed to contractures of the anconeus and epitrochlear is muscle or of the piriformis muscle, respectively. The vast majority of entrapment syndromes are caused by compression of fascial bands, ligaments, aponeuroses, or other rigid structures.[24]

The specific microenvironment around the nerves is increasingly highlighted as contributing a factor in these pathologies. This environment includes the perineurium,

TABLE 5.2

Entrapment Neuropathies That Are Associated with Modifications in Their Local Connective Tissue Environment

Upper Extremity Entrapment Neuropathies	Lower Extremity Entrapment Neuropathies
Median nerve entrapment	Common digital plantar nerve entrapment
Ulnar nerve entrapment	Tarsal tunnel syndrome
Radial nerve entrapment	Sural nerve entrapment
Superficial radial nerve entrapment	Saphenous nerve entrapment
(Wartenberg's syndrome)	Common peroneal nerve entrapment
Intrinsic constriction of suprascapular nerve	Superficial peroneal nerve entrapment
Thoracic outlet syndrome	Sciatic neuropathy
	Lateral femoral cutaneous nerve entrapment
	Obturator nerve entrapment
	Superior cluneal nerve entrapment

epineurium, intermuscular septa, and deep fascia. Modifications in these fascial structures can impact the mobility of the nerve in relating to the surrounding structures. Table 5.2 lists common dysfunctions that are at least partially influenced by such modifications in their surrounding tissue environment. Note that such entrapment neuropathies seem to be more frequent and/or be more easily recognized in the lower body region compared with the upper region.[24]

FASCIA-GENERATED LOW BACK PAIN

The lumbodorsal fascia has been proposed to represent a possible source of nonspecific low back pain.[25] Histological investigations revealed the presence of nociceptive free nerve endings within this fascial tissue.[2,26] *In vivo* elicitation of back pain via experimental stimulation of the lumbodorsal fascia—via hypertonic saline injection or via electrical high-frequency stimulation—suggests that dorsal horn neurons react by increasing their excitability.[9] In particular, the pain radiation and pain affect evoked by fascia injection exceeded those of the underlying muscle significantly. The most specific pain descriptors after fascia injection were burning, throbbing, and stinging sensations.

Subsequent to delayed onset muscle soreness, pain thresholds of the fascia decreased significantly more than those of the underlying muscle tissue.[27] Hoheisel et al.[28] demonstrated in rats that chronic irritation of the lumbodorsal fascia can induce sensitization phenomena at the spinal level. After experimentally induced chronic inflammation of this fascial tissue, the density of nociceptive fibers was significantly increased. Moreover, Pedersen et al.[29] were able to elicit spastic contractions in decerebrated cats by mechanically pinching their lumbodorsal fascia. These contractions occurred most at their ipsilateral back muscles, as well as on their contralateral back, their hamstring, and their gluteal muscles. When pinching the underlying muscles, the responses were much less pronounced compared with the fascial stimulation.

In addition, morphological changes in human lumbodorsal fascia have been demonstrated in chronic low back pain patients.[30] How exactly these characteristics relate to the etiology of low back pain is unclear. Wilke et al.[25] suggest that possibly microinjuries and/or inflammation in the lumbodorsal fascia may lead to or contribute to the above described sensitization of fascia-related dorsal horn neurons.

Greater understanding of the vast innervation of the fascial system as discussed above could open up opportunities to look at the management of chronic pain without using opioids. Perhaps providing novel mechanosensory stimulation or providing other kinds of novel afferent input to fascial tissues could be explored as alternative or complementary pathways to conventional pharmacological treatment. This holds promise of healing the fascia and breaking the cycle of chronic pain.

REFERENCES

1. Stecco, C., Gagey, O., Belloni, A., Pozzuoli, A., Porzionato, A., Macchi, V., Aldegheri, R., De Caro, R., Delmas, V. 2007. Anatomy of the deep fascia of the upper limb. Second part: Study of innervation. *Morphologie* 91:38–43.
2. Tesarz, J. 2010. Die Fascia thoracolumbalis als potenzielle Ursache für Rückenschmerzen: Anatomische Grundlagen und klinische Aspekte. *Osteopathische Medizin* 11(1):28–34.
3. Taguchi, T., Hoheisel, U., Mense, S. 2008. Dorsal horn neurons having input from low back structures in rats. *Pain* 138:119–129.
4. Grunwald, M. 2017. *Homo Hapticus.* Munich: Droemer Verlag, p. 54.
5. Tanaka, G., Kawamura, H. 1992. Reference man models based on normal data from human populations. Report of the Task Group on Reference Man, *The International Commission on Radiotogical Protection*, Nr. 23. http://www.irpa.net/irpa10/cdrom/00602.pdf
6. Schleip, R., Hedley, G., Yukesoy, C.A. 2019. Fascial nomenclature: Update on related consensus process. *Clin Anat.* online prepublication: https://doi.org/10.1002/ca.23423
7. Benetazzo, L., Bizzego, A., De Caro, R., Frigo, G., Guidolin, D., Stecco, C. 2011. 3D reconstruction of the crural and thoracolumbar fasciae. *Surg Radiol Anat* 33:855–862.
8. Taguchi, T., et al. 2013. Nociception originating from the crural fascia in rats. *Pain* 154:1103–1114.
9. Schilder, A., Magerl, U., Hoheisel, U., Klein, T., Treede, R. 2016. Electrical high-frequency stimulation of the human thoracolumbar fascia evokes long-term potentiation-like pain amplification. *Pain* 157:2309–2317.
10. Mense, S., Stahnke, M. 1983. Responses in muscle afferent fibres of slow conduction velocity to contractions and ischaemia in the cat. *J Physiol* 342:383–397.
11. Sakada, S. 1974. Mechanoreceptors in fascia, periosteum and periodontal ligament. *Bull Tokyo Med Dent Univ* 21 Suppl(0):11–13.
12. Fleury, M., et al. 1995. Weight judgment. The discrimination capacity of a deafferented subject. *Brain* 118:1149–1156.
13. Neuhuber, W.L, Jänig, W. 2017. The innervation of fascial tissues: Focus on thin-caliber afferents and sympathetic efferents. In *Fascia in the Osteopathic Field*, eds. Liem, T., Tozzi, P., Chila, A., pp. 339–350. Edinburgh: Handspring Publishing.
14. Yahia, L., Rhalmi, S., Newman, N., Isler, M. 1992. Sensory innervation of human thoracolumbar fascia. An immunohistochemical study. *Acta Orthop Scand* 63:195–197.

15. Giuriati, W., et al. 2018. Muscle spindles of the rat sternomastoid muscle. *Eur J Transl Myol* 28:7904.
16. Willard, F.H., Vleeming, A., Schuenke, M.D., Danneels, L., Schleip, R. 2012. The thoracolumbar fascia: Anatomy, function and clinical considerations. *J Anat* 221:507–536.
17. Stecco, C., et al. 2019. Dermatome and fasciatome. *Clin Anat.* https://doi.org/10.1002/ca.23408
18. Apok, V., Gurusinghe, N.T., Mitchell, J.D., Emsley, H.C. 2011. Dermatomes and dogma. *Pract Neurol* 11:100–105.
19. Stecco, C., et al. 2017. Microscopic anatomy of the visceral fasciae. *J Anat* 231:121–128.
20. Standring, S. (ed.). 2016. *Gray's Anatomy: The Anatomical Basis of Clinical Practice*, 41st ed., Edinburgh: Churchill Livingstone.
21. Craig, A.D. 2002. How do you feel? Interoception: The sense of the physiological condition of the body. *Nat Rev Neurosci* 3:655–666.
22. Damasio, A. 1999. *The Feeling of What Happens: Body and Emotion in the Making of Consciousness.* New York: Harcourt-Brace.
23. Bove, G.M. 2008. Epi-perineurial anatomy, innervation, and axonal nociceptive mechanisms. *J Bodyw Movem Ther* 12:185–190.
24. Stecco, A., Pirri, C., Stecco, C. 2019. Fascial entrapment neuropathy. *Clin Anat*: https://doi.org/10.1002/ca.23388.
25. Wilke, J., Schleip, R., Klingler, W., Stecco, C. 2017. The lumbodorsal fascia as a potential source of low back pain: A narrative review. *Biomed Res Int* 2017:5349620.
26. Tesarz, J., Hoheisel, U., Wiedenhöfer, B., Mense, S. 2011. Sensory innervation of the thoracolumbar fascia in rats and humans. *Neuroscience* 194:302–308.
27. Lau, W.Y., Blazevich, A.J., Newton, M.J., Wu, S.S., Nosaka, K. 2015. Changes in electrical pain threshold of fascia and muscle after initial and secondary bouts of elbow flexor eccentric exercise. *Eur J Appl Physiol* 115:959–968.
28. Hoheisel, U., Rosner, J., Mense, S. 2015. Innervation changes induced by inflammation of the rat thoracolumbar fascia. *Neuroscience* 300:351–359.
29. Pedersen, H.E., Blunck, F.J., Gardner, E. 1956. The anatomy of lumbosacral posterior rami and meningeal branches of spinal nerves (sinu-vertebral nerves). *J Bone Joint Surg* 38:377–391.
30. Langevin, H.M., et al. 2011. Reduced thoracolumbar fascia shear strain in human chronic low back pain. *BMC Musculoskelet Disord* 12:203.

6 Fascia and the Circulatory System

Anita Boser and Kirstin Schumaker

CONTENTS

INTRODUCTION

Our fascial system, including both the dense fibrous layers and the more loosely organized superficial layer, protects and supports joints, organs, nerves, blood vessels, and the lymphatic system. In doing so, it also facilitates movement and communication. When the structural support of the fascial system is altered, there are functional consequences for other body-wide systems—the neural and vascular networks—as well as the organ systems. The fascial network can be altered by injury and repair (severe ankle sprain), or through surgery (removal of a breast or repairing a broken bone), or disease (Duputryn's contracture), or when the fascial network is functioning atypically due to congenital reasons (Marfan's syndrome). In this chapter, we explore ways in which the organization of superficial and deep fascial layers facilitates the functioning of the vascular system, and we also present ways in which the fascial system impedes or interferes with the functioning of the vascular system, producing symptoms that are either vascular or neural.

We begin with the anatomy, describe the relationship between fascial layers and the circulatory system, then highlight and further describe some of the fascial structures that have been mentioned in other chapters of this book. Then we present what is known and

71

observed based on the available scientific evidence. While the evidence is limited, we can reasonably speculate about how vessel structure and its fascial context can either facilitate or limit fluid flow, and thereby effect somatic function. Finally, we will describe some interesting structural patterns and specific cases that have been observed by the authors (and other clinicians), with the goal of helping health care practitioners to understand the complex and varied relationship between the fascial network and the vascular system.

NEUROVASCULAR TRACTS

Blood vessels and nerves tend to travel through the body in bundles, surrounded and supported by fascial layers that include a fibrous matrix, fibroblasts and myofibroblasts, immune system cells, lymphatic vessels, microvessels, and the free nerve endings that sense tension within the matrix of the neurovascular tract. Collectively, all the elements of these tracts, outside of the vessels, is sometimes also referred to as the stroma. The diverse tissues of the bundles interact mechanically and biochemically. The neurovascular tract, a fascial corridor, houses many tissue types and provides passage for the body-wide network of the neural and vascular systems much in the way that the mediastinum is a region and a collection of all the tubes and vessels and nerves that pass through the thorax between the lungs.

VESSEL ANATOMY—LAYERS WITHIN THE VESSELS

Focusing on the vessels first, the walls of arteries and veins can be described as having three functional layers: the inner layer is endothelium (tunica intima or interna); the middle layer, tunica media, contains smooth muscle cells, collagen, and elastin; and the outer layer is the tunica externa or adventitia. We use the term adventitia. This outer layer is composed primarily of collagen arranged in helical patterns, but it also includes microvessels (vasa vasorum and lymphatic vessels) and cells that are important for artery health. The adventitia, described as having two layers by Witter, blends into the adjacent connective and adipose tissue, which is visible with immunohistochemical staining[1-4] (Figure 6.1). Some definitions of fascia include this outer layer of adventitia.[5]

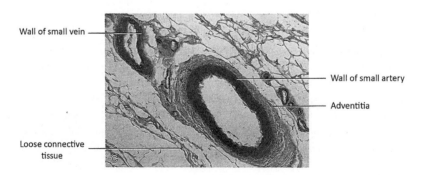

FIGURE 6.1 Immunohistochemical stain to show the presence and localization of collagen type III in small vessels. (Reprinted with permission from *Functional Atlas of the Human Fascial System* by Carla Stecco.)

Far from being inert, as previously assumed, current research suggests that the adventitia has a dynamic effect on the tunica media and endothelium, including the size of the lumen. Immune cells and progenitor cells reside in the adventitia, providing protection and repair for the vessels and possibly also the surrounding tissues.[6] Stenmark et al. describes the adventitia as a "biologic processing center" that may be the first to react to vessel injury.[7] Surrounding tissues also affect arteries through the adventitia. The cells of the adventitia respond to mechanical tension transmitted through the fibrous matrix around the vessels. Connective tissue fibers connect to nitric oxide receptors in arterioles and send signals that create vessel dilation in response to muscular contraction.[8]

VESSEL CONTEXT—LAYERS SUPPORTING THE VASCULATURE

The circulatory system, from the heart to the vascular beds, generally follows the framework of the fascial network, which provides support and protection. Long vessels are guided by canals, septa, and fibrous bands. Vessels are cushioned by loose connective tissue as they course through superficial fascia and intermuscular septa or alongside rigid or less mobile layers on their way from one layer to another. In places vessels are adhered to a fascial layer that lies adjacent to a rigid structure, such as where the fascia profundus lies over a bone, to stabilize the vessels during somatic activity. Where vessels traverse layers of loose connective tissue, they generally run at an angle from deep to shallow, so that there is independent movement between the freer outer layer and the less flexible deeper layer. Where the epidermal and epimysial layers lie close together, vessels run more perpendicular to the planes of profundus and epidermis. As they travel through the superficial fascial layer, where it is relatively thick and filled with adipose cells, collagen and elastin fibers create a supporting lattice with layers that divide to encompass the lymphatic vessels.[9–11] Divergent fascial layers, described as subcutaneous fascial bands, sometimes guide vessels through the more loosely organized subcutaneous adipose layer that is present just above and below the plane of superficial fascia.[11]

SUPERFICIAL LAYERS AND VESSELS

Arteries within the subcutis occur in two plexi: the subpapillary plexus just beneath the skin, and the deep arterial plexus that lies inside the superficial fascia. Shunts between the venules and arterioles of the deep plexus help to regulate blood flow to the subpapillary plexus, thus participating in thermoregulation. Only one-fifth of the subpapillary arteries are required to supply the skin—the rest are used for thermoregulation.[12]

Major superficial veins, such as the saphenous vein, run for long distances between layers within the superficial fascia. The superficial fascia splits into layers to create channels for major veins and lymphatic vessels with septa that attach to the vessel walls.[13–15] Fascial layers and bands associated with the veins may play an active role in vein dilation during exercise. The width of the fascial tunnel varies along the length of the vessel, depending on the arrangement of muscles and health of tissues, and in narrow spaces it can become a source of compression.[13,15]

Caggiati refers to the saphenous fascia as a "mechanical shield" that can offer protection from varicosity and notes that the tributary saphenous veins, with their smaller cell walls, fewer muscle cells, and less connective tissue protection, are at greater risk of varicosity.[13,16] However, there is evidence that defects of the vein wall, which may be due to injury and/or genetic deficiency in collagen synthesis, occur before varicosity develops.[17]

NEUROVASCULAR SHEATHS

In areas where the neurovascular tract passes around a bony or ligamentous edge—for example, the femoral bundle passing under the inguinal ligament, the axillary/brachial bundle passing under the clavicle, and the jugular vein, vagus nerve, and accessory nerve passing through the jugular foramen of the cranium—the neurovascular tract is wrapped in an extra layer of protection, a fascial sheath. Connective tissue is generally denser and stiffer in the proximal portion of the sheath, becoming thinner and looser as the vessels exit the sheath at the distal portion where it blends into fascia of adjacent muscles and septa. Studies have demonstrated that the sheath allows for mobility of vessels in relationship to each other and for the expansion of vessel size to allow for increased blood flow when needed.[18,19]

In general, sheaths are divided by septa which create tubular subcompartments for each vessel, making separate passages for nerve, artery, and vein. However, this is variable, and the septa do not necessarily isolate vessels along the entire length. For example, the axillary portion of the brachial plexus sheath has compartments for multiple nerves, blood, and lymphatic vessels, but in places the brachial artery is encased in the paraneural sheath and attaches to the brachial fascia. The iliopectineal arch separates the femoral nerve from the femoral sheath, allowing the femoral nerve greater range of motion and protecting the femoral vessels from compression by the iliacus muscle.[18,20]

VESSEL PATHWAYS TO THE VISCERA

Fascia that covers blood vessels interconnects with visceral fascia as well. The fasciae of these visceral vascular sheaths, which are similar to mesentery structures, is continuous with the visceral peritoneum that surrounds the organs, the parietal peritoneum that lines the organ cavities, and the fascia of the blood vessels as they enter and exit the organ. For example, the endopelvic fascia envelopes the visceral organs and creates conduits for vasculature through the hypogastric, umbilical-prevesical, and vesicorectal sheaths,[21] and Gibson's capsule includes the portal vein, hepatic artery, and bile duct.[22]

One of the most beautiful and obvious examples of connection between vascular and visceral fascia is the fibrous and serous pericardium. The adventitia of great vessels attaches directly to the serosal and fibrous pericardium. The serosal pericardium has two layers. The inner layer, also known as the epicardium, the visceral fascia of the heart, is separated by a thin layer of fluid from the second layer, which is the one-cell-wide, inner layer of the fibrous pericardium that connects to the pretracheal fascia, the posterior surface of the sternum, and the central tendon of the diaphragm.[23] (Figures 6.2 and 6.3) This connection between visceral, vascular, and myofascia is similar for all organs.

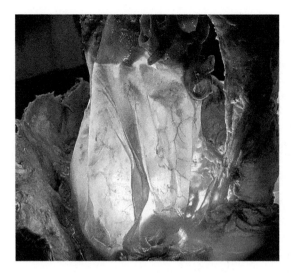

FIGURE 6.2 Up lit fibroserous pericardium with heart removed, still connected to the aorta (right), respiratory diaphragm, and ribs (left). (Courtesy of Andreas Hass. Image reproduced with permission from the Fascial Net Plastination Project, www.fasciaresearchsociety.org/plastination.)

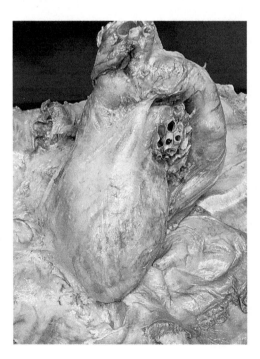

FIGURE 6.3 Pericardium highlighting its fascial continuity with the fascia of the aorta, left bronchus, pulmonary vessels, and respiratory diaphragm. (Courtesy of Rachelle Clauson. Image reproduced with permission from the Fascial Net Plastination Project, www.fasciare-searchsociety.org/plastination.)

VESSEL PATHWAYS FROM CORE OF THE BODY TO THE OUTER LAYERS

Arteries and veins perforate through multiple fascial layers in the course of nourishing tissues, from the core of the body to the outer layers. Perforations through the deep fascia often include a "triad" of artery, vein, and nerve and sometimes also a lymphatic vessel[24,25] (Figure 6.4). Taylor et al. notes the veins and arteries to the skin follow a connective tissue framework in sections called angiosomes and venosomes.[26] Perforations in the subcutaneous layer have been found to correspond to acupuncture points.[27] The deep fascia overlying epimysium includes a rich vascular and lymphatic network in addition to providing a conduit for vessel perforation passing through the epimysium and muscle. The gliding action of the fascia over the epimysium improves the mobility for muscles and vessels.[14,24]

To the extent that these fascial layers are healthy, the small vessels are mobile, supported by a loose web of hydrated connective tissue fibers that facilitates glide of the perforating neurovascular tract through the more densely structured fascia. This hydrated web allows the perforating vessel to glide in and out of the plane of dense fascia and through openings in fascial planes. Some of the hiatuses are large, while some are small in diameter, and the shape varies from slot-like to conical to pyramidal, or funnel-shaped.[25,28]

Epifascial veins, those just below the skin, and deep veins, which are below the muscular fascia, are interconnected with perforating veins that perforate the epimysium and deep fascia. Valves within the veins function to guide blood from the superficial veins to the deep veins. It is estimated that normally 90% of venous blood in the legs returns through the deeper veins.[29]

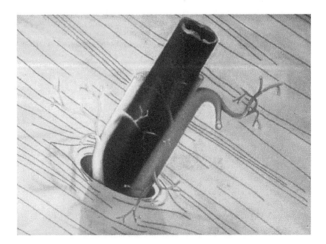

FIGURE 6.4 Passage of a triad through superficial fascial connective tissue. Left—nerve, middle—vein, right—artery. Most of these perforation points are topographically identical with traditional Chinese acupuncture points. (From Freiwald, J. et al., *Sports Orthop. Traumatol.*, 32, 258–266, 2016.)

RELATIONSHIP BETWEEN FASCIA AND VASCULATURE IN THE LEG

Fascia plays an important role in vascular regulation in the lower leg; the pressure created by fascia compartments and blood supply requires a stable balance. The deep fascia of the leg, especially that of the posterior compartment, constrains the muscles as they contract to generate pressure that pumps blood through the valved veins.[29] Muscular and fascial weakness can diminish the pump and result in venous insufficiency.[30] Conversely, compartment syndrome develops when venous drainage is impaired, but arterial flow remains normal. This can be due to acute or repetitive strain injury. Increased fascial thickness and stiffness has been found in conjunction with chronic anterior compartment syndrome.[31,32] Although fasciotomy is indicated in some cases of chronic exertional compartment syndrome, it does diminish the calf muscle pump action and may increase the risk for venous insufficiency.[33] Another interesting connection between fascia and the vasculature in the lower leg is the uncommon case of muscle herniation through the epimysium, suggested to occur at sites of vein perforation, which is often mistaken for varicosity or hematoma.[34] Although usually asymptomatic, a case report of peroneus longus herniation resulted in burning sensations.[35]

VESSEL PATHWAYS THAT CROSS JOINTS

Collateral vessels provide alternative pathways for blood supply needed to nourish joints when they are flexed and compressed or held in any functional position. Some collateral arteries are named "circumflex" in reference to the circumferential pathway that the artery takes, and others are simply named "collateral" indicating that they are alternative pathways. Motor nerves often follow partway along a circumflex arterial path, but these nerves do not make the complete loop around a joint or bone. In the feet and the hands, another category of collateral vessel is termed a perforating vessel, because these vessels connect the vascular network on the dorsum of the foot or hand with the plantar or palmar vascular network, or they connect a vessel in the extensor compartment with a vessel in the flexor compartment (in the forearm and lower leg, perforating the interosseous membrane). In the foot and hand, the perforating vessels pass from dorsal to plantar or palmar side at or near the joints, again helping ensure that the joints get adequate blood supply in any functional position.[23]

FASCIA AND SUBOPTIMAL VASCULAR FUNCTION
AND SOMATIC DYSFUNCTION

Blood vessels can be impinged or entrapped by fascia, similar to entrapment neuropathies. This can result in edema, occasional cramping, or less commonly, in intermittent claudication. For example, the femoral artery can be limited as it passes through the adductor hiatus and knee flexion can create deformation of the femoropopliteal artery.[28,36] An ultrasound study found that 72% of femoropopliteal artery occlusions occur at the adductor canal hiatus.[37] Noorani et al. describe a type of coeliac artery compression caused by impingement by the median arcuate ligament and detail six types of popliteal entrapment syndrome, two of which are caused by myofascial compression.[38] A study using magnetic resonance imaging showed that contraction of the medial gastrocnemius could displace and compress the popliteal neurovascular tract within the proximal tendon of the soleus.[39] A review study on popliteal cysts noted that compression of the popliteal vein is more common than compression of the artery, because arteries have stiffer walls and higher internal pressure.[40] However, De Oliveira et al. noted that symptoms due to compression of the femoral artery are more prevalent than those due to restriction of the saphenous nerve[28] (Figure 6.5).

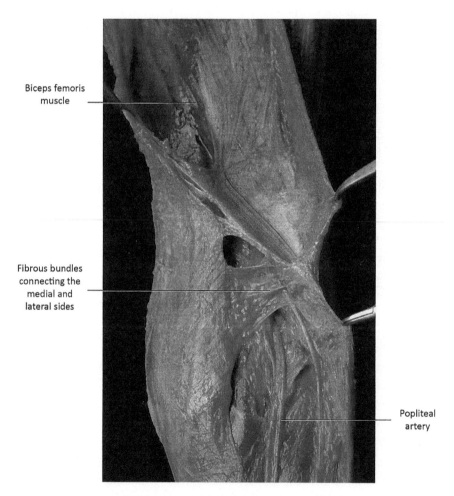

Biceps femoris muscle

Fibrous bundles connecting the medial and lateral sides

Popliteal artery

FIGURE 6.5 Fascial network of the popliteal region. The fascia lata was cut and is tractioned medially to show the complexity of fascial connections. Some fibrous bundles connect the fasciae of the medial and lateral heads of the gastrocnemius muscle and create a roof for the popliteal vessels. These bundles may cause compression syndrome. (Reprinted with permission from *Functional Atlas of the Human Fascial System* by Carla Stecco.)

More distally, McKeon describes how perforating arteries passing through the interosseous membrane of the lower leg can be damaged when an injury to the ankle extends from the tibiofibular syndesmosis up into the interosseous membrane.[41] Fascial restriction of arteries into the lower leg can cause patients who do not have the risk factors commonly associated with peripheral artery disease (PAD) to present with symptoms and signs of this disease, namely intermittent claudication and muscle stiffness of the lower legs experienced with exercise.[42]

Compression is not limited to the lower limbs. Perforating neurovascular tracts that pass through hypertonic brachialis muscle can be impinged by chronic muscle contraction or high muscle tone, creating nerve ischemia and nociception that leads to inhibition of movement that would lengthen or stretch the small neurovascular tract.[43] Other vascular entrapment syndromes involve the renal arteries, the superior mesenteric artery, celiac artery, and iliac vein.[38] We suggest that hypertonicity in other muscles, such as the coracobrachialis, extensor digitorum longus, and psoas, can also compress vessels that accompany the perforating nerves.

Multiple studies have investigated iliac vein compression syndrome, which is also called May–Thurner syndrome (MTS), and the anatomical variations within this syndrome have long been documented. In MTS, the left common iliac vein is chronically compressed by the right common iliac artery, possibly also by the left internal iliac artery (hypogastric artery). These vessels press the common iliac vein against the body of the fifth lumbar vertebra. Chronic pulsatile vein compression causes turbulent flow, which leads to development of intraluminal spurs and ridges and other endothelial changes, which further disrupt laminar flow and may lead to deep vein thrombosis and venous insufficiency. Some degree of iliac vein compression and occlusion, without symptoms of iliac vein compression, may be present in 66% of the general population. Moderate symptoms of iliac vein compression include swelling in the left lower limb, pain, varicosity, and skin changes that indicate venous insufficiency. Right iliac vein versus left iliac vein compression occurs at a rate of 1:3.[44–46] We are particularly interested in these studies for reasons that will be outlined next.

WORKING HYPOTHESIS BASED ON CLINICAL OBSERVATIONS

Fascial compartments become stiff and extremely pressurized when the venous return is impinged. Alteration of the superficial fascia is likely to restrict lymphatic flow and changes in lymphatic flow are likely to affect the superficial fascia.[12] Additionally, fibrovascular and vascular bands can create deep gluteal syndrome through compression of nerves in the gluteal compartment.[47] Speaking as clinicians, we offer that with a passive straight leg raise (patient supine), the practitioner may note that the limb feels heavy and they may perceive the resistance to be localized in the posterior hip or the posterior thigh. This perceived resistance is often assumed to come from the sciatic nerve or may be attributed to muscle hypertonicity. Another factor producing the impression of heaviness could be greater blood volume in the limb, resulting from venous outflow restriction. We regularly note that when we address fascial restriction of the vessels supplying the hypertonic tissues, the limb suddenly feels less heavy. Another observation: when performing a passive straight leg lift on both limbs, on a patient who presents primarily with nerve symptoms in the left lower extremity (left sciatica and/or neuropathy in the left foot or lower leg), we typically find the entire right lower extremity and the left gluteal area offer heaviness and resistance.

We posit that lumbosacral neural impingement could arise over time from consequences of fascial restriction of vasculature in the opposite limb and that treatment of fascial restriction in the right lower extremity is important for remediating neural issues in the left lower extremity. Common slip and fall incidents as well as high impact sports injuries involving unilateral overstretch could create asymmetrical injury to the vascular system.

We further suggest that research could be designed to investigate the hypothesis that nociception in the adventitia leads to vasodilation and blood profusion in the muscles adjacent to and distal to the neurovascular tract (suggesting a neuromotor protective response for threatened vasculature). We have found that when slack is provided to the neurovascular tract and then followed with a specific gentle stretch, tissue changes result in a lasting reduction in nociception and protective stiffening.

If muscular stiffening is a protective mechanism that prevents excessive overstretch and or impingement of vessels, and muscular stiffening either impinges nerves or leads to lumbar disc injury, then this proposed vascular protection mechanism may underlie many neural impingement patterns. Although there is no evidence for this, there are two manual therapy studies using fascial techniques that demonstrate positive effects on the circulatory system. For example, a study that used osteopathic fascial release techniques along arterial pathways for patients with knee osteoarthritis improved resistive index of the superficial femoral artery and active knee flexion.[48] Another study for patients with Type 2 Diabetes and PAD found that treatment of 15 weekly connective tissue massages resulted in improved circulation to both limbs with residual effects 6 months after treatment.[49] It should be noted that although manual therapy can be used to reduce the muscle stiffening that we attribute to venous impingement, and although peripheral neuropathy and sciatic nerve impingement may benefit from neurofascial manipulation and/or vascular-fascial manipulation, a conservative (non-surgical) manual approach of working with the neurovascular tracts will not reduce the intraluminal changes that develop over time in the vessels that have chronically disrupted blood flow. In particular, it is important to identify signs of common iliac vein compression early, before obstructive remodeling within the vessel has progressed.[45]

REFERRAL GUIDELINES

When surgical approaches are not indicated, and in addition to surgical treatment approaches, multiple manual therapy approaches could be used to address fascial restriction of vasculature: osteopathic manipulative therapy (OMT), connective tissue massage (CMT), strain/counter strain (SCS), neural manipulation (NM), and neurovascular release (NVR) can all produce a favorable tissue response, here defined as normalization of muscle tone and extensibility. Theoretical explanations for the results will vary, depending on the school of thought around the techniques. Other manual therapy approaches such as structural integration (SI), which classically utilize tissue differentiation techniques that involve deeper touch, may benefit patients with fascial restriction of vasculature given that vasculature generally runs through the fascial compartments and intermuscular septa that are released by SI practitioners. Such structural approaches will be especially beneficial to vasculature when the practitioner is able to utilize a lighter and/or a more specific touch. Therapeutic approaches that are less specific, such as dermoneuromodulation (DNM) and some forms of myofascial release (MFR) could also benefit the vascular network in general and neurovascular tracts specifically.

A few clinical pearls to pass on to referring physicians: In our experience, cramping of hamstrings or feet during yoga or stretching may indicate fascial restriction of the deeper vasculature. Stecco et al. suggest that deep fascia and epimysium should be targeted when there is cramping, and the superficial fascia should be addressed when there is dysfunction of the venous system or lymphatic system or when there is thermoregulatory dysfunction of the skin.[12] "Numbness" reported by a patient who does have discrimination of light touch, may be an experience of "dullness" that we propose to be the sensation of reduced blood flow to cutaneous nerves. Practitioners of the Jones Institute School of SCS consider a burning sensation to be a possible symptom of venous restriction. Patients with high elastin and low collagen in their connective tissue, those who are considered hypermobile, often benefit from vascular release (symptoms of discomfort are reduced and structure feels more balanced), with a caution to the practitioner that vessels should not be "overhandled", and specific work will be more beneficial than broad, pervasive applications of fascial work.

FINAL THOUGHTS

We offer this overview of the anatomical relationships between the vascular system and the fascial system as supportive background to our presentation of some structural patterns that could have their origin in fascial restriction of the peripheral vascular system. It is our intent for clinicians and researchers who read this chapter to draw upon these images and ideas when in their own initial stages of inquiry into the underlying causes of peripheral vascular or neural symptoms, and when considering possible therapeutic interventions. This chapter has highlighted the body's intelligent, adaptive capacity, and how the complex interrelationships among body-wide systems (neural, vascular, and fascial) can often mask the actual complexity of dysfunction.

For your further consideration, we close with a familiar adage among structural integration practitioners: "Where you think it is, it ain't". In other words, whether you are working to assess vascular dysfunction, improve physical function, or resolve other somatic complaints—the most helpful place to work may not be where the symptoms or the pain happen to be presenting.

REFERENCES

1. Witter, K., Tonar, Z., Schöpper, H. 2017. How many layers has the adventitia?— Structure of the arterial tunica externa revisited. *Anatomy Histology Embryology*, 46(2):110–120.
2. Gasser, T.C., Ogden R., Holzapfel, G. 2006. Hyperelastic modelling of arterial layers with distributed collagen fibre orientations. *Journal of the Royal Society Interface*, 3:15–35.
3. Willard, F. 2012. Somatic fascia. In *Fascia: The Tensional Network of the Human Body*, eds. Schleip, R., Findley, T., Chaitow, L., and Huijing, P., pp. 11–18, Edinburgh/London: Churchill Livingstone Elsevier.

4. Stecco, C. 2015. *Functional Atlas of the Human Fascial System*. pp. 5–43, 305. Edinburgh/London: Churchill Livingstone Elsevier.

5. Adstrum, S., Hedley, G., Schleip., R., Stecco., C. Yucesoy, C. 2017. Defining the fascial system. *Journal of Bodywork and Movement Therapies*, 21(1):173–177.

6. Majesky, M.W., Dong, X.R., Hoglund, R., et al. 2011. The adventitia a dynamic interface containing resident progenitor cells. In *ATVB in Focus Vascular Cell Lineage Determination and Differentiation*, ed. W. Eugene Chen, pp. 1530–1539. https://www.ahajournals.org/doi/pdf/10.1161/ATVBAHA.110.221549

7. Stenmark, K.R., Nozik-Grayck, E., Gerasimovskaya, E., et al. 2010. The adventitia: Essential role in pulmonary vascular remodeling. *Comprehensive Physiology*, 1(1):141–161.

8. Hocking, D., Titus, P., Sumagin, R., Sarelius, I. 2008. Extracellular matrix fibronectin mechanically couples skeletal muscle contraction with local vasodilation. *Circulation Research*, 102(3):372–379.

9. Schleip, R., Klingler, W., Wearing, S., et al. 2016. Functional *in vitro* tension measurements of fascial tissue—A novel modified superfusion approach. *Journal of Musculoskeletal and Neuronal Interactions*, 16(3):256–260.

10. Taylor, G.I., Palmer, J.H. 1987. The vascular territories (angiosomes) of the body: Experimental study and clinical applications. *British Journal of Plastic Surgery*, 40:113–141.

11. Li, W., Ahn, A. 2011. Subcutaneous fascial bands—A qualitative and morphometric analysis. *PLoS One*. https://journals.plos.org/plosone/article?id=10.1371/journal.pone.0023987

12. Stecco, A., Stern, R., Fantoni, I., De Caro, R., Stecco, C. 2016. Fascial disorders: Implications for treatment. *Physical Medicine and Rehabilitation, PMR*, 8(2):161–168.

13. Caggiati, A. 2000. Fascial relations and structure of the tributaries of the saphenous veins. *Surgery Radiology Anatomy*, 22:191–196.

14. Stecco, C., Tiengo, C., Stecco, A., Porzionato, A., Macchi, V., Stern, R., De Caro, R. 2012. Fascia redefined: Anatomical features and technical relevance in fascial flap surgery. *Surgical and Radiologic Anatomy*, 35(5):369–376.

15. Caggiati, A. 2001. Fascial relationships of the short saphenous vein. *Journal of Vascular Surgery*, 34(2):241–246.

16. Caggiati, A. 1999. Fascial relationships of the long saphenous vein. *Circulation*, 21(28):2547–2549.

17. Fan, C.M. 2005. Venous pathophysiology. *Seminars in Interventional Radiology*, 22(3):157–161.

18. Basinger, H., Hogg, J.P. 2019. Anatomy, abdomen and pelvis, femoral triangle. *StatPearls*. https://www.ncbi.nlm.nih.gov/books/NBK541140/#article-21683.s2

19. Retzi, G., Kapral, S., Greher, M., Walter, M. 2001. Ultrasonographic findings of the axillary part of the brachial plexus. *Anesthesia & Analgesia*, 92(5):1271–1275.

20. Stecco, C., Giordani, F., Fan, C., Chiara Frigo, A., Macci, V., Biz, C., De Caro, R. 2019. Role of fasciae around the median nerve in pathogenesis of carpal tunnel syndrome: Microscopic and ultrasound study. *Clinical Anatomy*, 22(4):846–847.

21. Bordoni, B., Sugumar, K., Leslie, S. 2019. Anatomy, abdomen and pelvis, pelvic floor. *StatPearls*. https://www.ncbi.nlm.nih.gov/books/NBK482200/

22. Lesondak, D. 2017. *Fascia: What It Is and Why It Matters*. Edinburgh: Handspring Publishing.

23. *Gray's Anatomy*, 38th ed. 1995. Edinburgh/London: Churchill Livingstone.

24. Bhattacharya, V., Barooah, P, Nag, T., et al. 2010. Detail microscopic analysis of deep fascia of lower limb and its surgical implication. *Indian Journal of Plastic Surgery*, 43(2):135–140.

25. Freiwald, J., Boumgart, C., Kuehnemann, M., Hoppe, M. 2016. Foam-rolling in sport and therapy—Potential benefits and risks. *Sports Orthopaedics and Traumatology*, 32:258–266.
26. Taylor, G.I., Caddy, C.M., Watterson, P.A., Crock, J.G. 1990. The venous territories (venosomes) of the human body: Experimental study and clinical implications. *Plastic and Reconstructive Surgery*, 86(2):185–213.
27. Langevin, H., Yandow, J. 2002. Relationship of acupuncture points and meridians to connective tissue planes. *The Anatomical Record*, 269(6):257–265.
28. De Oliveira, F., Fontes, R., da Silva Baptista, J., Mayer, W., Boldrini, S., Liberti, E. 2009. The connective tissue of the adductor canal—A morphological study in fetal and adult specimens. *Journal of Anatomy*, 214(3):388–395.
29. Meissner, J. 2005. Lower extremity venous anatomy. *Seminars in Interventional Radiology*, 22(3):147–156.
30. Meissner, M., Moneta, G., Burnand, K., et al. 2007. The hemodynamics and diagnosis of venous disease. *Journal of Vascular Surgery*, 46(6):S4–S24.
31. Benjamin, M. 2009. The fascia of the limbs and back—A review. *Journal of Anatomy*, 214(1):1–18.
32. Turnipseed, W., Hurschler, C., Vanderby, R. 1995. The effects of elevated compartment pressure on tibial arteriovenous flow and relationship of mechanical and biochemical characteristics of fascia to genesis of chronic anterior compartment syndrome. *Journal of Vascular Surgery*, 21(5):810–817.
33. Singh, N., Sidawy, A., Bottoni, C., Antedomenico, E., Gawley, T., Harada, D., Gillespie, D., Uyehara, C., Cordts, P. 2006. Physiological changes in venous hemodynamics associated with elective fasciotomy. *Annuals of Vascular Surgery*, 20(3):301–305.
34. Sharma, N., Kumar, J., Verma, R., Jhobta, A. 2017. Tibialis anterior muscle hernia: A case of chronic, dull pain and swelling in leg diagnosed by dynamic ultrasonography. *Polish Journal of Radiology*, 82:293–295.
35. Toms, A.F., Rushton, L.A., Kennedy, N.R. 2017. Muscle herniation of the peroneus longus muscle triggering superficial fibular nerve paresthesia. *Sonography*, 5(1):36–40.
36. MacTaggart, J., Phillips, N., Loneth, C., et al. 2014. Three-dimensional bending, torsion and axial compression of the femoropopliteal artery during limb flexion. *Journal of Biomechanics*, 47(10):2249–2256.
37. Scholten, F., Gonneke, A.O., Warnars, W.P., Mali, W., van Leeuwen, M. 1993. Femoropopliteal occlusions and the adductor canal hiatus, Duplex study. *European Journal of Vascular Surgery*, 7:680–683.
38. Noorani, A., Walsh, S.R., Cooper, D.B., Varta, K. 2008. Entrapment syndromes. *European Journal of Vascular and Endovascular Surgery*, 37:213–220.
39. Levein, L.J. 2003. Popliteal artery entrapment syndrome. *Seminars in Vascular Surgery*, 16(3):223–231.
40. Sanchez, J., Conkling, N., Labropoulos, N. 2011. Compression syndromes of the popliteal neurovascular bundle due to baker cyst. *Journal of Vascular Surgery*, 54(6):1821–1829.
41. McKoen, K.E., Wright, R.W., Johnson, J.E., et al. 2012. Vascular anatomy of the tibiofibular syndoesmosis. *Journal of Bone and Joint Surgery*, 94(10):931–938.
42. Koutakis, P., Myers, S., Cluff, K., et al. 2016. Abnormal myofiber morphology and limb dysfunction in claudication. *Journal of Surgical Research*, 196(1):172–179.
43. Mehta, V., Suri, R.K., Arora, J., Kumar, H., Yadav, Y., Rath, G. 2010. Crucial neurovascular structures entrapped in a brachial intramuscular tunnel. *Romanian Journal of Morphology and Embryology*, 51(1):199–201.
44. Raju, S., Neglen, P. 2006. High prevalence of nonthrombotic iliac vein lesions in chronic venous disease: A permissive role in pathogenicity. *Journal of Vascular Surgery*, 44(1):136–144.

45. Raju, S. 2008. Iliac vein outflow obstruction in "primary" chronic venous disease. *Phlebolymphology*, 15(1):12–15.

46. Brinegar, K.N., Sheth, R.A., Khademhosseini, A., et al. 2015. Iliac vein compression syndrome: Clinical, imaging and pathologic findings. *World Journal of Radiology*, 7(11):375–381.

47. Carro, L.P., Hernando, M.F., Curezal, L., et al. 2016. Deep gluteal space problems: Piriformis syndrome, ischiofemoral impingement and sciatic nerve release. *Muscle, Ligaments and Tendons Journal*, 6(3):384–396.

48. Jardine, W.M., Gillis, C., Rutherford, D. 2012. The effect of osteopathic manual therapy on the vascular supply to the lower extremity in individuals with knee osteoarthritis: A randomized trial. *International Journal of Osteopathic Medicine*, 15(4):125–133.

49. Castro-Sanchez, A.M., Morena-Lorenzo, C., Maratan-Penarrocha, G.A., et al. 2011. Connective tissue reflex massage for type 2 diabetic patients with peripheral arterial disease: Randomized controlled trial. *Evidence-Based Complementary and Alternative Medicine*. https://www.hindawi.com/journals/ecam/2011/804321/

7 Hormonal Effects on Fascia in Women

Angeli Maun Akey and Kathleen O'Neil-Smith

CONTENTS

INTRODUCTION

Recent research has revealed the clinical importance of hormones on fascia.[1–3] Hormones are important in maintaining female soft tissue integrity given the many structural changes a woman's body undergoes for successful reproduction. Clinically, soft tissue changes have been observed during menstruation, pregnancy, and with the use of estrogen blocking aromatase inhibitor medications for breast cancer. It is now known that as hormone levels vary throughout the menstrual cycle, the ratio of collagen and elastin is altered, causing changes in musculoskeletal tissue and function.[3]

This chapter will examine the likely effects of hormones—estrogen, progesterone, androgens [testosterone and dehydroepiandrosterone (DHEA)], and relaxin—on a woman's fascia. We will also review the preclinical and clinical research about these hormones. While more research is still needed to gain a full understanding of how hormones work in the body and to resolve some contradictions in research findings, we nonetheless hope to impress upon the clinician the importance of hormones for healthy fascial tissue in women, especially during the perimenopausal transition when sex steroid hormones sharply decline.

CURRENT UNDERSTANDING OF HORMONES ON FASCIA

ESTROGEN, PROGESTERONE, ANDROGENS (TESTOSTERONE AND DHEA), AND RELAXIN

There is emerging evidence from studies lead by Carla Stecco and others that sex steroid hormones and relaxin act to facilitate the soft tissue adaptions needed for successful reproduction and recovery.[1-3]

In one study, an examination of fascia collected from the leg, abdomen, and thigh of women participants revealed that all examined fibroblasts contained the relaxin receptor 1 (RXFP1) and estrogen receptor alpha (ERα), with a lower expression in postmenopausal women compared with premenopausal women.[4] It also demonstrated that all fibroblasts from different parts of the muscular fascia expressed sex hormone receptors.[4] Fibroblasts are a key component of fascia throughout the body.[3]

ESTROGEN AND FASCIA

Estrogen strengthens the muscle and connective tissue by increasing type I collagen expression, overall cross-link concentrations of collagen, and decreasing type III collagen.[5] Collagen determines the tensile strength of the connective tissue.[6] Though the overall amount of collagen decreases during the perimenopausal transition, there is an increase in type I collagen relative to type III collagen, so the net effect is tissue stiffness.[5,7] Fibrosis is the accumulation of excess connective tissue.[8] Studies demonstrate that estrogen protects the muscles and fascia from fibrogenesis.[4,9] Therefore, one could infer that once estrogen levels *diminish* during the perimenopausal transition, fibrogenesis prevails.[5,8]

Not only does estrogen stimulate type I collagen,[5] it also slows down the breakdown of collagen and elastin. Elastin is a connective tissue molecule that gives the tissue its property of resilience, allowing it to extend/recoil with ease and form elastic fibers.[5] Collagen and elastin breakdown is slowed by downregulating MMPs.[5] These MMPs are zinc-dependent endopeptidases that have been shown to denature endopelvic connective tissue.[5,10] Postmenopausal women have lower estrogen levels. As a result, they have relatively increased activity of these MMPs compared with their premenopausal states. Hence, diminished levels of collagen in postmenopausal women results in increased myofascial issues and rapid fascial sagging. Moreover, tissues derived from prolapsed organs show lower levels of elastin, stiffer extracellular matrices (ECMs), and decreased tissue strength.[5]

A limited number of studies demonstrate that estrogen replacement therapy (ERT) reduces fibrogenesis in the fascial system in postmenopausal women. One small study showed that the effects of ERT in postmenopausal women may influence tendon biomechanical properties and morphology.[11] Collagen fibrils are the so-called "building blocks" of tendons. These fibrils significantly contribute to the mechanical properties of the tendon that it forms.[11] A higher tendon fractional synthesis rate and higher fibril density and greater number of smaller fibrils were associated with ERT users versus controls not using ERT. The findings included lower relative stiffness during maximal isometric voluntary contraction (one-legged resistance exercises) seen in ERT users versus controls. The authors concluded that the participants using ERT had less tendon stiffness compared with the control group under load. This suggests a correlation between higher estradiol levels and reduced tendon strength.[11]

PROGESTERONE AND FASCIA

A study that focused on the function of progesterone in regulating the activity of collagenase and matrix metalloproteinases (MMPs) found that physiological concentrations of progesterone significantly impact the release of collagenase and total MMP activity.[10] Moreover, inhibition of the production and activation of MMP-1 (aka "procollagenase") by progesterone has been observed in other tissues and cells such as postpartum rat uterine explants,[12] smooth muscle cells in culture,[13] and guinea pig uterine cervical fibroblasts.[14] The inhibitory effect of progesterone on collagenase and related MMPs supports the hypothesis that progesterone influences the integrity and maintenance of the endometrial connective tissue.[10] Another important anatomical area where hormones affect fascia is the lower esophageal sphincter (LES).[15,16] An analysis of rising serum levels of estrone, estradiol, and progesterone during pregnancy, in relation to LES pressure changes, reveals a correlation between the reduction in LES pressure with the progressive rise in sex hormone levels. This suggests that elevated estrogen and progesterone during pregnancy reduce LES pressure by impairing the integrity of the lower esophageal sphincter.[16] The reduced LES pressure is thought to cause reduced acid clearance and gastric emptying.[17] This is an etiological factor that contributes to the high frequency of GERD symptoms seen in pregnancy.[17]

ANDROGENS: TESTOSTERONE, DHEA, AND FASCIA

TESTOSTERONE

Testosterone impacts men and women differently. Women naturally have approximately 10% of the testosterone levels of their male counterparts. Testosterone has been found to be lower in postmenopausal women.[18] It is known that men experience fewer anterior cruciate ligament (ACL) injuries than their female counterparts. It has been suggested that higher levels of testosterone in males increases their knee laxity and lowers ACL tear incidents.[19] However, it has not yet been determined if the increased knee laxity in males is due to their higher relative testosterone concentrations or if it is influenced by the presence of other hormones. This requires further studies.[18–20,24] Dupuytren's contractures characterized by palmar fascia shortening is most often seen in men.[21] It has been shown that this palmar fascia has higher levels of androgen receptors than normal fascia.[21] The clinical implications of this finding have yet to be determined.

DHEA

Although there is not much information on DHEA and its role on fascial tissue, local intravaginal application of DHEA to the epithelial layer has been shown to improve the sexual function of women experiencing sexual dysfunction.[22] Labrie et al. suggests that the androgenic hormone, DHEA, affects collagen formation and helps maintain the strength of the vaginal musculature. It appears that DHEA specifically treats the epithelial layer as well as the muscular layer of the aging vagina to help restore the health of the tissue.[22]

RELAXIN AND FASCIA

The discovery of relaxin's role in regulating the healthy turnover of collagen introduced new insights into the potential relationship between relaxin and fascia.[23] Relaxin is a small peptide hormone in the insulin superfamily with collagenolytic effects believed to be mediated by the release of collagenases, matrix metalloproteases, and plasminogen activator.[24] It remodels collagen to prevent fibrosis and inflammation.[4] Relaxin binds to relaxin family peptide receptors (RXFP1, RXFP2, RXFP3) that are found throughout the fascial system.[25] Relaxin-1 is well-known for its effects on collagen and ECM remodeling.[4] It promotes both a decrease in type I and III collagen and the synthesis of MMPs.[4] Relaxin-2 has been used to decrease collagen accumulation in several rodent models of induced fibrosis.[4] In such studies, treatment of relaxin-1-knockout mice with recombinant relaxin-2 in various stages of induced fibrosis lead to a complete reversal of collagen deposition in the lung[26] and heart.[27] The fundamental concept in these studies is that relaxin can prevent progressive collagen deposition in diseased states characterized by fibrosis. Relaxin's role in decreasing collagen formation and inhibiting excess collagen deposition suggests that it may also play a part in the incidence of female ACL tears. Studies focusing on the impact of sex hormones on female ACL cells indicate a statistically higher serum concentration of relaxin (SRC) in women who experience ACL tears than those who do not, finding a mean SRC for athletes without tears to be 1.8 ($\pm$3.4) pg/mL and for athletes with ACL tears to be 6.0 ($\pm$8.1) pg/mL.[24] Given that males were not found to have significant serum levels of relaxin, it is plausible that chronic relaxin exposure diminishes the integrity of the female ACL, contributing to the gender disparity in ACL injury prevalence (Table 7.1).[24]

TABLE 7.1
Specific Hormone Effects on Fascial Components

Hormones	Function on Fascia
Estrogen	• Increases collagen synthesis[4] • Increases tendon turnover[11] • Slows breakdown of collagen and elastin by downregulating MMPs[5] • Protects muscle and fascia from fibrogenesis[4,9]
Progesterone	• Induces synthesis of collagen and elastic fiber proteins[5] • Inhibits action of MMPs to maintain endometrial integrity[10]
Androgens (Testosterone and DHEA)	• Critical for development, growth, and maintenance of tissue during puberty[48] • Increase knee laxity[20] • Strengthens vaginal musculature[22]
Relaxin	• Remodels collagen to hinder fibrosis and inflammation[24] • Increases pelvic and pelvic joint laxity in pregnant women[24] • Promotes both a decrease in type I and III collagen and increase in synthesis of MMPs[23]

EVIDENCE OF HOW HORMONES MAY WORK TOGETHER TO AFFECT FASCIA *IN VIVO*: PREGNANCY AND MENSTRUAL CYCLE VARIATION

PREGNANCY

Fascia, at the microscopic level, has hormonal receptors that can affect the body's mechanical properties on a macroscopic level.[28] In pregnancy and at the end of the follicular phase of the menstrual cycle, the sex steroid hormones progesterone and estrogen induce components of the extracellular matrix (ECM), namely expression of collagen, elastin, and fibrillin 1.[29,30] Collagen is responsible for the stiffness of connective tissue while elastin and fibrillin are responsible for its stretchiness.[3] Both elastin and fibrillin are elastic fiber components.[30] Fibroblasts secrete the glycoprotein fibrillin, which increases fascial elasticity.[31] Recall the clinical consequences of tissue collagen weakness as seen in Ehlers-Danlos syndrome, which results from defects in the genetic coding of collagen synthesis,[31] and the hypermobility seen in Marfan syndrome, which results from a genetic mutation in the fibrillin-1 gene causing defects in fibrillin-1 synthesis.[32]

The ECM of the cervix contains type I and III collagens as well as proteoglycans, hyaluronan, and elastic fibers that are important in maintaining the cervix's mechanical function.[30] The ECM of the cervix is gradually relaxed through remodeling by progesterone and estrogen signals so that the cervix can prepare for labor.[30,33] High levels of estrogen and relaxin increase pelvic floor and pelvic joint laxity in pregnant women,[24] which also prepare a woman's body for childbirth.

Despite all these adjustments, detrimental alterations to the fascial system may occur.[7] Pregnancy and labor can cause trauma and pathological changes to the fascia of the abdomen and pelvic floor, low back pain, pelvic organ prolapse, pelvic girdle pain, and stress urinary incontinence among other complications.[7]

MENSTRUAL CYCLE VARIATION

How fascial fibroblasts exactly respond to hormonal stimuli is currently a topic of research. An *in vitro* study published in 2019 showed for the first time that fibroblasts isolated from the human fascia lata can modulate production of collagen and elastin via specialized hormone receptors.[3] These receptors respond to both estradiol and relaxin and these two hormones vary during the normal menstrual cycle. The researchers mimicked this menstrual variation *in vitro* and found that when fibroblasts were treated with estradiol alone in the follicular phase, type I collagen levels dropped in the periovulatory phase. However, with the addition of relaxin-1 to the cell culture, the production of collagen remained the same at both the follicular and periovulatory levels of hormones. The results confirm the antifibrotic function of relaxin-1 and its ability to decrease matrix synthesis. It also represents a "first step in how menstrual and other female hormonal dysfunctions can cause dysregulation of extracellular matrix production in the fasciae".[3]

CLINICAL CONSEQUENCES OF HORMONES AND FASCIA

1. Soft tissue changes during the menstrual cycle (plantar fascia and ACL data)
2. Myofascial pain is more common in women than men and more common in postmenopausal women than menopausal women
3. Pelvic organ prolapse (POP) and stress urinary incontinence (SUI) as examples of pelvic floor fascial aging
4. Aromatase induced musculoskeletal syndrome (AIMSS)

SOFT TISSUE CHANGES DURING MENSTRUAL CYCLE (PLANTAR FASCIA AND ACL DATA)

Lee and Petrofsky[34] demonstrated that plantar fascia elasticity changes during the menstrual cycle. In addition, women soccer players were more susceptible to anterior cruciate ligament (ACL) injuries than their male counterparts and most susceptible during premenstrual and menstrual periods.[35] Studies have found that when estrogen peaks during the preovulatory phase, there is more knee laxity, resulting in an increase in injury risk. As mentioned before, estrogen increases the synthesis of type I and type III collagen, therefore, it is plausible that the increase in production of collagen makes the ACL laxer, increasing the likelihood of injury. A determinant of laxity is the ratio of type I to type III collagen.[8] In females who are on oral contraceptive pills (OCPs), the estrogen levels are lower and more stable through-out the cycle.[36] This agrees with the theory and statistical evidence that females on OCPs have greater resistance to acquiring injury to the ACL because of the reduced hormonal fluctuations during the cycle.[37] In addition, there have been studies on the influence relaxin has on the ACL and its contribution to causing more injury. In a previously mentioned study,[24] serum relaxin concentration was at a much higher level in females who sustained an ACL injury versus those who did not. The mecha-nism by which relaxin alters the mechanical properties of the human ACL has yet to be fully elucidated. However relaxin, with its collagenolytic properties, may act to decrease the strength of the ACL, thus making the ACL weaker and more sus-ceptible to injury.[24] The data on the concept of hormonal influences on ACL tears in women is also inconclusive and, frankly, sometimes contradictory as to the specific hormonal influences and risk of injury during the different menstrual cycle phases. However, the key takeaway is that hormones have significant effect on the integrity of the ACL and soft tissue properties and the exact contribution of each hormone *in vivo* has yet to be clarified.

MYOFASCIAL PAIN

With emerging evidence about the fascial system and its relationship to pain,[37] clini-cians are encouraged to think about the etiology of pain rather than simply prescribing medication to alleviate the symptoms. When we take a deeper look at fascia as an organ system with all of its components, fascial pathology has to be considered as a contributor to the etiology for pain syndromes. Fascial inflammation and injury are hypothesized to have a role in the pathophysiology of fibromyalgia,[38] musculoskeletal disorders, and back pain.[40] Fascia has a mechanical role in assisting flow and move-ment in the musculoskeletal system. It allows for elasticity and contractility of both smooth and skeletal muscles. When the integrity of fascia is compromised, pathology can occur. With pelvic floor tissue and pathology, pain often occurs as a common symptom.[5]

In pregnancy, there is evidence of the effectiveness of myofascial therapy in preg-nant women with low back pain or pelvic floor pain.[39] Strain, pressure, and stretching of the visceral peritoneum, bladder, urethra, rectum, and fascial tissue can result in pain in 50%–80% of the women during pregnancy.[40,41] In a study demonstrating the efficacy of osteopathic treatment methods to heal pain during pregnancy, subjects were treated with visceral mobilization and myofascial techniques in the cervical, thoracic, and lumbar spine.[39] The series of osteopathic treatments showed signifi-cant effects in reducing pain and increasing the lumbar range of motion in pregnant women with low back pain. A clinically significant improvement in functional dis-ability, activity, and quality of life were also observed.[40,41]

Trindade et al. demonstrated a correlation between myofascial pain and age.[42] The study indicates that the human deep temporal fascia is stiffer among older par-ticipants than in people who are younger. Thus, increasing age creates stiffer and less flexible connective tissue.[43] When it comes to gender differences in myofascial pain, adult women have reported more instances of myofascial pain than men[4] and postmenopausal women report more instances than adult premenopausal women.[43]

In the pelvis, fascial aging can result in pelvic floor dysfunction, such as pelvic organ prolapse and stress urinary incontinence due to mechanical issues. Aging tissue can also result in painful conditions such as atrophic vaginitis.[43]

PELVIC ORGAN PROLAPSE AND STRESS URINARY INCONTINENCE

Pelvic organ prolapse (POP) is the downward movement of pelvic organs from their established sites of attachment due to a weakened support system.[5] In postmenopausal women, estrogen plays a key role in maintaining the structural integrity of the endopelvic fascial system.[5] A critical component of this system is called the arcus tendinosis fasciae pelvis (ATFP).[6] The ATFP is a connective tissue that upholds the anterior vagina and provides attachment to the supporting ligaments of the pelvis. Moalli et al.[6] determined that type I collagen in the ATFP decreased in postmenopausal women. Recall that type I collagen tends to confer stiffness.[5] Appropriate amount of stiffness is necessary especially in the pelvic region to hold up pelvic organs. When this is diminished due to menopause, the risk of POP increases.[5] Postmenopausal women who were not on hormone therapy had a decrease in collagen I/(III + V) ratio in their ATFP, affecting its tensile strength.[6] After a year of hormone therapy, the collagen composition ratio returned to the ideal levels found premenopausal women,[6] further providing evidence that hormones play an important role in healthy female fascial tissue.

Just caudal to the ATFP is the levator ani muscle complex. The levator ani muscle and the vagina are attached to each other by collagen and smooth muscle fibers.[44] Stress urinary incontinence occurs when increased intra-abdominal pressure causes involuntary urine leakage[45]. Altered fascial components can result in a dysfunctional levator ani muscle complex that can contribute to stress urinary incontinence.

AROMATASE INHIBITOR INDUCED MUSCULOSKELETAL SYNDROME

Postmenopausal women with breast cancer are often prescribed aromatase inhibitors (AIs), such as letrozole and anastrozole to block the conversion of androgens to estrogen.[46] These medications are known to cause aromatase induced musculoskeletal syndrome (AIMSS), which is characterized by joint stiffness, decreased grip strength, arthralgia, and myalgia.[48] These symptoms are likely caused by teno-synovial changes and intra-articular fluid retention.[47] Postmenopausal women have fewer relaxin and estrogen receptors on fascial fibroblasts compared with premenopausal women,[4] suggesting that postmenopausal women have fascia that does not respond to usual hormonal cues.[31] These hormonal cues prompt elastin synthesis. Without elastin, these women experience increased body and fascial stiffness. Increased fascial stiffness can sensitize myofascial pain receptors, making the muscles stiffer as well.[4] In addition, postmenopausal women taking AIs experience more vaginal dryness and sexual dysfunction compared with postmenopausal women without breast cancer.[44] Why is this important? Twenty-five percent of women taking AIs for breast cancer discontinue the medication because AIMSS adversely affects their quality of life.[48]

CONCLUSION

This chapter shows that hormones play an important role in supporting the healthy function of the fascial system in women. Clinicians should keep this in mind when assessing and treating female patients, especially those experiencing the perimenopausal transition. Even though we are just beginning to understand the exact details of how hormones affect fascial tissue, we know that they do.

REFERENCES

1. Stecco, C. et al. "Hyaluronan within fascia in the etiology of myofascial pain." *Surg and Rad Anatomy* 33, no. 10 (2011): 891–896.
2. Stecco, C. et al. "The fasciacytes: A new cell devoted to fascial gliding regulation." *Clinical Anatomy* 31, no. 5 (2018): 667–676.
3. Fede, C. et al. "Sensitivity of the fasciae to sex hormone levels: Modulation of collagen-I, collagen-III and fibrillin production." *PloS One* 14, no. 9 (2019): 1–12.
4. Fede, C. et al. "Hormone receptor expression in human fascial tissue." *EJH* 60, no. 4 (2016): 224–229.
5. Zhou, L. et al. "Estrogen and pelvic organ prolapse." *Journal of Molecular and Genetic Medicine* 10, no. 221 (2016). doi:10.4172/1747-0862.1000221.
6. Moalli, P.A. et al. "Impact of menopause on collagen subtypes in the arcus tendineous fasciae pelvis." *American Journal of Obstetrics and Gynecology* 190, no. 3 (2004): 620–627.
7. Lee, D.G., Lee, L.-J., and L. McLaughlin. "Stability, continence and breathing: The role of fascia following pregnancy and delivery." *Journal of Bodywork and Movement Therapies* 12, no. 4 (2008): 333–348.
8. Pavan, P.G. et al. "Painful connections: Densification versus fibrosis of fascia." *Current Pain and Headache Reports* 18, no. 8 (2014): 441.
9. Klair, J.S. et al. A longer duration of estrogen deficiency increases fibrosis risk among postmenopausal women with nonalcoholic fatty liver disease. *Hepatology* 64, no. 1 (2016): 85–91.
10. Marbaix, E. et al. "Progesterone regulates the activity of collagenase and related gelatinases A and B in human endometrial explants." *Proceedings of the National Academy of Sciences* 89, no. 24 (1992): 11789–11793.
11. Hansen, M. et al. "Effect of estrogen on tendon collagen synthesis, tendon structural characteristics, and biomechanical properties in postmenopausal women." *Journal Applied Physiology* 106, no. 4 (2009): 1385–1393.
12. Jeffrey, J.J., Coffey, R.J., and Eisen, A.Z. "Studies on uterine collagenase in tissue culture: II. Effect of steroid hormones on enzyme production." *Biochimica et Biophysica Acta (BBA)-General Subjects* 252, no. 1 (1971): 143–149.
13. Jeffrey, J.J., Roswit, W.T., and Ehlich, L.S. "Regulation of collagenase production by steroids in uterine smooth muscle cells: An enzymatic and immunologic study." *J cellular Physiology* 143, no. 2 (1990): 396–403.
14. Rajabi, M., Solomon, S., and Poole, A.R. "Hormonal regulation of interstitial collagenase in the uterine cervix of the pregnant guinea pig." *Endocrinology* 128, no. 2 (1991): 863–871.
15. Sumiyoshi, H. et al. "Esophageal muscle physiology and morphogenesis require assembly of a collagen XIX–rich basement membrane zone." *The Journal of Cell Biology* 166, no. 4 (2004): 591–600.
16. Jacobson, B.C. et al. "Postmenopausal hormone use and symptoms of gastroesophageal reflux." *Archives of Internal Medicine* 168, no. 16 (2008): 1798–1804.

17. Menon, S. et al. "Do differences in female sex hormone levels contribute to gastro-oesophageal reflux disease?" *European Journal Gastroenterology & Hepatology* 25, no. 7 (2013): 772–777.

18. Burger, H.G. et al. "A prospective longitudinal study of serum testosterone, dehydroepiandrosterone sulfate, and sex hormone-binding globulin levels through the menopause transition. *The Journal of Clinical Endocrinology and Metabolism* 85, no. 8 (2000): 2832–2838.

19. Shultz, S.J. et al. "Relationship between sex hormones and anterior knee laxity across the menstrual cycle." *Medicine & Science in Sports & Exercise* 36, no. 7 (2004): 1165–1174.

20. Rozzi, S.L. et al. "Knee joint laxity and neuromuscular characteristics of male and female soccer and basketball players." *The American Journal of Sports Medicine* 27, no. 3 (1999): 312–319.

21. Pagnotta, A., Specchia, N., and Greco, F. "Androgen receptors in Dupuytren's contracture." *Journal of Orthopaedic Research* 20, no. 1 (2002): 163–168.

22. Labrie, F. et al. "Effect of intravaginal dehydroepiandrosterone (Prasterone) on libido and sexual dysfunction in postmenopausal women." *Menopause* 16, no. 5 (2009): 923–931.

23. Bathgate, R.A.D. et al. "Relaxin: New peptides, receptors and novel actions." *Trends in Endocrinology & Metabolism* 14, no. 5 (2003): 207–213.

24. Dragoo, J.L. et al. "Prospective correlation between serum relaxin concentration and anterior cruciate ligament tears among elite collegiate female athletes." *The American Journal of Sports Medicine* 39, no. 10 (2011): 2175–2180.

25. Hanafy, S. et al. "Serum relaxin-3 hormone relationship to male delayed puberty." *Andrologia* 50, no. 2 (2018): e12882.

26. Samuel, C.S. et al. "Relaxin deficiency in mice is associated with an age-related progression of pulmonary fibrosis." *The FASEB Journal* 17, no. 1 (2003): 121–123.

27. Du, X.-J. et al. "Increased myocardial collagen and ventricular diastolic dysfunction in relaxin deficient mice: A gender-specific phenotype." *Cardiovascular Research* 57, no. 2 (2003): 395–404.

28. Zügel, M. et al. "Fascial tissue research in sports medicine: From molecules to tissue adaptation, injury and diagnostics: Consensus statement." *British Journal of Sports Medicine* 52, no. 23 (2018): 1497–1497.

29. Nallasamy, S. et al. "Steroid hormones are key modulators of tissue mechanical function via regulation of collagen and elastic fibers." *Endocrinology* 158, no. 4 (2017): 950–962.

30. Cambron, J. "Findings from the frontiers of fascia research: Insights into 'innerspace' and implications for health." *Journal of Bodywork & Movement Therapies* 23, no. 1 (2019): 101–107. doi:10.1016/j.jbmt.2018.12.005.

31. Micha, D. et al. "An in vitro model to evaluate the properties of matrices produced by fibroblasts from osteogenesis imperfecta and Ehlers-Danlos syndrome patients." *Biochemical and Biophysical Research Communications* 521, no. 2 (2020): 310–317.

32. Sakai, L.Y. et al. "FBN1: The disease-causing gene for Marfan syndrome and other genetic disorders." *Gene* 591, no. 1 (2016): 279–291.

33. Winn, R.J., Baker, M.D., and Sherwood, O.D. "Individual and combined effects of relaxin, estrogen, and progesterone in ovariectomized gilts. I. Effects on the growth, softening, and histological properties of the cervix." *Endocrinology* 135, no. 3 (1994): 1241–1249.

34. Lee, H. et al. "Differences in anterior cruciate ligament elasticity and force for knee flexion in women: Oral contraceptive users versus non-oral contraceptive users." *European Journal of Applied Physiology* 114, no. 2 (2014): 285–294.

35. Möller-Nielsen, J., and Hammar, M. "Women's soccer injuries in relation to the menstrual cycle and oral contraceptive use." *Medicine and Science in Sports and Exercise* 21, no. 2 (1989): 126–129.

36. Konopka, J.A. et al. "The intracellular effect of relaxin on female anterior cruciate ligament cells." *The American Journal of Sports Medicine* 44, no. 9 (2016): 2384–2392.

37. Schilder, A. et al. "Sensory findings after stimulation of the thoracolumbar fascia with hypertonic saline suggest its contribution to low back pain." *PAIN®* 155, no. 2 (2014): 222–231.

38. Liptan, G.L. "Fascia: A missing link in our understanding of the pathology of fibromyalgia." *Journal of Bodywork and Movement Therapies* 14, no. 1 (2010): 3–12.

39. Stuge, B. et al. "The efficacy of a treatment program focusing on specific stabilizing exercises for pelvic girdle pain after pregnancy: A randomized controlled trial." *Spine* 29, no. 4 (2004): 351–359.

40. Wiesner, A. et al. "Osteopathic intravaginal treatment in pregnant women with low back pain." *International Urogynecology Journal* 28, no. 1 (2017): S115. London.

41. Sabino, J., and Grauer, J.N. "Pregnancy and low back pain." *Current Reviews in Musculoskeletal Medicine* 1, no. 2 (2008): 137–141.

42. Trindade, V. et al. "Experimental study of the influence of senescence in the biomechanical properties of the temporal tendon and deep temporal fascia based on uniaxial tension tests." *Journal of Biomechanics* 45, no. 1 (2012): 199–201.

43. Kallak, T.K. et al. "Aromatase inhibitors affect vaginal proliferation and steroid hormone receptors." *Menopause* 21, no. 4 (2014): 383–390.

44. Arenholt, L.T.S. et al. "Paravaginal defect: Anatomy, clinical findings, and imaging." *International Urogynecology Journal* 28, no. 5 (2017): 661–673.

45. Bhattarai, A., and Staat, M. "Modelling of soft connective tissues to investigate female pelvic floor dysfunctions." *Computational and Mathematical Methods in Medicine* 2018 (2018): 1–16.

46. Usluogullari, B. et al. "Use of aromatase inhibitors in practice of gynecology." *Journal of Ovarian Research* 8, no. 1 (2015): 4.

47. Lintermans, A. et al. "Prospective study to assess fluid accumulation and tenosynovial changes in the aromatase inhibitor-induced musculoskeletal syndrome: 2-year follow-up data." *Annals of Oncology* 24, no. 2 (2012): 350–355.

48. Koskenniemi, J.J., Virtanen, H.E., and Toppari, J. "Testicular growth and development in puberty." *Current Opinion in Endocrinology, Diabetes and Obesity* 24, no. 3 (2017): 215–224.

Section II

Function

8 Biotensegrity— The Structure of Life

John Sharkey

CONTENTS

> There is nothing in a caterpillar that tells you it's going to be a butterfly.
>
> **R. Buckminster Fuller (1895–1983)**

PROLOGUE

In the twenty-first century, anatomy and biomechanics are moving away from the purely mechanistic observations made by Vesalius, Borelli, Descartes, and others. These explanations of human movement were based on man-made objects, such as millers' wheels, clocks, and watches and involved such constructs as levers, pulleys, inclined planes, screws, and pin-joints. Man-made objects must be fashioned in such a way that they obey the algorithm that guided their assembly. For man-made structures that algorithm is gravity.

Human beings belong to a different category. Gravity plays little or no role in the genesis of human embryology.[1]

A machine is not capable of constructing itself. We, however, are. For more than a century it has been averred that embryological structures are formed by internally generated mechanical force responses. Thompson succinctly described this, explaining organs and other structures as the "diagrams of underlying forces".[2] Human beings self-assemble. Immersed within a fluid nongravitational environment, embryos continuously adapt, responding to external and internally generated forces. This is not a quality of man-made structures.[3] Human beings can function in the air, at sea, under water, upside down, and downside up, even in outer space, with relative ease. This is something a building cannot do.[4] Given all that, is it accurate to continue to assume that complex living organisms are built using the same methods as a motor car, a bridge, or a building?

The human form is constantly changing, adapting, and repairing. This is supported by the research of Harris et al. who inform us that when fascia is required to function in tension, it will contain a softer morphology.[5] Conversely, if the fascia is necessitated to function predominantly under compression, it becomes harder/stiffer.[5] Fascia adapts to the role it is assigned to play in the body. The internal forces are the algorithms of growth and form.[2] If required to function in tension, it remains "soft", if required to function mostly under compression, fascia becomes "harder" (think tendon, ligament, and bone). Regardless of these changes and adaptions it is still the same tissue.

Biotensegrity provides new explanations concerning how we manage to stay upright in the field of gravity, pump blood, tolerate repetitive movements, and much more.[6] From the viewpoint of physics, biotensegrity is the force vector concept applied to biology.[7]

INTRODUCTION-ORIGINS OF TENSEGRITY

The word "tensegrity" was coined by the inventor and futurist R. Buckminster Fuller. Tensegrity is a portmanteau of two words: tension and integrity.[8] A description used by Fuller, as part of a patent submission,[9] described tensegrity as "Islands of compression inside an ocean of tension" (Figure 8.1). Almost concurrently, French architect David Emmerich was building *self-stressing* structures based on polyhedral configurations. In his patent submission he used a similar definition, adding: "The whole is maintained firmly like a self-supporting structure, hence the term self-stressing".[3]

Tensegrity structures have two elements: tension and compression.[7] Compression is provided by struts, dowels, or bars representing the *discontinuous* elements. In the body, this element is often, but somewhat inaccurately, compared with the bones. The tension element is supplied by wire, Dacron thread, etc. This element creates a *contiguous* tensional network, supporting the discontinuous elements in space. This tensional element comprises the fascia and other soft tissues. The end result is equilibrium (Figure 8.2), a stabilization and homeostasis of the overall structure.[10]

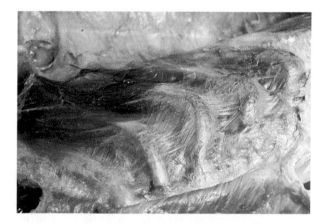

FIGURE 8.1 Fuller's poetic description of tensegrity as "islands of compression inside an ocean of tension" can be seen here as the costal bones provide the discontinuous compression strut "islands" amid the "sea" of tensional fascia/collagen fiber. (Image by author.)

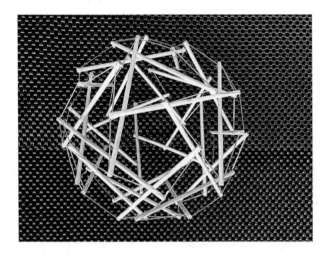

FIGURE 8.2 Tensegrities are composed of discontinuous compression member (or strut) and a contiguous tensional member (the wire). Note that none of the struts are touching and the space between the struts is maintained by the algorithm provided by the combined tension and compression forces. In made-man objects, the tensional member is contiguous; not so in organic structures, where this element is continuous.

Please understand that in man-made tensegrity structures, the contiguous element needs to be tied with a knot, welded, or secured with bolts. Not so in human beings.

Overall, tensegrity is an energy efficient force transmission system dissipating both internal and external forces via changes in tension and compression.[11] In a living structure, a biotensegrity, changes in tension and compression have been observed to be translated into changes in chemistry and metabolism.[12] Additionally, changes in electromagnetic forces, light and auditory emissions, weak biophoton emissions,[13] and overall cell expression through mechanosensitive pathways[14] have been observed. The popular term to describe this physiological process is *mechanotransduction*.[15] Mechanotransduction involves a series of biological processes that translate mechanical forces into signals sensed by specific cell receptors that convert mechanical signals into a biochemical cellular response resulting in gene activation.[13–15]

This process occurs through cellular force transmission via specialized transmembrane cell receptors called integrins. Integrins allow mechanical forces to be translated across and throughout the intercellular environment. Additionally, integrins work in conjunction with other associated proteins (i.e., fibronectin) to promote cell-to-cell information exchange throughout the extracellular and intercellular matrix, thus linking the outside with the inside.

For more than 30 years, Donald Ingber and his team at Harvard have focused on mechanotransduction. While genes are vital for cell function, Ingber's lab demonstrated how cells regulate metabolic processes and genetic transcriptions in response to changes of tension and compression in their environment. These results can include changes to physiology, metabolism, and collagen formation. Ingber states, "*Molecules, cells, tissues, organs, and our entire bodies use tensegrity architecture to mechanically stabilize their shape, and to seamlessly integrate structure and function at all size scales*".[15]

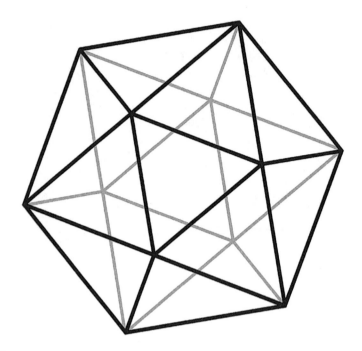

FIGURE 8.3   The icosahedron is recognized as the underlying physical construct of living cells. The truss-based, triangulated architecture provides the space-filling efficiency required to offer stability and mobility with minimal energy expenditure.

At this point it should also come as no surprise to the reader that Ingber has discovered the basic structure of a cell is a tensegrity structure (Figure 8.3).[12]

Biotensegrity offers a model that is hard to ignore. Prior to the biotensegrity model, the accepted paradigm for human movement was grounded in solid Newtonian physics, based on square-frame levers applied to rigid elements standing on solid ground. In a similar vein, classical anatomy continues to be taught as a system of mere muscle origins and insertions on a bony skeleton, another collaborator in this gross oversimplification of the human body.

WHEN IS A COLUMN NOT A COLUMN?

The names we give to things can shape the way we think about them. Generally, the language of anatomy and specifically the naming of structures fall short in providing even a hint of contribution that a structure plays in human motion, emotion, physiology, or metabolism. For example, the word "muscle" derives from the Latin *musculus* which means "*little mouse*". While this tells us nothing about the function of this specialized type of connective tissue, it is safe to say that no one thinks they have got hundreds of little mice running around under their skin helping them to move. Not so when we speak about the "*vertebral column*". That is exactly the way we see it. We view the spine as an axially loaded, compression loaded structure. This has been the norm for decades, if not centuries.

From a biotensegrity point of view this simply cannot be. A column is a structure of support: a rigid, immobile, base-heavy, and unidirectional structure of support; let alone a column composed of multiple rigid bodies, hinged together by flexible, virtually frictionless joints. With such a model even simple motions like forward flexion or squatting would tear tissues and crush bone (Figure 8.4a). If our spine is a "column" it would be one with a constantly shifting center of gravity on a quickly moving base (our pelvis and legs). This model would necessitate incalculable forces.[11,16]

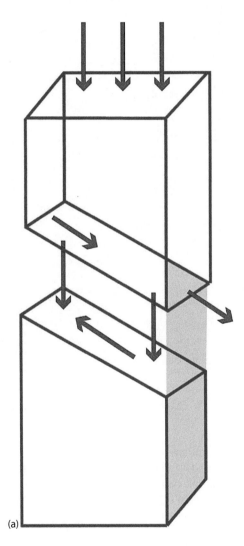

(a)

FIGURE 8.4 (a) This image demonstrates that if joints (e.g., a knee joint) were truly compressive structure's the femur would "slide off" the articulating surface of the tibia, especially when squatting. When simple compressive loads are applied, compressive and shear stress must exist on planes that are oriented obliquely to the line of application of the load. (Adapted from Levin, S.M., *Spine: State Art Rev.,* 9, 2, 1995.) (*Continued*)

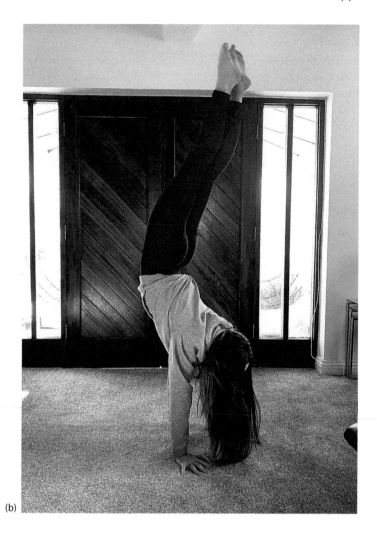

(b)

FIGURE 8.4 (Continued)   (b) When is a column not a column? When it is upside down.

As designed by nature, human spines are omnidirectional stable structures. Even when performing handstands (Figure 8.4b), cartwheels, or simply standing still, they facilitate motion and multiple degrees of freedom.

Recent research by Schleip et al.[17] established fascia as an active player in bio-mechanical activity. Fascia provides contractile forces that impact musculoskeletal mechanics. This continuous tensional force provided by the fascial network has been described as "pre-stress".[3] In addition, muscle fibers in continuity with the fascia dissipate internally generated forces in conjunction with the bones. We call them tendons. Using the biotensegrity algorithm nonlinear motion is achieved by use of a geometrically arranged, multi-bar closed kinematic chain (CKC). In nonorganic

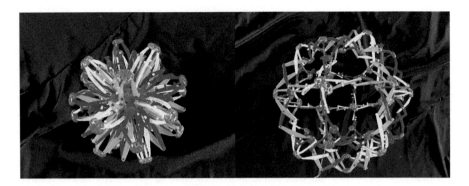

FIGURE 8.5 In a tensegrity, the focus is on shape-changing and deformation, the component "parts" move relative to each other without any part lengthening or shortening. Instead the entire structure shape changes similar to what we see when we expand a Hoberman sphere. Although the entire sphere can shrink, expand, and elongate, none of the individual component parts lengthen or shorten. (Images by author.)

matter it takes welding those two bars together, or joining them with a bolt or a pin. It is not possible to establish a two-bar CKC that is both stable and can provide motion. In human terms, a three-bar CKC (a triangle) would provide stability but no motion. To establish efficient motion with stability we need a minimum of four bars, with one bar acting as the stabilization element.

The principle of the four-bar (or more) CKC provides a satisfactory hypothesis for human motion. In a four-bar CKC, each bar offers a different angular relationship with variability in length that will influence, govern, and limit itself and other four-bar CKCs in the system.[18] The principle of the four-bar (or more, 8, 16, 32 and so on) CKC provides a satisfactory hypothesis for human motion. This moves us away from the centuries old, two-bar, pin-joint models of Borelli. Our joints are not constructed of overlapping bones with pins located at either end to fortify their positions and eliminate transverse shifting forces.[10] Our joints allow near frictionless articulating surfaces. Our vertebral bodies do not slide off each other when we bend or twist. In the biotensegrity model, component parts move relative to each other without any one part lengthening or shortening but, rather, changing shape. An excellent example of this is the multi-bar Hoberman sphere. This model demonstrates expansion and contraction without any of its components shortening or lengthening (Figure 8.5).

ARE LIVING CONSTRUCTS SOFT OR HARD MATTER?

Biotensegrities are governed by the laws of soft matter physics.[7] Because fascia and connective tissue are soft matter it should not be unreasonable to assume that we must use soft matter physics to explain human connective tissue. Hard matter physics explains solid man-made structures. Soft matter undergoes phase changes from more fluid to more solid, and from stiffer to softer. This occurs over varied timescales ranging from milliseconds to several years.[3]

In other words, what was once a compression member can, over time, become the tensional member. By operating in a nonlinear manner, it becomes stiffer and stronger with stress. An example of this is blood. Erythrocytes and other constituents of the blood can change their shape, deforming under a stimulus, such as temperature or mechanical pressure then return to their resting state after the stimulus has been removed.[19] Similar changes have been demonstrated in research studies described in *Direct Physical Formation of Anatomical Structures by Cell Traction Forces*.[20] This fact is essential in our understanding of fascia. Another time-dependent example can be seen in the slow thickening of fascia as a direct response to the continued presence of pain.[19]

Several studies have confirmed fascia not only as a tissue of force transmission in muscular dynamics but that fascia is also capable of generating active contraction.[21-25] In addition, connective tissues "glide" or move relative to thinner or thicker specialized structures around them, whether they are muscle fibers, endo-/peri-/epimysium, nerves, blood vessels, or lymphatic structures.[26]

Additionally, Blechschmidt and Gassers[27] spoke specifically concerning the movement of various fluids and their influence on structural development in the emerging embryo.

Fluids have an infinite range of volumes, vectors, and speed of flow influencing the local and global tension and compression specific to the environment (i.e., the matrix) due to differences in turbulent flow, resonance, and oscillations moment to moment. Breath must also be considered as having a significant impact and influence in this regard.

In biotensegrity pre-stress is contributed to by the self-generated forces of contractile cells and by osmotic dynamics of fluid flow leading to morphological diversity. Fluids including blood, lymph, urine, and interstitial fluids are influenced by the changing forces of breath, and vice versa.[28]

DISSECTION AND TENSEGRITY

The etymology of the word "anatomy" is derived from the Greek words "ana" (up) and "temnein" (to cut). Literally, it means "to cut up". Differentiating a tensegrity from a biotensegrity also requires a deconstruction.[27] A static tensegrity structure has no breath or nervous system. A biotensegrity is a living construct that cannot be reassembled to its original configuration once taken apart. Such interventions, like surgical interventions, result in body-wide adaptations leading to emergent properties that can have unwanted local and global consequences.

As the scalpel incises the skin one immediately witnesses the skin retract from the margins. This can be witnessed continuing some distance from the site of incision. This suggests evidence of pre-stress in the tissue, even in a cadaver.[29] In a tensegrity-informed anatomical dissection one can study tissue continuity by cutting apart that very continuity and carefully observing the changes to what was once whole. These changes in the skin and subcutaneous tissues reflect tensegrity-based architectural principles at play. Medical specialists witness this pre-stress during surgical interventions at the level of the skin and deeper in the areolar septal fascia.[30] Whereas the surgeon is required to put structures and tissues back together again in as a functional manner as possible, the dissector does not have this concern.

The process of dissection (Figure 8.1) provides unique opportunities to investigate connective tissue relationships in a manner that would not be compatible in living humans. It can reveal complex structural, architectural and *tensegrity-informed* functional relationships. Armed with this knowledge of fascial anatomy and the tensegrity viewpoint of the force vectors at play, the clinical anatomist can better inform medical and allied health specialists about the complex global synergies required to ensure the best possible functional outcomes of surgical interventions.[10] Fascia and tensegrity are inextricably interlinked. Fascia can be viewed as the ubiquitous heterogeneous fabric of the human body, while tensegrity can be viewed as the construction method underpinning our fascia. This construction is nurtured by nature, responding and adapting, not exclusively by genetic expression but also by the forces of the local environment or, if you will, epigenetics.

At the gross level, these forces can be explained using terms such as tension and compression. Forces acting at the cellular or nuclear level also could be described using the language of attraction and repulsion. Such forces could include electromagnetic forces, light and auditory emissions, weak biophoton emissions, and spontaneous chemiluminescence.[13] Medical and health specialties including (but not limited to) anatomy, surgery, pathology, occupational medicine, radiology, physical therapies, obstetrics, and gynecology can all benefit from a greater understanding of tensegrity as the main organizing principle of the human body.

Tensegrity provides a practical explanation concerning body-wide continuity and explains why movement in one part of the body has an impact/effect on more distant components of the overall structure. This is due to tensegrity being fractal, multiscale, and heterarchical.[3]

TUBES—HELICES, CHIRALITY, AND CONNECTIVE TISSUE STRUCTURES

Human biotensegrities have thousands of miles of pipe-like tubules and cylinder-like structures. They are ubiquitous throughout our form (Figure 8.6). These constructs are a specific consequence of the forces that act out in embryological development. There are no straight lines in any aspect of the human form. Every structure is spiraled into being.

Helical tubes are themselves tensegrity structures.[31] Responsible for transporting fluids and electromagnetic particles, we can include arteries, veins, arterioles, venules, lymphatics, nerves, muscle fibers, collagens, bronchioles, spinal cord, dura, stomach, intestines, trachea, esophagus, and ureters as examples of these helical "tubes". It is further hypothesized that many such structures remain to be discovered and described in anatomical terms.[32]

According to Benias et al.,[32] real-time histological images of living tissues at a depth of 60–70 μm are now a reality made possible by use of confocal laser endoscopy. These images show heretofore unseen reticular patterns throughout the tissues examined, revealing a previously unrecognized fluidic *interstitium* in the body. Other bespoke research is providing fertile ground for new discoveries, such as the newly described tubular lymphatic vessels identified in the brain using

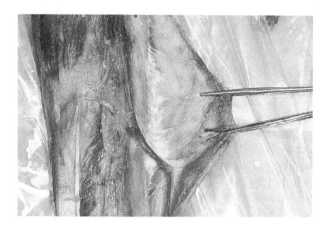

FIGURE 8.6   In this image we see neurovascular tubes evident within, and deep, to the skin of the lower limb. (Image by author.)

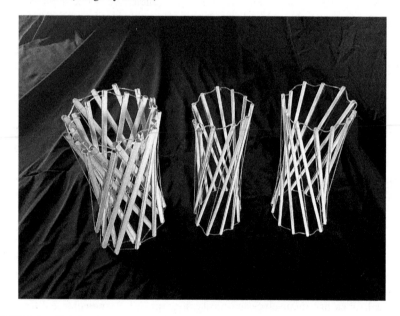

FIGURE 8.7   This image shows, on the right side of the picture, both a right and a left chiral structure. The structure on the left side of the picture shows a combination of the two, creating a chiral arrangement that models the pattern of how collagen fibers orient themselves. The arrangement provides integrity and stability to the tube. Based on this chirality, any stress exerted on micro- or macrotubules would not be longitudinal but, rather, spiral.

in vivo multiphoton microscopy imaging.[33] The bursting of such tubules or pipes (e.g., blood vessels, nerves, and collagens) within us is a rare occurrence and it can be seen in diseased or genetically weakened, helical tubes. These tubules are also tensegrity-based helical structures and move us farther away from linear, mechanical thinking (Figure 8.7).

In the paper "Space, Stars, C60, and Soot", Kroto[34] shows that carbon-based exceptionally stable, C60 clusters (think of a 60-sided soccer ball shape) both self-assemble and effortlessly go on to form helical structures. C60 is essentially a tensegrity icosahedron or *buckminsterfullerene*. While this conformation has yet to be unequivocally confirmed, when applied here it does suggest that stress exerted on such micro- or macro-tubules would not be longitudinal but rather spiral, based on its chirality.

Figure 8.8 provides a visual account of the chiral orientation. Chiral orientation refers to asymmetrical molecular structures whose mirror image is not superimposable. Collagen fibers, themselves tubular, exhibit chirality and are at the heart of the architectural arrangement and functional behavior of all tubular structures throughout the body.

Collagen provides tensile strength due to its triple helical protein, which is the most abundant structural element of the ECM.[35] Tensegrity, underlain by chirality provides stable, nonlinear counterbalances of mechanical forces within living tissues. These forces maintain, generate, and repair the mechanical and geometric structures of living tissues. The forces are dealt with via an *auxetic* expansion and contraction, an increase in both length and width of the helical tube.[36] Recent research by Gatt et al.[37] reported that not only the Achilles tendon but all tendons exhibit the very unusual mechanical property of getting fatter rather than thinner when stretched. This property is a first principle of tensegrity-based structures.

In the specific twenty-first century model of biotensegrity,[8] the focus is on shape-changing and plastic deformation. Connective tissue architecture allows for the apparent elongation or stretching of tissue and additionally, of elements within the tissue. Specifically in muscle, this refers to a 55° angle of crossed collagen fiber orientation. This orientation is referred to as *crimp*. In the heart and vessels, it is facilitated by a counter orientation of helical fibers also running at 55° to each other.[32,38]

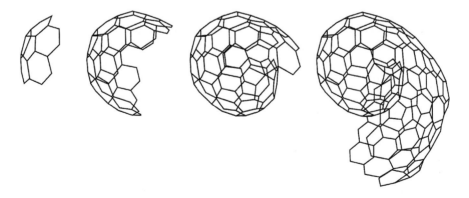

FIGURE 8.8 Tubules are tensegrity-based helical structures with their center being the inside of that helix (i.e., a tube). Any stress exerted on such micro- or macro-tubules would not be longitudinal but rather spiral, based on its chirality.

Does that mean the heart is yet another spiraling tube? Many anatomists have pondered on the heart as a helical structure, but try as they may, no one could uncoil the true helical nature of our hearts' anatomy. Enter Spanish cardiologist Dr. Torrent-Guasp, a Spaniard who investigated the anatomy of the heart over his long career and successfully unfolded this "Gordian knot" of cardiology by unveiling to the world the ventricular myocardial band.[38] Unwinding this cardiac structure into its natural biologic configuration confirms that the spiral motion of heart muscle to allow for the ejection and filling of blood. This is possible only by the helical and chiral nature of its architecture.

The development of tensegrity-based helical structures is energy efficient as seen at the micro level in the double-helix of DNA. We also see this form at the macro level within the collagen abundant in myofascial tissues.[3] These tissues include endomysium, which envelopes each muscle fiber; perimysium, enclosing and transfusing clusters of muscle fibers; and the all-embracing epimysium. The epimysium not only wraps up individual muscles but also shares, in continuous/contiguous fashion, in synergy with local and distant muscles in nonlinear expressions of force transmission.

The biotensegrity model has the potential to be transformative across multiple medical disciplines, bearing in mind (as mentioned previously) the global synergy and integrated relationship of the body as a complete, albeit nonlinear, whole.[11]

Accurately perceiving one's position in space and time (i.e., haptic perception, as opposed to tactile perception) based on a tensegrity model has been well-described by Turvey and Fonseca.[39] As a model, they employed both mechanical disturbances and tissue deformation. One only has to touch the surface of the skin in any location of the soma and the entire organism is aware of that touch. Individuals can further perceive its precise location, depth, force, and speed as well as its static or dynamic nature and more. While large numbers of patients worldwide suffer with inexplicable postsurgical pain,[40] modern medicine can now confidently turn to the new field of mechanobiology and biotensegrity to help explain, and potentially obviate, the physical forces at play. When fascia and other connective tissues are disrupted, due to surgery or other invasive disruptive treatment modalities, changes to the biotensegral architecture can result in changes to intracellular biochemistry, gene expression, gross physical function, and symptomatic pain.

It is further proposed that minimally invasive surgery, based on fascia-sparing approaches[41] and bloodless planes, requires detailed knowledge of fascial anatomy supported by biotensegrity principles. This understanding can specifically quantify and qualify the behavior of the local tissues' mechanics, kinematics, shape, stability, and global force transfers;[42] potentially improving overall patient outcomes.

CONCLUSION

Fascia provides an uninterrupted tensional network that is ubiquitous throughout the human form. The architectural principles that underlay the structural basis of fascia are now established as tensegrity based. Because the importance of fascia in human movement (both motion and emotion), shock absorption, metabolic and physiological processes, proprioception, healing and repair is now well established,[43] knowledge of tensegrity, and specifically biotensegrity, is essential for all medical, health care, and allied health practitioners.

In spite of the fact that the human body will adapt to injuries and surgeries, within an individual's capacity, insults to the fascial network can have undesirable consequences anywhere at the local and/or global level. The human body does not work "in-series". For this to be so would mean that if one component part were to be damaged, or no longer functioned, the entire organism would fail, similar to the old-fashioned, pre-LED, fairy lights on a Christmas tree.

From the micro to the macro humans are a tensegrity within tensegrity. We are scale-free, from the micro to the macro, with emerging properties evident at various levels of complexity. Biotensegrity provides a greater understanding of the geometry of the human form, as well as the microscopic, modular, connected, continuous elements of this closed system we call the body.

Simply put, biotensegrity is emerging as the new, twenty-first century paradigm for anatomy and physiology.

REFERENCES

1. Rydze, R., Schutt, A., Gibbons, W., Nodler, J. 2017. Gravity and embryo development. *Curr Obstet Gynecol Rep* 6, 51–54.
2. Thompson, D.A., Wentworth, A. *On Growth and Form*. Dover reprint of 1942, 2nd ed. (1st ed.). Mineola, NY: Dover Books on Biology.
3. Scarr, G. 2018. *Biotensegrity: The Structural Basis of Life*. Edinburgh: Handspring Publishing.
4. Valero-Cuevas, F.J. et. al. 2007. "The tendon network of the fingers performs anatomical computation at a macroscopic scale". *IEEE Trans Biomed Eng* 54, Number 6, Part 2.
5. Harris, A.K., Wild, P., Stopak, D. 1980. Silicone rubber substrata: A new wrinkle in the study of cell locomotion. *Science* 208, 177–179.
6. Mammoto, T., Ingber, D. 2010. Mechanical control of tissue and organ development. *Development* 137(9), 1407–1420.
7. Levin, S. The icosahedron as a biologic support system. 1981. *34th Annual Conference on Engineering in Medicine and Biology*, Volume 23, September 21–23, Houston, TX.
8. Sharkey, J. 2018. Biotensegrity—Anatomy for the 21st century informing yoga and physiotherapy concerning new findings in fascia research. *J Yoga Physiother* 6(1). doi:10.19080/JYP2018.06.555680.
9. Fuller, R., November 1962. *Tensile-Integrity Structures*. United States Patent 3063521.
10. Sharkey, J. 2016. Biotensegrity—Fascia and the fallacy of biomechanics. Parts 1,2,3. *AAMT J.* Summer Edition 2015.
11. Levin, S.M., 1995. The importance of soft tissues for structural support of the body. *Spine: State Art Rev* 9, 2.
12. Ingber, D.E. 2008. Tensegrity-based mechanosensing from macro to micro. *Prog Biophys Mol Biol* 97(2–3), 163–179.
13. Cifra, M., Pospíšil, P. 2014. Ultra-weak photon emission from biological samples: Definition, mechanisms, properties, detection and applications. *J Photoch Photobio B* 139, 2–10.
14. Saucerman, J.J., Tan, P.M., Buchholz, K.S., McCulloch, A.D., Omens, J.H. 2019. Mechanical regulation of gene expression in cardiac myocytes and fibroblasts. *Nat Rev Cardiol* 16, 361–378.
15. Ingber, D. 2009. Tensegrity and mechanotransduction. *J Bodyw Mov Ther* 12(3), 198–200.
16. Levin, S. 2002. The tensegrity–truss as a model for spine mechanics: Biotensegrity. *J Mech Med Biol* 2(3&4), 375–378.

17. Schleip, R. et al. 2019. Fascia is able to actively contract and may thereby influence musculoskeletal dynamics: A histochemical and mechanographic investigation. *Front Physiol* 10, 336.
18. Levin, S., de Solórzano, S.L., Scarr, G. 2017. The significance of closed kinematic chains to biological movement and dynamic stability. *J Bodyw Mov Ther* 21(3), 664–672.
19. Stecco, A., Gesi, M., Stecco, C., Stern, R. 2013. Fascial components of the myofascial pain syndrome. *Curr Pain Headache Rep* 17, 352.
20. Beloussov, L. 2006. Direct physical formation of anatomical structures by cell traction forces. An interview with Albert Harris. *Int J Dev Biol* 50(4), 93–101.
21. Stecco, C. et al. 2006. Histological characteristics of the deep fascia of the upper limb. *Ital J Anat Embryol* 111, 105–110.
22. Huijing, P.A. 2009. Epimuscular myofascial force transmission: A historical review and implications for new research. International Society of Biomechanics Muybridge Award lecture, Taipei, 2007. *J Biomech* 42, 9–21. doi:10.1016/j.jbiomech.2008.09.027.
23. Pavan, P.G., Pachera, P., Stecco, C., Natali, A.N. 2015. Biomechanical behavior of human crural fascia in anterior and posterior regions of the lower limb. *Med Biol Eng Comput* 53, 951–959. doi:10.1007/s11517-015-1308-5.
24. Krause, F., Wilke, J., Vogt, L., Banzer, W. 2016. Intermuscular force transmission along myofascial chains: A systematic review. *J Anat* 228, 910–918. doi:10.1111/joa.12464.
25. Schleip, R., Gabbiani, G., Wilke, J., Naylor, I., Hinz, B., Zorn, A., Jäger, H., Breul, R., Schreiner, S., Klingler, W. 2019. Fascia is able to actively contract and may thereby influence musculoskeletal dynamics: A histochemical and mechanographic investigation. *Front Physiol* 10, 336. doi:10.3389/fphys.2019.00336.
26. Guimberteau, J.C., Delage, J.P., McGrouther, D.A., Wong, J.K. 2010. The microvacuolar system: How connective tissue sliding works. *J Hand Surgery Eur* 35(8), 614–622.
27. Blechschmidt, E., Gasser, R.F. 2012. *Biokinetics and Biodynamics of Human Differentiation: Principles and Applications*. Berkeley, CA: North Atlantic Books.
28. Fronius, M., Wolfgang, C., Althaus, M. 2012. Why do we have to move fluid to be able to breathe? *Front Physiol*. Review Article, published: 22 May doi:10.3389/fphys.00146.
29. Sharkey, J. 2019. *Biotensegrity focused Thiel Soft Fixed Dissection Course*. Department of Anatomy and Human Identification, College of Life Sciences, University of Dundee, Scotland. https://www.ntc.ie/dissection-scotland/
30. Guimberteau, J.-C. 2005. Strolling under the skin. Endovivo. www.endovivo.com
31. Purslow, P.P. 2010. Muscle fascia and force transmission. *J Bodyw Mov Ther (JBMT)* 14(4), 411–417.
32. Benias, C.P. et al. 2018. Structure and distribution of an unrecognized interstitium in human tissues. *Scientific Reports* 8, Article number: 4947.
33. Louveau, A. et al. 2015. Structural and functional features of central nervous system lymphatic vessels. *Nature* 523, 337–341.
34. Kroto, H. 1988. Space, stars, C60, and soot. *Science* 242(4882), 1139–1145.
35. Golaraei, A. et al. 2018. Collagen chirality and three-dimensional orientation studied with polarimetric second-harmonic generation microscopy. *J Biophotonics* 12(1).
36. Sharkey, J. 2015. Letter to the editor. Transmission of muscle force to fascia during exercise. *J Bodyw Mov Ther* 19(3), 391.
37. Gatt, R. et al. 2015. Negative poisson's ratios in tendons: An unexpected mechanical response. *Acta Biomater* 24, 201–208.
38. Buckberg, B.G. 2002. Basic science review: The helix and the heart. *J Thora Cardiovasc Surg* 124(5), 863–883.
39. Turvey, M., Fonseca, S. 2014. The medium of haptic perception: A tensegrity hypothesis. *J Mot Behav* 46, 143–187.

40. Correl, D. 2017. Chronic postoperative pain: Recent findings in understanding and management. *Research* 6, 1054.
41. van der Wal, J. 2009. The architecture of the connective tissue in the musculoskeletal system—An often overlooked functional parameter as to proprioception in the locomotor apparatus. *Int J Ther Massage Bodyw* 2(4), 9–23.
42. Tomasek, J.J., Gabbiani, G., Hinz, B., Chaponnier, C., Brown, R.A. 2002. Myofibroblasts and mechanoregulation of connective tissue remodelling. *Nat Rev Mol Cell Biol* 3, 349–363. doi:10.1038/nrm809.
43. Lesondak, D. 2017. *Fascia: What It Is and Why It Matters.* Edinburgh: Handspring Publishing.

9 Effects of Loading and Nutrition on Fascia

Danielle Steffen and Keith Baar

CONTENTS

INTRODUCTION

Connective tissues including bone, cartilage, tendon, ligaments, and fascia, are critical components of a functioning musculoskeletal system. These tissues serve to absorb, transmit, and dissipate the forces applied to the body during movement. Each one is specialized for one or more mechanical functions based on the location in the body and the resulting amount and type of force applied to the cells within the tissue. Tendons, ligaments, and fascia function primarily to transfer force within the musculoskeletal system. Fascia has the added function of facilitating movements by lubricating the interface between tissues. To facilitate the transfer of force, these connective tissues are composed of an extracellular matrix (ECM) composed of structural proteins, which give them a high tensile strength,[1] and ground substance. The primary structural proteins are collagen, laminin, and elastin, with collagen contributing ~80% of the total protein. There are 28 different collagen proteins.[2] Within the musculoskeletal connective tissues, type I collagen makes up more than 90% of the collagen fraction, with type III collagen comprising much of the remaining fraction. Therefore, types I and III collagen are the major fibrillar collagens that provide tensile strength to the musculoskeletal connective tissues.[1]

By contrast, the major proteins of the ground substance are proteoglycans, proteins that have highly charged glycosaminoglycan (GAG) side chains. These charged GAGs serve to bring water into the tissue.[3] In bringing water into the tissue, the ground substance provides compressive strength. Compressive strength is utilized both during tensile loading (as the tissue is stretched), when the water within the tissue resists compression as the collagen molecules are squeezed together, and during compressive loading, such as when tissues wrap around bones or retinacula. Together, the dense collagen fiber matrix and proteoglycan-rich ground substance provide the mechanical strength of the tissues and, therefore, specific connective tissues use different ratios of these substances to meet their specific mechanical requirements.

In contrast to the classical view of the musculoskeletal connective tissues being relatively inert, stabile tissues where the collagen has a half-life of >105 years,[4] more recent data suggests that connective tissues are highly dynamic. Smeets and colleagues gave subjects undergoing knee replacement surgery phenylalanine containing a heavy isotope of carbon 2 h before and then throughout the operation. During the surgery, they collected samples of all the tissues of the knee and measured how much of the heavy phenylalanine had been incorporated into the proteins contained in those tissues in order to determine the rate of protein synthesis. As a control, the authors took a muscle biopsy at the time of surgery so that they could compare the tissues of the knee to more highly dynamic tissue. In contrast to expectation, protein turnover in the anterior cruciate ligament (ACL) and patellar tendon was greater than the muscle tissue, cartilage protein turnover was similar to muscle, and synovial tissue turned over almost three times faster than muscle.[5] In support of the findings of Smeets and colleagues, Myrick et al. recently showed that, over the course of an 8-month soccer season, the ACL of young women increased in size, suggesting that there was an increase in collagen in the tissue.[6] Together, this suggests that the musculoskeletal connective tissues are highly dynamic in their response to load.

The primary forces within the musculoskeletal system are *tension*, i.e., when the Achilles tendon is pulled in one direction during plantar flexion (Figure 9.1); *compression*, i.e., when the meniscus absorbs the impact force of a step (Figure 9.1b); and *shear*, i.e., when the superior extensor retinaculum allows the tendons of the tibialis anterior to slide beneath it during dorsiflexion (Figure 9.1c). When the musculoskeletal system is working properly, the specific load placed on the tissue results in a

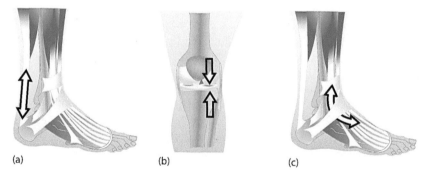

(a)   (b)   (c)

FIGURE 9.1   Loads within the musculoskeletal system. The three major loads in the musculoskeletal system are (a) *Tension*, when a tissue is pulled in one direction; (b) *Compression*, when a tissue is pushed in on itself; and (c) *Shear*, when two tissues slide past each other.

stimulus that orchestrates a cascade of events within the cell that results in changes to the proteins that make up the ECM. This molecular response is critical to the growth, differentiation, and development of the cells and dictates the resulting function of the tissue.

The connective tissues are largely made from a population of fibroblast cells that contain the high mobility group (HMG) box transcription factor SOX9.[7] Even though the cells have a similar origin, once the cells migrate into position and begin being loaded, they differentiate to fit their mechanical environment. In fact, fibroblast cells isolated from connective tissues at different locations in the body become transcriptionally distinct cell types.[8] These data suggest that the mechanical environment is essential to driving cell fate. Therefore, understanding the mechanical environment, and the cellular response to load, is essential for maximizing musculoskeletal cell and tissue function.

Beyond the mechanical environment, connective tissues are dependent on nutritional cues. As stated above, the primary protein within connective tissues is collagen, the most abundant protein in the body. In order for the collagen made in the cells to be released into the ECM, it has to be modified by the enzyme prolyl hydroxylase.[9] During the hydroxylation reaction, prolyl hydroxylase consumes vitamin C. Since humans lack the enzyme L-gulono-γ-lactone oxidase,[10] we are unable to make vitamin C and, therefore, we must consume enough of this micronutrient to support normal collagen turnover. Although this is the most direct nutritional input needed for healthy connective tissues, other foods are suggested to be important in connective tissue function. These foods and how they interact with loading to promote tendon, ligament, and fascial structure and function will be the focus of this chapter.

CELLULAR AND MOLECULAR RESPONSE TO LOADING

Tendons, ligaments, and fascia are formed by a dense and aligned collagen matrix. Although these three tissues are structurally similar, they can undergo regional specialization based on their mechanical environment. For example, retinacular fascial tissues, which need to lubricate the constant sliding of underlying tendons, have more than 10-fold higher levels of hyaluronan, a glycosaminoglycan (GAG) that functions as a lubricant, than the epimysial fascia, which surrounds muscles where shear forces are lower.[11] Similarly, the flexor digitorum profundus tendon of rabbits is structurally and functionally two distinct tendons: the tendon proper, that is loaded in tension, and a fibrocartilage portion, where the tendon is compressed as it passes through the carpal tunnel. Even though the cells of the two regions have the same origin, the total GAG content of the tendon varies from 0.2% of the dry weight in the tendon, up to 6.5% as the tissue takes on a fibrocartilage phenotype.[12] When the compressed region is experimentally released from the carpal tunnel, the GAG content within the tendon rapidly drops from 6.5% to 2.5% after only eight days and further decreases to below 1% within six months after the experimental release surgery.[12] To determine whether compressive load was sufficient to induce a fibrocartilage phenotype, Robbins and colleagues removed deep flexor tendons from cows, subjected them to 72 h of cyclic compressive load, and then measured markers of cartilage gene expression.[13] Just three days of compressive loading was enough to increase the expression of cartilage-enriched proteoglycans (PGs) such as aggrecan up to 4.5-fold.[13]

Unlike PGs and GAGs, lubricating proteins such as Prg4/lubricin are regulated by shear stress.[14] Simply applying a shear stress to cells for 24 h results in a three-fold increase in lubricin secretion. Because knocking out lubricin makes tendons stick together more tightly,[15] this suggests that shear forces are necessary to maintain the lubrication between tendons/fascial layers. Together, these data suggest that compressive and shear loads rapidly increase the expression of genes involved in cartilage formation and lubrication, respectively (Figure 9.2b and c).

Where compression and shear increase GAGs and lubrication, tensional forces are necessary for the production of an aligned collagen matrix.[16] The requirement for tension in the synthesis of a robust and aligned matrix is best seen when the load is removed. For example, when Majima and colleagues inserted a stainless steel wire between the tibial plateau and the base of the patella to release tension from the patellar tendon, the number of nuclei per square millimeter increased ~seven-fold, collagen fibril diameter decreased ~40%, and collagen bundles became less well oriented.[17] These data indicate that without tensional load, healthy connective tissues take on a scarred phenotype, becoming more cellular with smaller, less aligned collagen fibrils. By contrast, 1 h of kicking exercise resulted in a dynamic increase in patellar tendon collagen synthesis.[18] Collagen synthesis, as measured using stabile isotope infusion followed by tendon biopsies, was elevated ~40% 6 h after the exercise bout, peaked at 80% greater 24 h after the exercise, and was still 40% higher 72 h after.[18] Interestingly, the same group found that the 1-h kicking exercise did

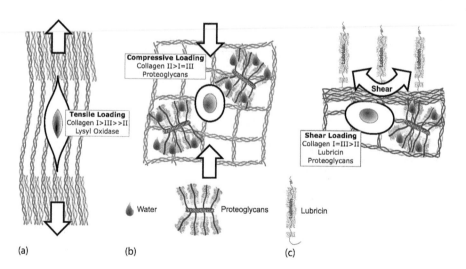

FIGURE 9.2 Different loads result in different cellular responses. In response to (a) tensile loading, cells secrete type I collagen and make lysyl oxidase, resulting in a stiff, aligned collagen matrix. In contrast, (b) compressive loads on the same cells make proteoglycans that contain a protein such as hyaluronic acid and gylcosaminoglycans (GAGs) such as chondroitin and keratin sulfate. Over time, this results in a decrease in collagen alignment and an increase in water in the tissue (held by the GAGs). Last, (c) shear loads lead to the production of proteoglycans and lubricin at the edge of the tissue, resulting in a collagen matrix that contains high amounts of fluid at the edge of the tissue to lubricate movement.

not increase collagen synthesis in women;[19] however, this could be a result of the time point of measurement—72 h in the women, which is 48 h after the peak of collagen synthesis in men.[18] An even greater increase in collagen synthesis is seen in muscle with tensile loading where collagen synthesis increases ~185% 6 h after exercise, stays at that level 18 h later, before returning to baseline 72 h after finishing the exercise bout.[18] In chicken muscle, tensional loading increases collagen protein synthesis by five-fold, resulting in a ten-fold increase in the amount of collagen within the muscle after as few as two days.[20] These data suggest that tensile loading increases collagen synthesis, resulting in an increase in collagen within connective tissues (Figure 9.2a).

In order to understand what about tensile loading drives an increase in collagen synthesis, we turned to an *in vitro* model of a ligament.[21] Three-dimensional engineered ligaments are structurally and functionally very similar to embryonic ligaments. Using these cultured ligaments and a molecular marker that is necessary for the load-induced increase in collagen synthesis [the extracellular-regulated kinase (ERK)],[22] we characterized what aspects of tensile loading connective tissue cells transduce into a signal that results in more collagen production.[23] These experiments demonstrated that the frequency and amplitude of the stretch on a ligament had similar effects on the cellular response, as even very small loads fully activated ERK. In contrast, the duration of an exercise bout was very important: The cellular response to tensile loading peaked between 5 and 10 min and then returned to baseline levels by 90 min (Figure 9.3a).[23]

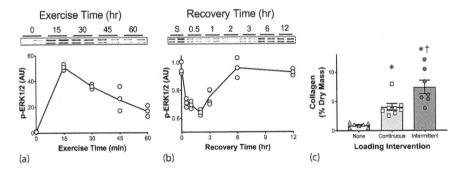

(a)   (b)   (c)

FIGURE 9.3 Short loads and long rest periods are optimal for musculoskeletal connective tissues. Data are presented from engineered ligaments undergoing load[36]. (a) The cellular response to loading [activation of the extracellular regulated kinase (ERK)] peaks at 10 min of loading (not shown) and progressively decreases even though the tissue is still being loaded. In (b), ligaments were stretched for 10 min (S/0 time) and then rested for 0.5, 1, 3, 6, or 12 h before another 10-min stretch, and ERK phosphorylation was determined. The data show that it takes 6 h of rest before the cells can respond completely to a second bout of load. (c) Ligaments were stretched either continuously (24 h a day) or intermittently (10 min of stretch, 6 h of rest, 10 min of stretch, …) for 5 days and the collagen content of the ligaments was determined. Continuous loading increased collagen ~4-fold, whereas an intermittent loading protocol increased collagen ~7.5-fold. This indicates that short bouts of loading (~10 min) with long periods of rest (≥6 h) is optimal for building musculoskeletal connective tissues.

These data suggested that the cells were quickly becoming refractory (resistant) to the tensile load. To determine how long it took to regain the capacity to signal, ligaments were loaded for 10 min and then rested for 0.5, 1, 3, 6, or 12 h (Figure 9.3b). Full signaling returned to the ligament cells only after resting for 6 h.[23] Last, an intermittent tensile loading program (4 × 10 min separated by 6 h) was compared with a continuous loading program, and the ligaments that received 40 min of tensile load each day in short bouts increased collagen synthesis twice as much as those being loaded 24 h a day. These data are similar to the response in bone where cells become refractory after ~40 loads and take 6–8 h to regain the ability to signal.[24] Together, these data suggest that musculoskeletal connective tissues increase collagen synthesis in response to short periods (~10 min) of tensile load separated by load period (~6 h) of rest (Figure 9.3c).

NUTRITION FOR CONNECTIVE TISSUES

As discussed above, the structure and function of tendons, ligaments, and fascia can be directly affected by nutrition. In the following sections, specific nutrients are discussed with regard to their ability to improve collagen synthesis.

Vitamin C

Vitamin C is a water-soluble vitamin, meaning that we need to consume an adequate amount every day. In industrialized societies, daily consumption of the 46 mg per day is not difficult for most people. This was not the case 250 years ago when British seamen on long voyages would routinely get scurvy, a disease characterized by easy bruising, tooth loss, the opening of old wounds, and the stiffening of tendons. In the first controlled nutrition study ever reported, the Scottish physician James Lind fed 12 sailors with scurvy one of six different interventions.[25] The two sailors who ate two oranges and one lemon each recovered completely within a week, whereas in the other sailors the symptoms continued. It took another 200 years before Jerome Gross showed that guinea pigs on a vitamin C-deficient diet did not synthesize collagen,[26] finally making the molecular connection between vitamin C, collagen synthesis, and scurvy. Vitamin C is consumed by the enzyme prolyl hydroxylase in the first posttranslational reaction following the synthesis of collagen. Without vitamin C, prolyl hydroxylase is inactivated and the collagen triple helices become unstable and can no longer be exported.[9] Because vitamin C is consumed in the hydroxylation reaction, it must be replaced every day. This also means that vitamin C levels are low in the morning and need to be replenished before the body can synthesize collagen in response to loading.[27] Even though the requirement for vitamin C in the synthesis of collagen has been recognized for 250 years, whether adding extra vitamin C increases collagen synthesis has yet to be determined.

Glycine

The proteins within tendons, ligaments, and fascia contain ~40% glycine by weight.[5] Because of the amount of glycine in these tissues, some researchers have hypothesized that increasing dietary glycine would benefit tendon healing. To test this hypothesis, Vieira and colleagues injured the Achilles tendon of rats using collagenase and then fed half of the rats a diet containing 5% glycine. After three weeks, the rats on the 5% glycine diet had greater collagen and glycosaminoglycan content than those on the control diet.[28] This increase in collagen and GAGs resulted in improved mechanical strength both in this study and in the follow up study where they added green tea to the nutritional supplement,[29] suggesting that glycine may aid in the recovery of tendon function after injury. It is important to note that these studies have yet to be repeated in human subjects and that most people would find it difficult to consume ~25 g of glycine a day. This is equivalent to a quarter of the bottle of most popular glycine supplements. However, given the success of the rodent data, human studies in this area are warranted.

GELATIN/HYDROLYZED COLLAGEN

A natural source of glycine is dietary collagen. As of 2019, dietary collagen is the fastest growing supplement, with sales topping $45 million in the United States in 2018. As described above, collagen is ~35% glycine and, therefore, consuming collagen could improve collagen synthesis within the connective tissues. The two most popular ways to consume collagen in the diet are gelatin and hydrolyzed collagen. Gelatin is released from the skin, bones, and other connective tissues of animals, such as cows, pig, and fish as a result of boiling (Figure 9.4). As a result, bone broths (soups made by boiling an animal carcass) are rich in gelatin; however, the amount of gelatin in a given bone broth varies from 432 to 9,000 mg per serving depending on how it is made.[30] For more consistent gelatin levels, commercial products from Jell-O® to Knox® gelatin can be found in most grocery stores. These products are normally used to make desserts because dissolving gelatin in hot water and then cooling it for ~4 h results in the formation of jelly. For those looking to dissolve dietary collagen in a liquid, hydrolyzed collagen dissolves better than gelatin. For hydrolyzed collagen, gelatin is further processed using either acid or enzymes such as pepsin, papain, bromelain, and protease.[31] These proteins are proteases, enzymes that cut proteins into smaller pieces called peptides. Because processing with acids or enzymes cuts the gelatin into smaller pieces (called peptides), hydrolyzed collagen is unable to form a gel and is more soluble in room temperature water. Even though different companies use different processes that result in different collagen peptides, whether this has any biological significance has yet to be determined.

To determine whether dietary collagen could increase collagen synthesis in connective tissues, we performed a randomized double-blinded placebo-controlled crossover designed study on subjects who consumed 0, 5, or 15 g of gelatin.[32] Over a three-day period, young men took a supplement containing 48 mg of vitamin C and either a placebo, 5 or 15 g of gelatin. The subjects took the supplement every 6 h between 7 a.m. and 7 p.m. One hour after taking the supplement, the subjects jumped rope to stimulate bone collagen synthesis. Interestingly, consuming 15 g of gelatin doubled the amount of collagen synthesized in either the placebo or 5-g groups. Furthermore, when blood was taken from the subjects an hour after taking the supplement and the serum was added to engineered ligaments, the engineered ligaments increased their collagen content in a dose-dependent manner. These data suggest that dietary collagen together with sufficient vitamin C increases collagen synthesis in tendons and ligaments. Repeating the

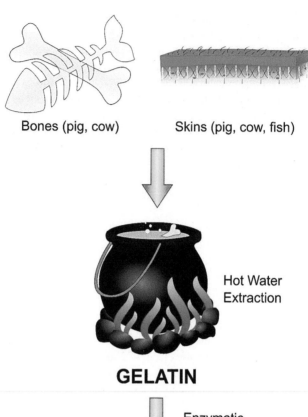

Bones (pig, cow)   Skins (pig, cow, fish)

Hot Water
Extraction

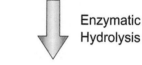

GELATIN

Enzymatic
Hydrolysis

Hydrolyzed Collagen

FIGURE 9.4   Boiling the skin, bones, and other connective tissues of cows, pigs, fish, and other animals results in the release of the collagen from within the tissues in the form of gelatin (denatured but mostly intact collagen protein). To make hydrolyzed collagen, the gelatin is further broken down using acid or enzymes such as pepsin, papain, bromelain, or protease. Therefore, the amino acid content of gelatin and hydrolyzed collagen is the same. The main difference is that one forms a gel and the other does not.

study with gelatin, hydrolyzed collagen, or a gummy made with half gelatin and half hydrolyzed collagen demonstrated that the gelatin and hydrolyzed collagen increased collagen synthesis equivalently, whereas the gummy had no effect.[27] The lack of an effect of the gummy is likely the result of boiling the juice and killing the vitamin C, because amino acid content in the blood was similar between the three feeding groups. Because dietary collagen can increase musculoskeletal collagen synthesis, it is not surprising that consumption of 10 g of hydrolyzed collagen decreased knee pain from standing and walking in a randomized double-blinded placebo-controlled study in athletes.[33] The decrease in knee pain could be the result of improved collagen synthesis in cartilage because cartilage thickness, measured using gadolinium labeled magnetic resonance imaging (MRI), increases with long-term consumption of hydrolyzed collagen.[34] In support of this work, a prospective double-blinded placebo-controlled clinical trial with a cross-over design showed that runners experiencing Achilles pain benefited from collagen supplementation.[35] In the study, injured runners were placed on an exercise rehabilitation program with or without supplementation with hydrolyzed collagen. Those runners in the collagen supplementation group had a significantly better outcome than those in the placebo group. Together, these data suggest that consuming gelatin or hydrolyzed collagen may increase collagen synthesis; however, much of the work is still preliminary and needs more research to support its widespread use.

OTHER NUTRIENTS

Because musculoskeletal sprains, strains, and pulls account for a third of all missed workdays and the only outcome measure in many studies is pain, a myriad of other nutrients are purported to improve tendon/ligament function. These, and other nutraceuticals, have recently been expertly reviewed by Fusini and colleagues[36] and we would encourage readers to go there for details on most of these agents. Many of the nutrients reviewed by Fusini and colleagues are thought to be anti-inflammatory. These agents may, therefore, work by decreasing pain rather than affecting the structure and function of the musculoskeletal connective tissues. Therefore, much more work is needed to validate these purported nutraceuticals.

COMBINING LOADING AND NUTRITION FOR CONNECTIVE TISSUES

Tendons and ligaments have relatively low blood flow, instead using diffusion from the environment to provide nutrients and remove waste products.[37,38] Most oxygen and nutrients come from the myotendinous junction,[39] the fat pad at the enthesis,[40] and the paratenon or the synovial sheath.[37,41–43] Similar to a sponge, fluid within connective tissues moves out as the tissue is loaded and when the tissue relaxes the fluid flows back into the tissue, increasing nutrient update.[41] Given that loading of connective tissue increases nutrient delivery, the timing of nutrition relative to load is an important consideration. Therefore, optimal time point for exercise following intake of supplement is related to the rate of digestion, adsorption, and delivery of the nutrient. For 15 g of vitamin C-enriched gelatin, amino acid levels in the blood peak approximately 1 h after ingestion. The blood isolated from subjects an hour after feeding is sufficient to increase collagen synthesis in engineered ligaments, and eating the vitamin C-enriched gelatin an hour before loading results in an increase in collagen synthesis in people.[32] These data suggest that loading the target tendons at approximately the peak of appearance in the blood can increase collagen production in musculoskeletal connective tissues.

Three case/limited participant studies have utilized this combined loading and nutrition protocol to improve connective tissue function and return to play. In the first, a professional basketball player with a central core patellar tendinopathy was provided 15 g of gelatin in orange juice an hour before a 10-min exercise protocol.[44] This rehabilitation protocol was added on top of his normal training and game schedule and contributed to the complete restoration of patellar tendon structure, as determined by MRI, and elimination of pain. In the second, nutrition and short periods of loading were used to accelerate return to play in two elite rugby players following ACL rupture.[45] Soon after reconstructive surgery, the athletes performed two to three range-of-motion/loading sessions per day, separated by 6 h and each session preceded by the ingestion of 10 g of gelatin with 250 mg vitamin C. The rehab sessions used the idea of a minimal effect dose of load[23] to maximally active collagen synthesis within the newly grafted ligament and to repair the hamstring tendon that was partially used as the graft, and the timed delivery of nutrients was thought to provide necessary substrates for collagen synthesis.[45] The result was a return to full hamstring strength in under 15 weeks and a return to international rugby in ~30 weeks. The last study using load and nutrition to maximize return to play was the cross-over design study on runners with Achilles pain described above. In this study, the 19 injured runners all performed 2×90 one-legged slow eccentric drops daily for 6 months with the leg both straight and bent. Half of the runners were supplemented with a hydrolyzed collagen for the first 3 months, while the others got the placebo. At the halfway point, the groups were switched. In the first three months, twice as many participants returned to running from the hydrolyzed collagen group than the placebo group. After the cross over, the collagen group again had twice as many people return to running. In the end, eight subjects returned to running from the hydrolyzed collagen group, whereas only four returned to running while in the placebo group.[35]

CONCLUSIONS AND FUTURE FOCUS

There is a clear relationship between load, nutrition, and tendon/ligament/fascia function. In response to tension, compression, and shear loads these tissues increase collagen, cartilage, and lubrication gene expression, respectively. The positive effect of loading is best seen in recovery from injury. Starting a loading program within two days after injury decreases return to play time by 25% when compared with a group that immobilized the injured area for nine days.[46] This means that the proper application of load is essential to the development of healthy musculoskeletal connective tissues. When these loads are combined with nutritional interventions such as vitamin C and gelatin or other nutrients like glycine, the result is an improvement in tissue structure and function. Even though there is strong evidence for how load alters tissue function, the role of nutrition in this process is in its infancy. Larger clinical studies are needed to determine whether dietary collagen has clinical efficacy or is simply the result of small sample sizes and a strong belief effect.

REFERENCES

1. Kjaer M. Role of extracellular matrix in adaptation of tendon and skeletal muscle to mechanical loading. 2004. doi:10.1152/physrev.00031.2003.
2. Ricard-Blum S. The collagen family. *Cold Spring Harb Perspect Biol* 3: 1–19, 2011.
3. Sasarman F, Maftei C, Campeau PM, Brunel-Guitton C, Mitchell GA, Allard P. Biosynthesis of glycosaminoglycans: Associated disorders and biochemical tests. *J Inherit Metab Dis* 39: 173–188, 2016.

4. Heinemeier KM, Schjerling P, Heinemeier J, Magnusson SP, Kjaer M. Lack of tissue renewal in human adult achilles tendon is revealed by nuclear bomb (14)C. *FASEB J* 27: 2074–2079, 2013.

5. Smeets JSJ, Horstman AMH, Vles GF, Emans PJ, Goessens JPB, Gijsen AP, van Kranenburg JMX, van Loon LJC. Protein synthesis rates of muscle, tendon, ligament, cartilage, and bone tissue in vivo in humans. *PLoS One* 14: e0224745, 2019.

6. Myrick KM, Voss A, Feinn RS, Martin T, Mele BM, Garbalosa JC. Effects of season long participation on ACL volume in female intercollegiate soccer athletes. *J Exp Orthop* 6, 2019.

7. Asou Y, Nifuji A, Tsuji K, Shinomiya K, Olson EN, Koopman P, Noda M. Coordinated expression of scleraxis and Sox9 genes during embryonic development of tendons and cartilage. *J Orthop Res* 20: 827–833, 2002.

8. Chang HY, Chi JT, Dudoit S, Bondre C, Van De Rijn M, Botstein D, Brown PO. Diversity, topographic differentiation, and positional memory in human fibroblasts. *Proc Natl Acad Sci USA* 99(20): 12877–12882, 2002.

9. Mussini E, Hutton J, Udenfriend S. Collagen proline hydroxylase in wound healing, granuloma formation, scurvy, and growth. *Science* 157(80): 927–929, 1967.

10. Nishikimi M, Koshizaka T, Ozawa T, Yagi K. Occurrence in humans and guinea pigs of the gene related to their missing enzyme L-gulono-γ-lactone oxidase. *Arch Biochem Biophys* 267: 842–846, 1988.

11. Fede C, Angelini A, Stern R, Macchi V, Porzionato A, Ruggieri P, De Caro R, Stecco C. Quantification of hyaluronan in human fasciae: Variations with function and anatomical site. *J Anat* 233: 552–556, 2018.

12. Gillard GC, Reilly HC, Bell-Booth PG, Flint MH. The influence of mechanical forces on the glycosaminoglycan content of the rabbit flexor digitorum profundus tendon. *Connect Tissue Res* 7: 37–46, 1979.

13. Robbins JR, Evanko SP, Vogel KG. Mechanical loading and TGF-β regulate proteoglycan synthesis in tendon. *Arch Biochem Biophys* 342: 203–211, 1997.

14. Nugent GE, Aneloski NM, Schmidt TA, Schumacher BL, Voegtline MS, Sah RL. Dynamic shear stimulation of bovine cartilage biosynthesis of proteoglycan 4. *Arthritis Rheum* 54: 1888–1896, 2006.

15. Hayashi M, Zhao C, Thoreson AR, Chikenji T, Jay GD, An K-N, Amadio PC. The effect of lubricin on the gliding resistance of mouse intrasynovial tendon. *PLoS One* 8: e83836, 2013.

16. Kapacee Z, Richardson SH, Lu Y, Starborg T, Holmes DF, Baar K, Kadler KE. Tension is required for fibripositor formation. *Matrix Biol* 27: 371–375, 2008.

17. Majima T, Yasuda K, Tsuchida T, Tanaka K, Miyakawa K, Minami A, Hayashi K. Stress shielding of patellar tendon: Effect on small-diameter collagen fibrils in a rabbit model. *J Orthop Sci* 8: 836–41, 2003.

18. Miller BF, Olesen JL, Hansen M, Døssing S, Crameri RM, Welling RJ, Langberg H, Flyvbjerg A, Kjaer M, Babraj JA, Smith K, Rennie MJ. Coordinated collagen and muscle protein synthesis in human patella tendon and quadriceps muscle after exercise. *J Physiol* 567: 1021–1033, 2005.

19. Miller BF, Hansen M, Olesen JL, Schwarz P, Babraj JA, Smith K, Rennie MJ, Kjaer M. Tendon collagen synthesis at rest and after exercise in women. *J Appl Physiol* 102: 541–546, 2007.

20. Laurent GJ, McAnulty RJ, Gibson J. Changes in collagen synthesis and degradation during skeletal muscle growth. *Am J Physiol—Cell Physiol* 18: 1–4, 1985.

21. Paxton JZ, Grover LM, Baar K. Engineering an in vitro model of a functional ligament from bone to bone. *Tissue Eng Part A* 16: 3515–3525, 2010.

22. Papakrivopoulou J, Lindahl GE, Bishop JE, Laurent GJ. Differential roles of extracellular signal-regulated kinase 1/2 and p38MAPK in mechanical load-induced procollagen α1(I) gene expression in cardiac fibroblasts. *Cardiovasc Res* 61: 736–744, 2004.

23. Paxton JZ, Hagerty P, Andrick JJ, Baar K. Optimizing an intermittent stretch paradigm using ERK1/2 phosphorylation results in increased collagen synthesis in engineered ligaments. *Tissue Eng Part A* 18: 277–284, 2012.
24. Burr DB, Robling AG, Turner CH. Effects of biomechanical stress on bones in animals. *Bone* 30: 781–786, 2002.
25. Lind J. *A Treatise of the Scurvy in Three Parts*. Edinburgh: Sands, Murray, and Cochrain, 1753.
26. Gross J. Studies on the formation of collagen: IV. Effect of vitamin C deficiency on the neutral salt-extractible collagen of skin. *J Exp Med* 109: 555–569, 1959.
27. Lis DM, Baar K. Effects of different vitamin C–enriched collagen derivatives on collagen synthesis. *Int J Sport Nutr Exerc Metab.* 2019. doi:10.1123/ijsnem.2018-0385.
28. Vieira CP, De Oliveira LP, Da Ré Guerra F, Dos Santos De Almeida M, Marcondes MC, Pimentel ER. Glycine improves biochemical and biomechanical properties following inflammation of the achilles tendon. *Anat Rec (Hoboken)* 298: 538–545, 2015.
29. Vieira CP, Da Ré Guerra F, De Oliveira LP, Almeida MS, Marcondes MCC, Pimentell ER. Green tea and glycine aid in the recovery of tendinitis of the Achilles tendon of rats. *Connect Tissue Res* 56: 50–58, 2015.
30. Alcock RD, Shaw GC, Burke LM. Bone broth unlikely to provide reliable concentrations of collagen precursors compared with supplemental sources of collagen used in collagen research. *Int J Sport Nutr Exerc Metab* 29: 265–272, 2019.
31. Hema GS, Joshy CG, Shyni K, Chatterjee NS, Ninan G, Mathew S. Optimization of process parameters for the production of collagen peptides from fish skin (*Epinephelus malabaricus*) using response surface methodology and its characterization. *J Food Sci Technol* 54: 488–496, 2017.
32. Shaw G, Lee-Barthel A, Ross MLR, Wang B, Baar K. Vitamin C-enriched gelatin supplementation before intermittent activity augments collagen synthesis. *Am J Clin Nutr* 105: 136–143, 2017.
33. Clark KL, Sebastianelli W, Flechsenhar KR, Aukermann DF, Meza F, Millard RL, Deitch JR, Sherbondy PS, Albert A. 24-Week study on the use of collagen hydrolysate as a dietary supplement in athletes with activity-related joint pain. *Curr Med Res Opin.* 2008. doi:10.1185/030079908x291967.
34. McAlindon TE, Nuite M, Krishnan N, Ruthazer R, Price LL, Burstein D, Griffith J, Flechsenhar K. Change in knee osteoarthritis cartilage detected by delayed gadolinium enhanced magnetic resonance imaging following treatment with collagen hydrolysate: A pilot randomized controlled trial. *Osteoarthr Cartil* 19: 399–405, 2011.
35. Praet SFE, Purdam CR, Welvaert M, Vlahovich N, Lovell G, Burke LM, Gaida JE, Manzanero S, Hughes D, Waddington G. Oral supplementation of specific collagen peptides combined with calf-strengthening exercises enhances function and reduces pain in Achilles tendinopathy patients. *Nutrients* 11: 1–16, 2019.
36. Fusini F, Bisicchia S, Bottegoni C, Gigante A, Zanchini F, Busilacchi A. Nutraceutical supplement in the management of tendinopathies: A systematic review. *Muscles Ligaments Tendons J* 6: 48–57, 2016.
37. Amiel D, Akeson WH, Renzoni S, Harwood F, Abel M. Nutrition of cruciate ligament reconstruction by diffusion: Collagen synthesis studied in rabbits. *Acta Orthop Scand* 57: 201–203, 1986.
38. Skyhar MJ, Danzig LA, Hargens AR, Akeson WH. Nutrition of the anterior cruciate ligament. Effects of continuous passive motion. *Am J Sports Med* 13: 415–418, 1985.
39. Manske PR, Lesker PA. Nutrient pathways of flexor tendons in primates. *J Hand Surg Am* 7: 436–444, 1982.

40. Benjamin M, Redman S, Milz S, Büttner A, Amin A, Moriggl B, Brenner E, Emery P, McGonagle D, Bydder G. Adipose tissue at entheses: The rheumatological implications of its distribution. A potential site of pain and stress dissipation? *Ann Rheum Dis* 63: 1549–1555, 2004.

41. Lundborg G, Holm S, Myrhage R. The role of the synovial fluid and tendon sheath for flexor tendon nutrition. *Scand J Plast Reconstr Surg Hand Surg* 14: 99–107, 1980.

42. Manske PR, Bridwell K, Lesker PA. Nutrient pathways to flexor tendons of chickens using tritiated praline. *J Hand Surg Am* 3: 352–357, 1978.

43. Whiteside LA, Sweeney RE. Nutrient pathways of the cruciate ligaments. An experimental study using the hydrogen wash-out technique. *J Bone Joint Surg Am* 62: 1176–80, 1980. http://www.ncbi.nlm.nih.gov/pubmed/7430206 [June 10, 2019].

44. Baar K. Stress relaxation and targeted nutrition to treat patellar tendinopathy. *Int J Sport Nutr Exerc Metab.* 2019. doi:10.1123/ijsnem.2018–0231.

45. Shaw G, Serpell B, Baar K. Rehabilitation and nutrition protocols for optimising return to play from traditional ACL reconstruction in elite rugby union players: A case study. *J Sports Sci* 37: 1794–1803, 2019.

46. Bayer ML, Magnusson SP, Kjaer M. Early versus delayed rehabilitation after acute muscle injury. *N Engl J Med* 377: 1300–1301, 2017.

10 Does Fascia Stretch?

Chris Frederick

CONTENTS

In order to properly answer the question, "Does fascia stretch?", it is important to establish at the outset what definitions to use. There are presently two definitions of the word fascia that have been submitted for acceptance to the Federative International Programme on Anatomical Terminologies (FIPAT): (1) "A fascia is a sheath, a sheet, or any other dissectible aggregations of connective tissue that forms beneath the skin to attach, enclose, and separate muscles and other internal organs", and (2) "The fascial system consists of the three-dimensional continuum of soft, collagen containing, loose and dense fibrous connective tissues that permeate the body. It incorporates elements such as adipose tissue, adventitiae and neurovascular sheaths, aponeuroses, deep and superficial fasciae, epineurium, joint capsules, ligaments, membranes, meninges, myofascial expansions, periostea, retinacula, septa, tendons, visceral fasciae, and all the intramuscular and intermuscular connective tissues including endo-/peri-/epimysium. The fascial system interpenetrates and surrounds all organs, muscles, bones, and nerve fibers, endowing the body with a functional structure, and providing an environment that enables all body systems to operate in an integrated manner".[1]

If we use the first, tissue-specific definition of fascia for the moment, then we would be obligated to restrict ourselves to considering only the kind of research designed to study the effects of mechanical stress and strain of connective tissue. Let's start with the beginning of a two-part article in 2003 that may well have initiated a long-standing debate about whether fascia has the ability to stretch that still reverberates today.[2] In it, the author Schleip states at the outset, "…studies have shown that either much stronger forces or longer durations would be required for a permanent viscoelastic deformation of fascia".

From this, the author determined that the thixotrophic (AKA "gel to sol") model of connective tissue plasticity could no longer suffice as a valid explanation as to what occurs when either or both practitioner and client feel what many described as "a release". That is, the colloid part of fascia—in the extracellular matrix, or

ECM—does not in fact become more fluid during commonly applied short phases of manual therapy technique. Piezoelectricity was another model that tried to explain that therapeutic "release" was due to applied manual therapy pressure that created an electric charge that then stimulated fibroblasts to produce more collagen. When placed under the scrutiny of research, both models failed to adequately explain or otherwise account for short-term tissue change that practitioners claimed to feel and observe. Some writers of popular blogs and articles took this to mean that the evidence has shown that all fascia cannot be stretched: "Manual therapists need not feel threatened by the news that we cannot stretch fascia".[3]

This new perspective—that fascia cannot be stretched, seemed to be further supported with a notable study in 2008,[4] with Schleip listed as an author along with Chaudry and others. The authors commented in that article that they came across other studies where some research authors reported evidence that supported practitioners' observations and explanations of a tissue "release" while finding other studies that argued against it. Therefore, Schleip et al. stated that they undertook their own study to resolve a fundamental question underlying such diverse findings. That question was whether the applied force and duration for a typical, average amount of time of a given manual myofascial technique could be sufficient to induce palpable viscoelastic changes such as tissue deformation in human fasciae.[4]

They developed a three-dimensional mathematical model with equations revealing very large forces, "that outside the normal physiologic range, are required to produce even 1% compression and 1% shear in fascia lata and plantar fascia". Their conclusion was,

> The palpable sensations of tissue release that are often reported by osteopathic physicians and other manual therapists cannot be due to deformations produced in the firm tissues of plantar fascia and fascia lata. However, palpable tissue release could result from deformation in softer tissues, such as superficial nasal fascia.[4]

Those authors chose a common manual therapy technique used by osteopaths and other practitioners who, "report local tissue release after the application of a slow manual force to tight fascial areas".[4] Reduced to its basic mechanical components, the technique used in this study—often called myofascial or fascial release—employed pressure and shear together to treat movement restrictions in specific dense (less elastic) fascial tissues and then in other softer (more elastic) fascial tissues. The combination of pressure and shear produces a stretch of the tissue, often directly into the barrier of restriction that has been variously described by practitioners as getting a plastic, permanent deformation of restricted tissues.

After that study was published, many more articles appeared online with definitive sounding headlines and titles like, "If We Cannot Stretch Fascia, What Are We Doing?", or even more succinctly, "Reasons not to stretch".[3,5] From the sound of those titles, it appeared that the controversy of whether fascia can stretch or not was settled. In fact, this is very much not the case.

The 2008 article previously mentioned appeared to provide valid evidence for the case against certain kinds of fascia—plantar fascia and fascia lata—being able to be therapeutically stretched for permanent treatment effect. However, that article also stated at the outset that "palpable tissue release could result from deformation in softer tissues".[4] Research that "investigated the potential importance of uniaxial tension in a variety of therapies involving mechanical stretch" was considered.[4] This fact—that less dense or "softer" connective tissues could indeed get the release effect from tissue deformation that many practitioners observe—was largely missing from the many articles and blogs that this author came across that questioned or advised whether stretching is necessary.

So although research explained and cited in that 2008 article that determined tissues such as the iliotibial band and the plantar fascia cannot be stretched to get a therapeutic effect without damaging the tissue, that was only true for a certain type of "dense connective tissue" in a specific location that endured peculiar biomechanical forces unique to it. Here are the quotations supporting that fascia does stretch from the original 2003 article by Schleip:[3]

1. Golgi receptors found throughout dense connective tissues "respond to slow stretch by influencing the alpha motor neurons via the spinal cord to lower their firing rate, i.e., to soften related muscle fibers". However, "such a stimulation happens only when the muscle fibers are actively contracting".
2. Ruffini type II receptors are found in "tissues associated with regular stretching" and associated with decreasing muscle tone via "inhibition of sympathetic activity".
3. "The majority of sensory nerves to muscles are types III and IV and abundantly exist in the interstitium and myofasciae. The majority of these interstitial receptors function as mechanoreceptors, which means they respond to mechanical tension [or stretch] and/or pressure".
4. "...a Japanese study had already revealed that types III and IV receptors in the fascia of temporalis, masseter and infrahyoid muscles show 'responses to the mandibular movement and the stretching of the fascia and the skin' ".
5. "Myofascial manipulation involves a stimulation of intrafascial mechanoreceptors. Their stimulation leads to an altered proprioceptive input to the central nervous system, which then results in a changed tonus regulation of motor units associated with this tissue".

In summary, while we discussed evidence that supports certain types of fascia cannot be therapeutically stretched, we also presented evidence that other types do stretch, via the different kinds of mechanoreceptors that are stimulated when the fascia in which they are embedded is stretched. One cannot stretch a mechanoreceptor in isolation and apart from the connective tissue in which it lies. More about this will be explained in the next section.

MECHANOBIOLOGY

More recently, biology has provided much well-established evidence that mammals, including humans, have many examples of stretch-dependent mechanisms that are essential for survival. If we start with just about any cell, the concept of tensegrity is a given in the burgeoning and fascinating field of mechanobiology.[6] Mechanobiology "centers on how cells control their mechanical properties, and how physical forces regulate cellular biochemical responses, a process that is known as mechanotransduction".[7] Tensegrity (a portmanteau of tension-integrity) depends on tensile prestress for its mechanical stability in biological structures and the physiological systems they drive. As Ingber states, "tensional prestress is a critical governor of cell mechanics and function, and how use of tensegrity by cells contributes to mechanotransduction".[7]

There is also evidence that the stretch-dependent tensegrity model may be applied to the extra cellular matrix:

> The ECM, a polymer network consisted [sic] of many different protein polymers, may be viewed as an extended cytoskeleton that connects cells within living tissues and organs. In many soft tissues, the ECM is tensed by adherent living cells that exert traction forces on their adhesions, ...this prestressed network essentially stabilizes itself like a tensegrity structure.[7]

In short, from nanoscale to macroscale, evidence shows that cells and the tissues, organs, systems, and organisms they differentiate into are all under a normal state of tension or stretch in the unperturbed steady state at rest that fosters homeostasis, as well as in the more active state of homeokinesis.

Earlier, the fascial system was described as a "three-dimensional continuum of soft, collagen containing, loose and dense fibrous connective tissues that permeate the body".[1] All of the neural receptors that communicate to the brain and the rest of the central and peripheral nervous systems about gamma and alpha muscle tone (and much more) are embedded within this system that is under tension or stretch at rest as well as during movement. Studies noted previously as well as many more include findings that a majority of those neural receptors fundamentally respond to mechanical stretch to drive cellular communication and physiology that activates life and function in the human body.

After just reviewing a number of previous citations that provided evidence for cell and tissue stretching, we turn to the stretching studies of larger regions of myofasciae of the human body, that is, the "muscles".

TO STRETCH OR NOT TO STRETCH—A BRIEF HISTORY

In 1999, a critical review of the clinical and basic science literature arguably started a debate among professionals in health, fitness, and sports about the merits of stretching that continues to this day. Titled, "Stretching before exercise does not reduce the risk of local muscle injury", it raised the hackles of many practitioners who also incorporated stretching into their work.[8]

Prior to that article, many generally assumed that stretching improved functional and athletic performance, increased flexibility, and reduced injuries.[9] Many practitioners from diverse disciplines were convinced about the importance of stretching as a necessary part of their protocols for successful outcomes. The article questioned belief systems with scientific evidence, which started a tide of controversy and dispute about the actual benefits of stretching.

This tide surged in 2002, when an article that stirred even more controversy appeared.[10] It was a systematic review of research that evaluated the benefits (or lack thereof) associated with stretching procedures in relation to protection from injury and post exercise soreness. Conclusions taken directly from the study were as follows:

> Stretching before or after exercising does not confer protection from muscle soreness. Stretching before exercising does not seem to confer a practically useful reduction in the risk of injury, but the generality of this finding needs testing.

In 2003, an article titled, "The stretching debate" surfaced in direct response to the previously discussed review.[11] It featured invited commentary by respected clinicians about the review that was largely negative on the benefits of stretching. Opinions were at times emotionally charged and reflected the conflicts between what many practitioners believed worked for them and what some researchers were claiming was really happening in stretching. Adamant pro and anti-stretch camps formed within professions practicing varietal therapies and also included fitness and sports coaches and trainers. This acrimonious climate was covered by the media, adding more fuel to the fire.[5] The public who was following this controversy were confused about whether they should stretch at all. Their practitioners, coaches, and trainers were not all in agreement about whether stretching should be implemented or if utilized, how to design an appropriate program.

For the next decade, there were published a multitude of studies comparing a variety of set parameters that established poor outcomes when static stretching is done up to an hour before athletic activity requiring power or strength.[12] Yet even as the case for the negative impact of stretching persisted, new studies showing specific benefits began to surface.

One systematic review on multiple studies indicated the following positive outcomes from stretching:[13]

1. Increased [range of motion (ROM)].
2. ROM increases bilaterally from unilateral stretch.
3. Static and dynamic warm ups are equally effective at increasing ROM prior to exercise.
4. Pre-contraction stretching [e.g., proprioceptive neuromuscular facilitation (PNF)] lowers excitability of muscle.
5. A pre-stretch contraction has been associated with greater acute gains in ROM compared with static stretching in many studies.
6. In contrast to static stretching, dynamic stretching is not associated with strength or performance deficits.
7. Dynamic stretching improved dynamometer measured power as well as jumping and running performance.
8. Static stretching performed before or after warm up does not decrease strength.
9. Four repetitions of 15-s holds of static stretching did not affect vertical jump.

Since the above systematic review was published in 2012, there have been many more studies on stretching that have come out. If we discuss just those studies that are in the "high-quality category", the choices are unfortunately few. And examples of the practical application of favorable outcomes are severely limited. The following are examples of high quality, starting with the highest: meta analyses, systematic reviews, and randomized controlled trials (RCTs).

CURRENT RESEARCH ON STRETCHING

This section is limited to discussing the relatively few high-quality studies that present research relevant to practitioners. As stated earlier, there is an abundant of lesser-quality studies available to peruse that have come out in the last 5–10 years.

An analysis of the current literature on the acute effects of dynamic stretching (DS) determined that, "there is a substantial amount of evidence pointing out the positive effects on range of motion (ROM) and subsequent performance" as determined by the measured production of force, power, sprint and jump.[14] As opposed to static stretching which commonly entails holding a position of stretch for a defined period of time, DS is performed with constant motion, into and out of the stretch position. DS in sports is commonly performed at faster tempos pre activity to aid performance and slower tempos post activity to aid recovery.

After years of debate about whether stretching was even appropriate for athletes to engage in, growing numbers of studies were finally pointing to the benefits. Despite a recent systematic review finding minimal evidence presented as to how DS actually affects the neuromuscular system,[15] DS is now considered an essential element of athletic preparation.[9]

Despite substantial amounts of evidence favoring individual and group dynamic stretching, the previously noted analysis also found numerous studies reporting no alteration or even performance impairment. Possible mitigating factors such as stretch duration, amplitude, or velocity were highlighted. However, it may be easily extrapolated that other additional factors such as stretch intensity, frequency, and tempo are also relevant.

A recent collaboration between top stretching researchers produced a systematic review summarizing the results of the high quality RCTs published to date.[15] This review produced a summary of stretching outcomes that provides one a comprehensive impression of where the science of acute, pre activity self stretching may be today.

ACUTE EFFECTS OF MUSCLE STRETCHING ON PHYSICAL PERFORMANCE, RANGE OF MOTION, AND INJURY INCIDENCE IN HEALTHY ACTIVE INDIVIDUALS: A SYSTEMATIC REVIEW

In this review, "an overview of the literature was performed citing the effects of pre activity stretching on physical performance, injury risk, and ROM, as well as the physiological mechanisms, with the objective of investigating, analyzing, and interpreting the acute physical responses to a variety of stretching techniques to provide clarity regarding the impact on performance, ROM, and injury".[15]

Limitations described by the authors that were encountered when reviewing the literature included, "issues related to internal validity (i.e., bias caused by expectancy effects) and external validity (i.e., stretch durations and warm up components, description detail of stretches, reporting bias against non-significant results)".

Based on this systematic review, the authors produced the following position statement for the Canadian Society For Exercise Physiology that has been paraphrased and condensed[15]:

> Muscle stretching pre activity (done by solitary individuals to themselves or in a group) in some form appears to be of greater benefit than deficit (in terms of performance, ROM, and injury outcomes) but the type of stretching chosen and the make up of the stretch routine will depend on the context within which it is used.

The following contexts were enumerated in the position statement and are followed by this author's comments:

1. "Regarding stretch duration: [Static stretch (SS)] and PNF stretching >60 s total per individual muscle are not recommended immediately before training or competition unless one is willing to sacrifice optimum physical performance for a decreased risk of specific muscle injury and/or a specific need for increased ROM".

   Comment: Setting individual circumstances aside, this conclusion seems mostly useful for those engaged in rehabilitation to full function that need to make steady progress while simultaneously keeping risk low to none for reinjury. It is the author's experience with athlete patients, and with colleagues and students working with athletes, that both SS and PNF >60 s per muscle is not done at all. Instead DS is used for all pre activity preparation.

2. "Regarding injury: injury reduction appears to require more than 5 min of total stretching of multiple task related muscle groups. However, when an optimal pre-event warm up with an appropriate duration of stretching is completed … the benefits of SS and PNF stretching for increasing ROM and reducing muscle injury risk at least balance, or may outweigh, any possible cost of performance decrements".

   Comment: (a) This statement confirms what is commonly practiced today in sport training, i.e., pre activity self stretching with best outcomes for performance is dynamic or DS.[9] However, if an individual is engaged in rehabilitation in order to return to sport activity, the guidelines indicate that if the person has decreased ROM or is recovering from a muscle injury, then an SS and/or PNF program may be indicated while DS is avoided until fully recovered. This author has had success with programs that are often combined, i.e., they address the target tissue or involved region that is recovering with SS or PNF first, then do DS before an activity that is paced and progressed according to the healing phase and ability of the person. (b) It is not clear what the statement, "more than 5 min" means, i.e., there is no defined termination point at which time it can be deemed that there is no benefit to a longer duration stretch. (c) Even if multiple muscle

groups are engaged in say a sport-specific manner, does it make a difference in what order those movements are produced, and if so, what are those
movements for each sport, each team player, an individual with specific or
unique needs?

3. "Regarding muscle length position: SS appears to enhance performance
   in activities performed at long muscle lengths. In this review, '5 studies
   demonstrated marked strength loss at short muscle lengths (−10.2%), which
   contrasted with moderate strength gains at the longest muscle lengths tested
   (+ 2.2%)' ".

   Comment: Because the totality of functional movement in sports entails
   patterns characteristic of combining concentric shortening with eccentric
   lengthening, and sometime isometric positioning, a 10% loss in strength
   in a shortened position seems hardly a reasonable trade-off for a 2% gain
   in a lengthened position. However, if an athlete is engaged in a sport or
   in specific training that requires more eccentric strength, it may be determined that SS may be indicated at longer muscle lengths functional for that
   activity.

4. "Regarding dynamic stretching: DS may induce moderate performance
   enhancements and may be included in the stretching component to
   provide task specific ROM increases and facilitation of dynamic performance when performed soon before an activity; however, there is no
   evidence as to whether it influences injury risk. Furthermore, while the
   literature examining the effect of stretching on physical performance is
   extensive, the literature examining injury risk is much smaller...".

   Comment: This statement indicates that it is still not known what precise type or manner of stretching may increase or decrease risk of injury.
   Therefore, more studies are needed.

5. "Regarding muscle soreness: There is conflicting evidence as to whether
   stretching in any form before exercise can reduce exercise induced muscle
   soreness".

   Comment: This author has clinical experience and testimonials from many
   students that has confirmed repeatedly that at least one specific type of
   assisted stretching does reduce and eliminate muscle soreness depending
   on many factors, including but not limited to sleep deprivation, dehydration, malnutrition, and chronic low-level systemic inflammation. It may
   be considered that the positive results noted may be from various combinations of parameters peculiar to the specific assisted stretching cited.[12]
   Further research is warranted to verify.

From reviewing this systematic study as well as the author's position statement on
guidelines for the Canadian Society for Exercise Physiology, this author concludes
that there is still insufficient tangible, concrete, or practical information from evidence-based research alone, to design a comprehensive sport- or athlete-specific
acute self stretch program.

Another opinion offered by a contemporary author who also recently reviewed much of the literature on stretching science has come to a similar, though differently worded conclusion: "There is still much we do not understand and, for now, the conclusions lie somewhere in the middle—stretching is sometimes good, but not that good, and when good, only under certain conditions".[16]

Coming around full circle from the beginning of this chapter when the controversy of whether fascia could be stretched or not was posited, a high-quality systematic literature review of randomized controlled trials was conducted that looked at the effectiveness of myofascial release, a form of direct and indirect stretching of restricted fasciae.[17] It was concluded that, "MFR is emerging as a strategy with a solid evidence base for the future trials".

CONCLUSION

While studies about macro stretching, that is, those that focus on whole body and muscle groups are voluminous, they are of mostly poor quality in terms of research design. Unfortunately, the few that are high quality do not currently offer precise enough guidelines for practitioners to plan complete valid and reliable assisted stretch therapy or self stretch programs for their patients and clients.

While not currently offering practical guidelines either, studies on micro and nano stretching of cells, tissues, and mammals (much of it about fascial tissues) are gathering specific data that will eventually evolve future design of high-quality macro stretch studies.

The burgeoning field of mechanobiology provides a logical reason for this prediction given that it examines fundamental questions of how living cells physically organize themselves from individual molecules to whole organisms and, as some researchers state, "that this provides a mechanism to channel forces from the macroscale to the nanoscale, and to facilitate mechanochemical conversion in living organisms".[7]

Mechanobiologists have determined that the design principles of tensegrity structure is inherently a tension (or stretch)-based system with functions that govern life-sustaining principles in various organic structures such as polypeptides in proteins; microfilaments, microtubules, and intermediate filaments in the cytoskeleton; cells and ECM in tissues; and bones and muscles. As the authors state,

The shape stability and immediate mechanical responsiveness of all these structures depends on the prestress that is transmitted across their structural elements. Because cells use tensegrity to structure themselves, mechanical forces and physical cues applied at the macroscale can be channeled over stiffened structural elements, and concentrated on individual structures (e.g., focal adhesions) and molecules at the micrometer and nanometer scales. Specifically, the use of structural hierarchies (systems within systems) that span several size scales and are composed of a tensed network of muscles, bones, ECMs, cells, and cytoskeletal filaments that focus stresses in specific mechanotransducer molecules is key to how living cells carry out mechanochemical transduction, which is critical for their growth and function.[7]

Based on the findings and conclusions of researcher Ingber and many others who have worked for decades investigating and applying tensegrity principles in mechanobiology, it can be stated that the human tensional network is a force transmission, mechanotransducive dependent system in which stretching plays a large and crucial role along with other forces to drive most of the physiological processes of life, much less to drive physical movement of the entire body.

Hopefully, this is the kind of science that will enable researchers to comprehensively study stretching from systemic, whole-body effects of the fascial system, to specific fascial tissues, down to cells and molecules that drive those processes of life.

REFERENCES

1. Adstrum, S., Hedley, G., Schleip, R., Stecco, C., Yucesoy, C.A. 2017. Defining the fascial system. *Journal of Bodywork & Movement Therapies*, 21: 173–177. www.bodyworkmovementtherapies.com/article/S1360-8592(16)30259-5/fulltext.
2. Schleip, R. 2003. Fascial plasticity a new neurobiological explanation. *Journal of Bodywork and Movement Therapies*, 7(1): 11–19. https://doi.org/10.1016/S1360-8592(02)00067-0.
3. Sanvito, A. 2012. If We Cannot Stretch Fascia, What Are We Doing? www.massage-stlouis.com/blog/if-we-cannot-stretch-fascia-what-are-we-doing (accessed August 12, 2019).
4. Chaudhry, H., Schleip, R., Ji, Z., Bukiet, B., Maney, M., Findley, T. 2008. Three-dimensional mathematical model for deformation of human fasciae in manual therapy. *The Journal of the American Osteopathic Association*, 108: 379–390.
5. Reynolds, G. 2013 Reasons Not to Stretch. *New York Times*. well.blogs.nytimes.com/2013/04/03/reasons-not-to-stretch (accessed August 13, 2019).
6. Wall, M., Butler, D., El Haj, A., Bodle, J.C., Loboa, E.G., Banes, A.J. 2018. Key developments that impacted the field of mechanobiology and mechanotransduction. *Journal of Orthopaedic Research*, 36(2): 605–619. www.doi.org/10.1002/jor.23707.
7. Ingber, D.E., Wang, N., Stamenović, D. 2014. Tensegrity, cellular biophysics, and the mechanics of living systems. *Reports on Progress in Physics*, 77(4): 1–42. https://doi.org/10.1088/0034-4885/77/4/046603.
8. Shrier, I. 1999. Stretching before exercise does not reduce the risk of local muscle injury: A critical review of the clinical and basic science literature. *Clinical Journal of Sport Medicine*, 9(4): 221–227.
9. Jeffreys, I. 2016. Warm up and flexibility training. In *Essentials of Strength Training and Conditioning*, 4th ed., Haff, G.G., Triplett, Triplett, N.T. eds., Kindle location 8518–8533 of 18512. Kindle Edition, Human Kinetics.
10. Herbert, R. Gabriel, M. 2002. Effects of stretching before and after exercising on muscle soreness and risk of injury: Systematic review. *British Medical Journal*, 325: 468–472. https://doi.org/10.1136/bmj.325.7362.468.
11. Chaitow, L., ed. 2003. The stretching debate. *Journal of Bodywork and Movement Therapies*, 7(2): 80–96.
12. Frederick, A., Frederick, C. 2020. *Fascial Stretch Therapy*, 2nd ed. Edinburgh: Handspring Publishing Ltd.
13. Page, P. 2012. Current concepts in muscle stretching for exercise and rehabilitation. *International Journal of Sports Physical Therapy*, 7(1): 109–119.
14. Opplert, J., Babault, N. 2018. Acute effects of dynamic stretching on muscle flexibility and performance: An analysis of the current literature. *Sports Medicine*, 48(2): 299–325.

15. Behm, D.G., Blazevich, A.J., Kay, A.D., McHugh, M. 2016. Acute effects of muscle stretching on physical performance, range of motion, and injury incidence in healthy active individuals: A systematic review. *Applied Physiology, Nutrition, and Metabolism*, 41(1): 1–11. https://doi.org/10.1139/apnm-2015-0235.
16. Mitchell, J. 2019. *Yoga Biomechanics Stretching Redefined*. London: Handspring Publishing Ltd.
17. Ajimsha, M.S., Al-Mudahka, N.R., Al-Madzhar, J.A. 2015. Effectiveness of myofascial release: Systematic review of randomized controlled trials. *Journal of Bodywork & Movement Therapies*, 19: 102–112.

11 The Fascial System in Walking

James Earls

CONTENTS

INTRODUCTION

This chapter will give a brief introduction to the roles of fascial tissues during repeated rhythmical movements experienced during gait. The chapter will pay particular focus to the issues surrounding older people, but the implications equally apply to the rest of the population. Reduced mobility causes issues around independence and the ability to complete activities of daily living. Decreased mobility can lead individuals toward social isolation which further challenges physical strength and self-esteem.

Issues that have been highlighted for people over 65 years of age include decreased stride length and decreased speed alongside the threat that one limitation opens the "disablement pathway"—a negative spiral of increasingly reduced mobility and strength accelerated by sarcopenia.[1] A global prescription of "getting out and walking more" is often prescribed and has been known to delay sarcopenia and give a sense of well-being, but is it always the correct advice?

Reduced mobility and its links with decreased walking speed and stability has implications for road safety[2] and may also lead to secondary soft tissues dysfunctions if appropriate gait mechanics cannot be achieved.

This chapter blends findings from literature on walking issues for the elderly with myofascial mechanics to search for novel interventions that may alleviate some of the issues through treatment and prevention. By switching onto the positive spiral through aerobic exercise of walking, the patient can benefit from "improved cognitive performance, memory and mood…thought to be a result of increased hippocampal neurogenesis".[3] However, making correct interventions to support efficiency of gait can be enhanced by appreciating interdependent relationships between joints, their ranges, and related tissue dynamics. Below, the practitioner will gain insight into issues that may affect older people but also appreciate aspects of gait that apply to all ages.

A PROBLEM WITH GAIT?

The many benefits of walking have been known for centuries. The peripatetic philosophers of Ancient Greece and the twentieth century showed walking assists contemplation, following the steps of Thoreau and numerous civil rights marches around the world walking can be an act of resistance, and it can be a progress toward health with practitioners of all levels and styles recommending it for patients.

Walking has been shown to improve neurogenesis, slow down sarcopenia, and assist with social integration (for a review, see O'Mara, 2019)[4] and much of its value comes from being accessible and free to everyone. Little more than time and space are needed to walk and there may even be benefit from not even using shoes while walking, which makes it exceedingly affordable.[5] However, it should be noted that a full foot health screen to rule out any form of neuropathy should be performed before any patient is advised to walk barefoot outside.

One tool that has influenced our perception and involvement with walking has been the increased use of pedometers, which are now contained in the workings of watches and phones and generally encourage us toward a 10,000 steps per day goal. Although some papers challenge the value of the worldwide recommendation of 10,000 steps per day as an arbitrary number, there are many benefits to getting up and getting out and including approximately 30 min per day to aerobic exercise.[6]

However, is this prescription suitable for the elderly? One of the advantages of walking as an exercise is the almost universal capability to walk, but studies have shown older people to be slower than ideal for road safety and to have a high rate of walking impairments—85% of men and 93% of women could not walk 2 m at a speed that was considered safe to cross roads.[2] Although the study was performed only in England, the results matched those of studies performed in the United States, Ireland, South Africa, and Spain, which all showed lower walking speeds for older people than the accepted 1.2 m/s for pedestrian crossings.

Gait is a complex action requiring healthy cooperation between numerous body parts from the obvious musculoskeletal tissues to the more discrete vestibulo-ocular system. As such, gait cannot be condensed into a few pages, but we will touch on a number of principles that assist the practitioner to see beyond simple prescriptions for any patient, and this chapter should act as a call for more attention to the aging process and the roles of fascial tissues.

GAIT MECHANICS

A common approach to understanding the mechanics of gait was based on the so-called inverted-pendulum model but recent work has improved on the accuracy of the model by including the spring-like action of the collagenous tissues.[7] The inverted-pendulum model assumes efficiency of human gait is achieved by our relatively straight-legged style that allows the skeletal system to absorb much of the force at heel strike and during single leg support, while the forward swing of the rear leg is assisted by gravity. The inverted-pendulum model ignores collagenous tissues that can be recruited for movement efficiency.

Over the last few decades numerous researchers have found the locomotor system incorporates elastic soft tissue elements that recycle energy through the use of momentum and elastic tissues.[7] Recruitment of the elastic elements within our locomotor system provides an efficiency that is enhanced by the joint ranges available during the human gait pattern. It has been found that our long stride, not only facilitates the use of gravity to swing the rear leg forward again but it also recruits numerous elastic mechanisms that temporarily capture kinetic energy of momentum and recycle it back into the system.

Movement efficiency is optimized by the interactions between muscle and the deep fascia that holds it in place. Research has shown in-series and in-parallel collagenous tissues interact with the muscle tissue during repeated rhythmical movement to reduce eccentric and concentric and concentric muscle.[8] For example, the in-series tendons of the plantar flexor group use the body's momentum as it "vaults" over the foot to bring the foot out of pronation (the windlass effect) while the tendons simultaneously lengthen and the muscle fibers remain isometrically contracted.[8] Using ultrasound, Fukunaga's group demonstrated the Achilles' tendon performs a stretch-shortening cycle (SSC) during gait. During SSC-type movements, the muscle fibers remain close to isometric while the elastic tissues (in-series and in-parallel) are strained by the associated kinetic energy. The energy contained within the strained tissues is then released to feed kinetic energy into the return movement and reduce the active contraction of muscle fiber.

If the Achilles tendon and its associated muscles use SSC mechanics, it is safe to assume that other plantar flexor tendons will do the same to reduce the metabolic expense of concentric or eccentric contractions. Allowing the elastic tissue to strain rather than lengthening the muscle fibers optimizes the force–length relationship of the muscle fibers, which further produces more efficiency within the soft tissue system.[9] However, the use of SSC requires adequate movement at each joint to allow momentum to strain the elastic tissues. Joint range of motion aids stiffening of the soft tissues acting to decelerate momentum and, if inadequate range of motion is available, other tissues will have to compensate. In the example of the windlass mechanism described above, if reduced ankle motion or toe extension is present, the foot will lose some aspects of the windlass mechanism, inhibiting the foot's return to a rigid lever and place extra stress on the plantar and calf tissues. However, the implications of decreased foot stiffness might not be limited to the foot and leg.

Joint and tissue interrelationships were confirmed through computer modeling by Dean and Kuo[10] that showed biarticular coupling between the hips and knees improved economy, speed, and stability of gait. The body's position at toe-off during a long stride requires simultaneous toe, knee, hip, and spinal extension. Loss of extension in any one of these joints will influence the extension and/or the alignment of the others. A simple experiment of walking with a restriction in any one of the named joints (toe, ankle, knee, hip or spine) will reaffirm the important interrelationships through the body—we must be able to couple each of those joint extensions simultaneously to maximize the efficiencies provided by the fascial system.

In doing the walking experiment above, one often feels the extra workload placed on the musculature around the hip and low back. Decreased range of motion creates a need for more active concentric positive work, the work performed during acceleration. The hip flexors tension during hip extension as the limb progresses into late stance toward toe-off, thereby providing deceleration and control of the movement while also loading elastic strain into the anterior hip region. Although the hip does not have the same collection of long tendons available to the foot and ankle, 40% of the net negative work (i.e., work involved in deceleration) during extension is performed by passive elastic tissues (single and two-joint muscles, joint capsule, ligament, and skin)[11] and they provide approximately 50% of the net positive work during the hip flexor power burst for toe-off.[12]

Achieving the idealized toe-off position (commonly achieved at 60% of gait cycle) requires the interplay between a number of joint ranges and tissue tensioning. Immediately prior to toe-off, the toes, knee, hip, and lumbar spine are all extended. The increased range at each joint allows the range of collagen-based tissues to strain and they are all ready to release the energy contained within the strained tissues at toe-off in a catapult-type mechanism.

Catapult and trigger mechanisms are common movement strategies for ballistic feeders and high-jumpers, like the flea, but each of these has an obvious locking mechanism that allows the build-up of muscle tension to lengthen the elastic springs.[13] Ballistic feeders and athletic jumpers of the animal kingdom release tissue locks to unleash the energy, and it appears we use a similar mechanism as we roll over our toes to achieve the same end.

Rather than using an internal tissue lock, human gait uses the friction between foot and ground to allow the capture of energy through momentum as the body passes over the foot and ankle complex into the extended toe-off position. A portion of the energy provided by body's momentum is then used for the SSC to provide efficiency, speed, and stability for the forward swing of the leg when the trigger is released at toe-off.

Issues that may affect the efficiency, timing, or aim of the trigger and catapult mechanism of toe-off should be investigated in patients presenting with low back and hip soft tissue dysfunction and with walking impairments of almost any nature. Range of motion of the great toe joint should be functionally assessed to ensure it can contribute during gait with differential tests to check for hallux rigidus and limitus. As in most cases, conservative treatment should be attempted first to alleviate hallux limitus. Knee, hip, and low back issues may be relieved through the use of rocker type shoes in cases of hallux rigidus.

MUSCLE FORCE AND TIMING

Even though the collagenous elastic tissues lengthen as they capture energy, the muscle fibers directly associated with any tendon can be contracting eccentrically, concentrically, or isometrically depending on the associated forces and the stiffness inherent within the tendon.[7] For example, if the tendon is more compliant and momentum is high, the muscle may need to shorten to control the movement, and, conversely, if the tendon is stiff, the muscle will need to lengthen to allow an appropriate range of movement to occur. Efficient loading of calf musculature requires enough range of the ankle and toe joints during a stride. But, as pointed out above, being able to take a long enough stride to facilitate tissue strain also requires adequate range of the same-side knee, hip, and lumbar spine.[12]

Not only do the fasciae provide elastic recoil during SSC movements, but they also assist muscle force output during contraction. Rubenson et al.[14] investigated muscle–tendon mechanics and found fascicle length optimizes for force production during walking and running to within a narrow range on the ascending limb of its force–length curve. Rubenson and colleagues concluded that the regulation of muscle strain is probably regulated by tendon stretch. Just as joint ranges are interdependent during gait, so too is the interaction between muscle and fascial tissue length; therefore, if we lose some tendon strain due to reduced range of motion, we are less able to modulate muscle effort.

Sawicki and colleagues[15] drew similar conclusions when showing elastic tissue strain and fascicle length attune to one another in a complex system that optimizes force production. The tissue strain and fiber length relationship are significant because force output is reduced when muscle fibers contract from shortened or lengthened positions. Contractions initiated from a mid-range of muscle fiber length allow myosin and actin fibrils to optimally align for force production. So maintaining both elastic and contractile tissue length within certain limits—neither too long nor too short—will minimize metabolic cost while optimizing force output.

Elastic loading also optimizes muscle force–velocity by allowing a slower contraction of the muscle when the load is released.[13] The initial momentum of the movement is produced by elastic energy released from the fascial tissues, and the muscle then contracts at a speed that maximizes its force–velocity relationship.

To summarize the tissue strain dynamics outlined, fascial strain contributes directly to the movement in a number of ways:

1. It reduces the negative work required of muscle tissue experiencing momentum.
2. Elastic strain optimizes the force–length relationship.
3. Fascial tissues use the stress provided by momentum to strain the tissue which it can then release to assist the return movement.
4. Because the release of elastic energy is faster than the muscle contraction, fascial tissues assist with the force–velocity relationship.

The cyclical nature of walking provides the human movement system with a range of energy efficiencies. The efficiency of the long striding human gait results from a mosaic of factors that include overall better alignment with gravity and a series of joints that facilitate extension to assist the simultaneous loading and release of kinetic energy in a range of elastic tissues which, in turn, also optimizes muscle force output.

SOFT TISSUE DYSFUNCTION

The late Leon Chaitow often summarized the causes of soft tissue dysfunction as being due to "overuse, misuse, disuse and abuse"[16] but we have yet to fully understand the complexities involved in the correct "use" of soft tissues. For example, as alluded to above, we need to explore the implications of restricted toe extension on hip flexors and many other similar interdependent relationships that play out in the moving body whereby the loss of one range affects the potential efficiency of another area.

Maintenance of mobility and strength is obviously important for those approaching their later years to ward off the descent down the "disablement pathway". By acknowledging the interrelationships between joints and the force and speed benefits of the fascial tissue, perhaps we can create novel strategies to maintain mobility of the foot/ankle complex and the hip joint in particular.

Limited hip extension was found to be associated with reduced speed and increased falls for older walkers.[17] Joint coupling was also explored by Lewis and Ferris[18] who investigated the effect of giving the extension instruction to actively "push-off" at toe-off. Their results found that during the more active push-off condition, subjects achieved fewer degrees of hip extension.

The attentive reader may have noticed that I have deliberately referred to "toe-off" in this chapter in preference to the more common "push-off" for numerous reasons. One, is the potentially negative affect of the commonly prescribed movement cue, but the other is that the image "push-off" creates. "Pushing-off" implies an active concentric contraction on the part of the plantar flexors and, although it is something we can choose to do when required to walk uphill or more quickly, it is not the body's natural tendency. When walking on a neutral incline at a regular and preferred speed, the body prefers the efficiency of the stretch-shortening mechanics, which allow the muscle fibers to remain isometric.

Lewis and Ferris' work had the intention to find alternative strategies to reduce the workload on the hip flexors, but it also shows that there may be wider implications of any instruction we give to patients. By influencing workload in one area or joint, we may be increasing or decreasing it in another. Altering the natural workload of soft tissues will invoke one of the four causes of soft tissue dysfunction according to Chaitow and to appropriately load and challenge each soft tissue group, we need to be aware of the coupling relationships. The degree to which efficiency is affected is variable and may correlate with age, tissue health, and degree or style of movement compensation—but there will be some form of compensation somewhere.

The full body tensioning we see at toe-off position has developed through anatomical changes made during our evolutionary adaptations. The skeletal changes have allowed movement at one joint to couple into another through cooperative alignment. For example, toe extension, ankle dorsi- and plantar flexion, knee, hip, and lumbar extension all occur on the parasagittal plane. This is not the case with our primate cousins with their abducted great toes. The alignment of human joint angles allows numerous joints to simultaneously extend in response to momentum. The tissues associated with each joint are thereby strained prior to toe-off and can contribute to the forward swing of the leg.

Developing a wider view of tissue and joint interactions is essential when considering soft tissue dysfunctions as described above, the foot, hip and spine are all interdependent for their appropriate loading. Joint interrelationships are particularly important during retraining of healthy movement patterns, especially when using any forms of environmental intervention such as orthoses or changes in footwear—the practitioner must consider the cumulative effect(s) farther along the chain.

CONCLUSION

To minimize the chances of soft tissue dysfunction there are a number of guidelines that could be investigated:

1. Long steps are required to transfer kinetic energy into the elastic tissues, the stride tensions the tendon and assists the force output of the muscles. However, there are many factors that could shorten the stride. It can be as simple as inability to heel strike on the forward leg, but the overall length of stride is more likely to be affected by the joints of the extended limb. Reduced ankle dorsiflexion, or extension of the toes, knee, hip, or lumbars on the side of the trailing limb the stride will also shorten and reduce SSC benefits.
2. If there is hip dysfunction, the practitioner should investigate ankle mobility and toe extension range. Consider conservative interventions first if either is affected. They can include manual therapy, stretching programs, adaptations to footwear, and the use of expertly prescribed orthotics. Toe extension is related to functional hip extension during gait; if joint mobility cannot be restored, rocker type shoes could be considered. A balance must be struck between the mobility of the ankle, the front of the hip and lumbar spine, and the strength of each associated tissue needed to control those events. Ideally, each should be harmoniously aligned with adequate range of motion.
3. Maintenance of mobility for older patients should include investigations of stride length to enhance stability and speed of gait.
4. Of course, a full mobility and strength screen should be included as part of any holistic health plan to ensure any advice on increasing activity levels is appropriate and safe.

REFERENCES

1. Bean, J., Kiely, D., Herman, S., Leveille, S., Mizer, K., Frontera, W. and Fielding, R. (2002). The relationship between leg power and physical performance in mobility-limited older people. *Journal of the American Geriatrics Society*, 50(3), pp. 461–467.
2. Asher, L., Aresu, M., Falaschetti, E. and Mindell, J. (2012). Most older pedestrians are unable to cross the road in time: A cross-sectional study. *Age and Ageing*, 41(5), pp. 690–694.
3. Vonderwalde, I. and Kovacs-Litman, A. (2018). Aerobic exercise promotes hippocampal neurogenesis through skeletal myofiber-derived vascular endothelial growth factor. *The Journal of Physiology*, 596(5), pp. 761–763.
4. O'Mara, S. (2019). *In Praise of Walking*. 1st ed. London: Bodley Head.
5. Holowka, N., Wallace, I. and Lieberman, D. (2018). Foot strength and stiffness are related to footwear use in a comparison of minimally- vs. conventionally-shod populations. *Scientific Reports*, 8(1), pp. 1–12.

6. Tudor-Locke, C., Hatano, Y., Pangrazi, R. and Kang, M. (2008). Revisiting "How many steps are enough?" *Medicine & Science in Sports & Exercise*, 40(Supplement), pp. S537–S543.

7. Roberts, T. and Azizi, E. (2011). Flexible mechanisms: The diverse roles of biological springs in vertebrate movement. *Journal of Experimental Biology*, 214(3), pp. 353–361.

8. Fukunaga, T., Kawakami, Y., Kubo, K. and Kanehisa, H. (2002). Muscle and tendon interaction during human movements. *Exercise and Sport Sciences Reviews*, 30(3), pp. 106–110.

9. Biewener, A. (2016). Locomotion as an emergent property of muscle contractile dynamics. *The Journal of Experimental Biology*, 219(2), pp. 285–294.

10. Dean, J. and Kuo, A. (2008). Elastic coupling of limb joints enables faster bipedal walking. *Journal of The Royal Society Interface*, 6(35), pp. 561–573.

11. Silder, A., Whittington, B., Heiderscheit, B. and Thelen, D. (2007). Identification of passive elastic joint moment-angle relationships in the lower extremity. *Journal of Biomechanics*, 40(12), pp. 2628–2635.

12. Whittington, B., Silder, A., Heiderscheit, B. and Thelen, D. (2008). The contribution of passive-elastic mechanisms to lower extremity joint kinetics during human walking. *Gait & Posture*, 27(4), pp. 628–634.

13. Vogel, S. (2013). *Comparative Biomechanics*. Princeton, NJ: Princeton University Press.

14. Rubenson, J., Pires, N., Loi, H., Pinniger, G. and Shannon, D. (2012). On the ascent: The soleus operating length is conserved to the ascending limb of the force-length curve across gait mechanics in humans. *Journal of Experimental Biology*, 215(20), pp. 3539–3551.

15. Sawicki, G., Lewis, C. and Ferris, D. (2009). It pays to have a spring in your step. *Exercise and Sport Sciences Reviews*, 37(3), pp. 130–138.

16. Chaitow, L. (2011). Adaptation perspectives and low back pain. *Massage Today*, 11(11).

17. Kerrigan, D., Lee, L., Collins, J., Riley, P. and Lipsitz, L. (2001). Reduced hip extension during walking: Healthy elderly and fallers versus young adults. *Archives of Physical Medicine and Rehabilitation*, 82(1), pp. 26–30.

18. Lewis, C. and Ferris, D. (2008). Walking with increased ankle pushoff decreases hip muscle moments. *Journal of Biomechanics*, 41(10), pp. 2082–2089.

12 Visual Assessment of Postural Antecedents to Nonspecific Low Back Pain

Thomas W. Myers

CONTENTS

INTRODUCTION

Myofascial force transmission extends beyond the usual proximal and distal muscle attachments via the parietal myofasciae.[1–3] A map of "myofascial meridians" is proposed to trace common patterns of postural compensation via myofascial force transmission.[4] Contributions from these fascial kinetic chains to nonspecific low-back pain (NSLBP) are tracked to the lumbopelvic junction on five of these myofascial chains. Three common postural patterns—anterior pelvic shift, pelvic tilt, and posterior rib cage shift—are delineated, and visual assessment protocols are presented. Generalized strategies toward more functional balance in gait, stance, and functional movement are outlined.

MYOFASCIAL FORCE TRANSMISSION

The connective tissue matrix is the mechanical environment in which all our 70 trillion cells work and live.[5–7] Although the word "fascia" has been used to describe this ubiquitous milieu,[8,9] it is not entirely correct, as our biomechanical, auto-regulatory system has now been conclusively shown to extend below the dissectible level to link the fascia via transmembranous proteins to the cytoskeleton[10–14] (Figure 12.1). Even though *in vivo* the fascia is intimately connected to the periarticular connective tissues such as ligaments and periostea, as well as the visceral fasciae and meninges, here we limit ourselves to the myofascial connections.

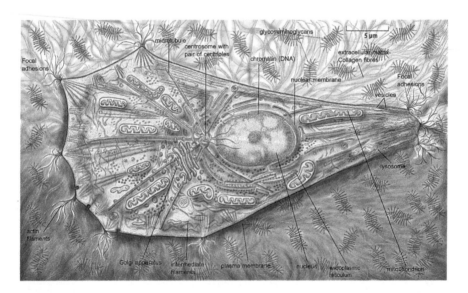

FIGURE 12.1 Our "biomechanical auto-regulatory system" extends beyond the musculoskeletal system into the environment around every cell. The nucleus, cytoskeleton, and membrane of each cell is so intimately connected and responsive to mechanical changes in the local environment (glycocalyx and other hydrophilic proteins) that the traditional view of cells as rounded, freely floating, and water balloons floating is obsolete.

BEYOND ORIGIN AND INSERTION

Given all the interconnections, can we find evidence for myofascial force transmission beyond the usually imposed limits of a muscle's origin and insertion?

Anyone who has done even casual stretching has experienced that a deep stretch is not confined to a single muscle but spreads out into an entire area or along a line to other parts of the body. In research, however, this phenomenon has been largely ignored. Perhaps that is because we are so intellectually married to classical anatomy and "isolated muscle theory"[15–18] Most of our analysis of muscle function involves asking, "What would this muscle do if it were the only muscle on the body?" For example, if we remove all the muscles except the biceps brachii, what would it do (Fig. 12.2a)? By such a process, we would conclude that the biceps is a radio-ulnar supinator, an ulnohumeral flexor, and a stabilizer of the glenohumeral joint. But have we thoroughly analyzed the biceps' function?

No muscle ever works alone in the body, so we have not considered the movements the biceps could assist working in conjunction with synergists. More salient—our single-muscle analysis ignored relevant attachments beyond the origin and insertion.

- Muscles have clinically significant attachments to neighboring muscles via intermuscular areolar tissue.[19] In the biceps' case, this would include brachialis and coracobrachialis in the same fascial compartment. The biceps can also distributes strain, via the intermuscular septa on either side of the humerus, to the triceps.
- Muscles also attach to the ligaments beneath them, providing reinforcement to ligaments when they tense. In the biceps' case, this would include both the capsular cuff around the shoulder and the flexor ligaments of the elbow. Very few of the body's ligaments are not reinforced by muscles, the cruciate and odontoid ligaments being notable exceptions.[20]
- Muscles are supplied by neurovascular bundles, in which the vessels and nerves are wrapped in fascial tunics called adventitia in this case, the brachial plexus, which need sufficient glide not to be impinged by local muscle contraction, especially when under heavy joint load. Trauma, inflammation, or overuse issues can engender adhesions, which limit the movement of that nerve causing "pins and needles" as circulation is restricted in nearby vessels.[21]

Looked at in this way, muscles contract not only from origin to insertion but metaphorically can also be seen as "fish" contracting within the larger fascial "net". They will pull or push on all local tissues that accommodate the contraction in normal movement but have unwanted effects if there is not accommodation.[22] This is very relevant to visually assessing possible biomechanical factors in NSLBP:

- Muscles also have effects up and down the body from one "myofascial unit", or muscle, to the next.[2,23] The biceps brachii is part of a myofascial continuity that stretches from ribs three to five to the lateral aspect of the thumb. The biceps operate within this myofascial continuity to connect our aim with our grip (Figure 12.2b).

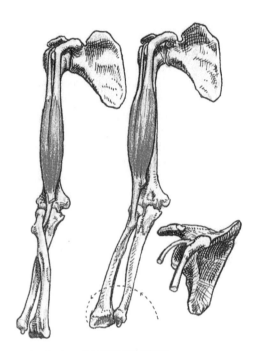

Anterior views of the right Biceps showing its
function in helping supination of forearm with
(a) the elbow slightly flexed

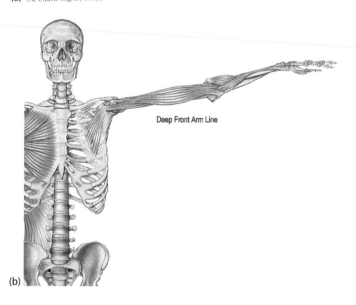

Deep Front Arm Line

(b)

FIGURE 12.2 The biceps are often considered in isolation (a), however the biceps are also part of a myofascial continuity that stretches from the axial ribs to the distal thumb (b & c). ([a] Taken from human structure and shape by John Hull Grundy, used with permission; [b] Courtesy of Elsevier.)   (*Continued*)

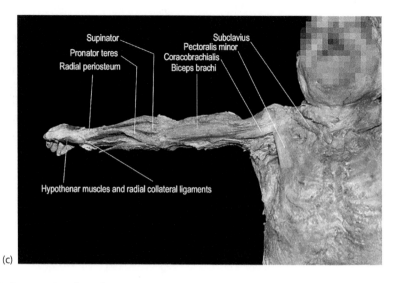

FIGURE 12.2 (Continued)   The Deep Front Arm Line continuity *in situ* (c). (Courtesy of the author.)

Though research into the clinical relevance of longitudinal myofascial force transmission is new, early indications are positive.[3,4] Most of the study has been on immediate transmission, for example, when one performs the common straight-leg lift test, where does the strain go? Not just into the hamstrings as is commonly supposed, but studies clearly demonstrate force transmission beyond the origin and insertion.[24,25] Other early studies point to the existence of sustained force transmission that can pull through the various planes of fascia. This can pull the skeleton into less than efficient patterns of use.[2]

MUSCLE ATTACHMENTS RECONSIDERED

To review muscle attachments in terms of the fascial net, the common misconception that "muscles attach to bones" is so ubiquitous as to be stuck in the minds of medical and clinical professionals. A more accurate statement would be as follows: a tendon arises from the periosteum or ligamentous capsule, spreads and opens its weave to accommodate the muscle cells in the middle, and binds tightly again into a tendon; this tendon blends with the periosteum around the insertional bone—this is an unbroken continuity, with no separation among the individually named units. Although certain muscles, the psoas major, for instance, do have fibers that continue beyond the periosteum to anchor into the collagen matrix of the bone itself, these tendons are subject to avulsion fractures when suddenly overloaded.[26] However, despite our common assumption, most tendons do not attach to bones but rather blend with the surrounding layer of periostea only.

A careful dissection of this common form of attachment shows that the fascial structures within are layered. Although the deeper layers are more attached to the periosteum, the more superficial layers of tendons and epimysium communicate directly with the next myofascial unit (muscle) along the same path. For a common example, the hamstring group is commonly shown as attaching to the posterior aspect of the ischial tuberosity. The deeper part of the tendon certainly does blend with the periosteum of the ischium, but the majority of fibers pass directly into the sacrotuberous ligament (Figure 12.3). Thus, within the sacrotuberous ligament, the more superficial fibers can be seen both to provide a medial attachment for the

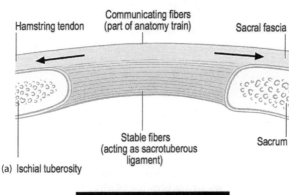

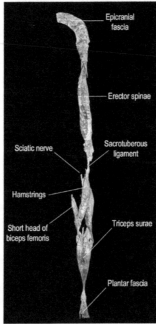

FIGURE 12.3 (a) The deep fibers of a ligamentous or periosteal muscle attachment includes fibers communicating bone-to-bone, as well as more superficial fibers communicating from myofascial unit to myofascial unit, as can be seen in (b) a myofascial continuity from top to toe, the Superficial Back Line. [a] Courtesy of Elsevier, [b] Courtesy of the author.

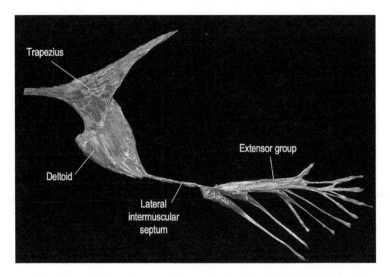

FIGURE 12.4   The superficial back arm line dissected intact in untreated tissue. The fabric connection holds together independent of the bones, from the proximal trapezius to the backs of the fingers.

gluteus maximus and to cross over the edge of the sacrum onto the inferior portion of the sacral and thoracolumbar fascia. The more superficial fibers of this fascial complex communicate strain over time from the hamstrings to the erector spinae and vice versa.

As Figure 12.4 shows, there is a dissectible, continuous myofascial layer that "touches in" and blends in its deeper aspect to the periosteal/ligamentous layer, but with the more superficial layers communicating beyond these attachments. If sustained muscle contraction can have effects beyond the confines of their listed attachments, this pull must be sustained by strong collagen fibers aligned with the line of pull. Fascia has a grain, like wood, and repetitive patterns of myofascial force transmission occur mainly along these pathways. Sudden forces that occur oblique to these pathways can cause injury.

Not all myofascial force distribution pathways are created equal. Fortunately, there are maps of these pathways, so we can make clinically relevant choices about where to intervene.

THE ANATOMY TRAINS MAP OF MYOFASCIAL MERIDIANS

Preliminary as these maps may be, we have been able to dissect all of the following chains of myofascia, most of them in both fixed and untreated cadavers. The method consists of turning the scalpel 90°, thereby using the blunt edge to separate each layer of myofascia from the overlying or underlying musculature, and then running the scalpel between the continuous myofascial layer and the deeper continuous periosteal/ligamentous layer that surrounds the bones themselves (Fig. 12.4).

Crucially, the fiber direction must align so that a continuous pull can be demonstrated. Connections from the hamstrings to the sacrotuberous ligament to the erector spinae is allowed given that all these have continuous fibers that run in a straight line and can thus transfer force. A connection from the hamstrings to the quadratus lumborum would not be allowed because that would involve a radical shift of layers. Similarly, connecting the hamstrings with the quadratus femoris is also out, despite their apposition, because it involves a radical change of direction. When one considers the potential longitudinal fascial slings that traverse the body, with these rules, we can identify 12 myofascial meridians running longitudinally along the trunk and limbs.

To summarize briefly, as this system is fully explained elsewhere,[4] there are three myofascial continuities that traverse the cardinal planes of the body—ventral, dorsal, and lateral. Four lines traverse the four quadrants of the arm. There are four helical lines that connect contralateral girdles and function in rotation.

Centered within all these is the deep front line (DFL), which encompasses all the structures commonly assigned to the body's "core", as in "core strength" and "core stability".[27,28] A three-dimensional understanding of the role and dysfunction of the DFL is essential to both the immediate and sustained relief from NSLBP.

Let us briefly track the anatomy of the lines from the feet to the low back, culminating in the many connections of the DFL to low back function and stability.

SUPERFICIAL FRONT LINE

The lower superficial front line (SFL; Figure 12.5a) includes the dorsal tendons and muscles of the foot, the retinacula on the front of the ankle, the anterior crural compartment with the tibialis anterior, and long toe extensors. This continuity, plus the fascial fabric on the surface of the tibia blends into the fascia that comprise the bridle for the patella and into the quadriceps complex.

While the vastus intermedius affects the hip through its connection to the iliofemoral ligament, only the rectus femoris crosses the hip to attach to the anterior ilium. Although this position would make the rectus femoris an obvious candidate for maintaining the pelvis in an anterior tilt (hip flexion), the fact that it is a polyarticular muscle makes it a bad candidate to stabilize posture because it would have to simultaneously steady both hip and knee joints to work in this way. Thus, the effect of the lower SFL on NSLBP is indirect.

SUPERFICIAL BACK LINE

The superficial back line (SBL; Figure 12.5b and 12.3b) includes the plantar surface of the foot, the triceps surae, hamstrings, sacrotuberous ligament, the entire erector spinae, and the galea aponeurotica. Although chronic tension in the SBL seems ubiquitous in the modern era, its ability to create posterior pelvic tilt (hip extension) and thus contribute to NSLBP is limited by the same two-joint problem with the hamstrings as we saw in the rectus femoris. Thus, the SBL often plays a supporting role, not a starring one, in low back pain (LBP). This supporting role often travels to the low back—sacral multifidus and the sacroiliac joint specifically—from faulty foot placement or chronic misuse of the suboccipital group.

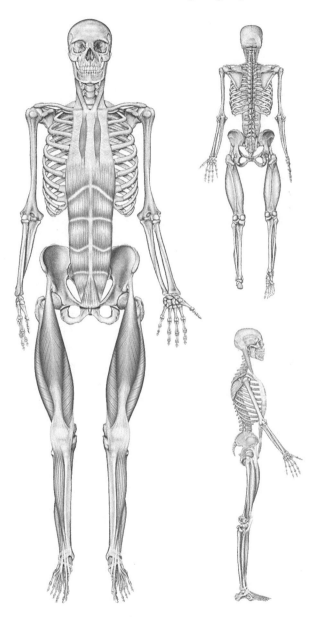

FIGURE 12.5   (a) The superficial front line (SFL).   (*Continued*)

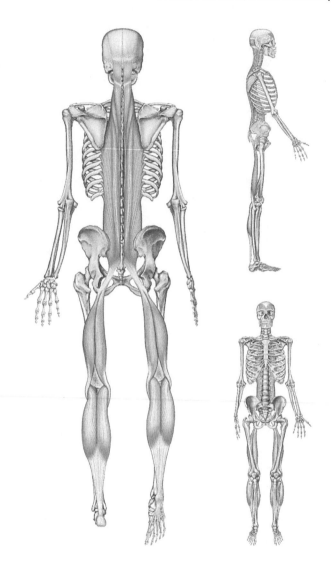

FIGURE 12.5 (Continued)   (b) the superficial back line (SBL).   *(Continued)*

LATERAL LINE

The two lateral lines (LLs; Figure 12.5c) begin with the fibularii muscles supporting the lateral arch, continuing up onto the iliotibial tract and the abducting gluteals, appearing like the letter "Y" when viewed from the side. From the iliac crest to the upper neck, the LLs appear as a series of Xs comprising the lateral abdominal obliques and intercostals, culminating in the X of the sternocleidomastoid and splenius to control head swing in gait. The LLs will always be implicated in one-sided LBP, especially via the extensions of the LL into the quadratus lumborum and

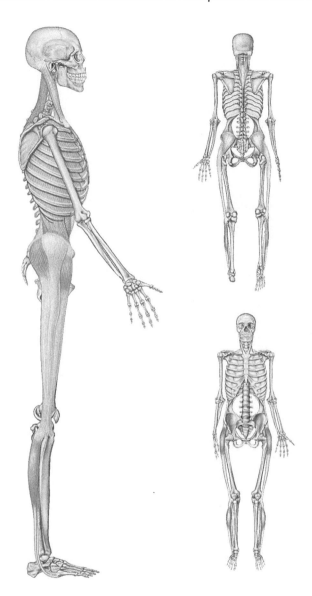

FIGURE 12.5 (Continued)   (c) the lateral line (LL).   (*Continued*)

the iliolumbar ligament, but again plays only a supporting role in NSLBP. True leg length discrepancies can have a role in NSLBP, which will definitely require compensation in both lateral lines.

Spiral Line

The two spiral lines (SLs; Figure 12.5d) wrap the trunk in a double lattice running from the side of the skull across to the contralateral scapula and around the trunk

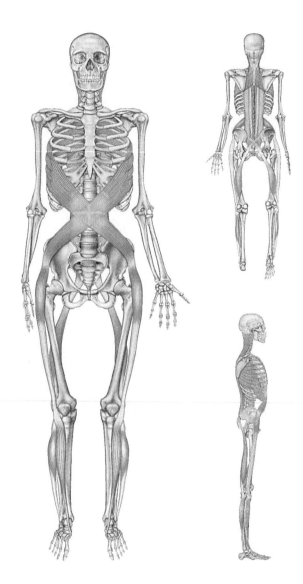

FIGURE 12.5 (Continued)   (d) the spiral line (SL).   (*Continued*)

to the original side's ASIS (Anterior Superior Iliac Spine), acting to stabilize and modulate rotational and oblique planar movements. The lower SL makes a sling, like a jump rope, from anterior ilium to posterior ischium by way of the arches. Given the legs' role in setting the position of the pelvis, the SLs do participate in NSLBP but are more likely to contribute to one-sided pain by pushing a knee to medially rotate or one arch to pronate more than the other.

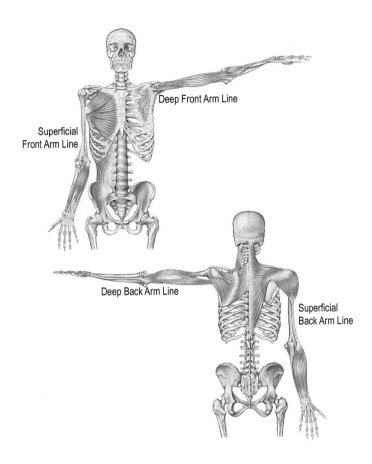

FIGURE 12.5 (Continued)   (e) the four arm lines.   (*Continued*)

ARM LINES

The four arm lines (ALs; Figure 12.5e) traverse the arm from axial skeleton to fingertips, essentially filling in the four quadrants of the arm. The weight of a misaligned shoulder girdle can impinge on breathing (common) which could contribute to LBP (less common).

FUNCTIONAL LINES

The three functional lines (Figure 12.5f) act to extend the arm lines down to the pelvic girdle, and therefore can be complicit in NSLBP, and increase efficiency in throwing, pushing, and stabilizing. The back functional line (BFL) links the humerus to the contralateral femur by way of the latissimus dorsi, superficial layers of the thoracolumbar fascia, and on into the gluteus maximus and its fascial extensions.

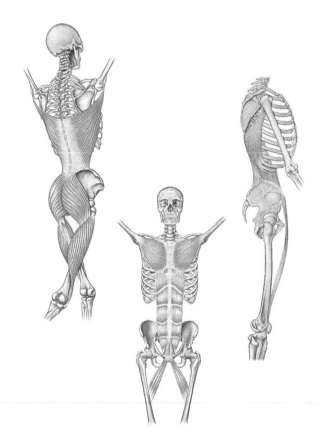

FIGURE 12.5 (Continued) (f) the three functional lines. *(Continued)*

The front functional line (FFL) makes a similar connection across the front via the pectoralis major, linking into the rectus abdominis and accompanying fascia, across the public symphysis to the adductor group, principally the longus, linking it to the femur on the opposite side.

The weaker ipsilateral functional line (IFL) connects the lateral edge of the latissimus to the posterior edge of the external abdominal oblique and on into the sartorius, which attaches in the pes anserinus of the medial knee.

DEEP FRONT LINE

If the previous myofascial continuities play supporting roles postural strain leading to NSLBP, the star of the show is the deep front line (DFL; Figure 12.5g). This "core" line begins deep in the tarsum of the foot with the tibialis posterior and long toe flexors, runs up the back of the leg deep to the soleus, crosses the posterior aspect of the knee, and follows the adductor group to the ischiopubic ramus. Then it fascially connects into the pelvic floor and deep lateral rotator group posteriorly. The DFL also connects

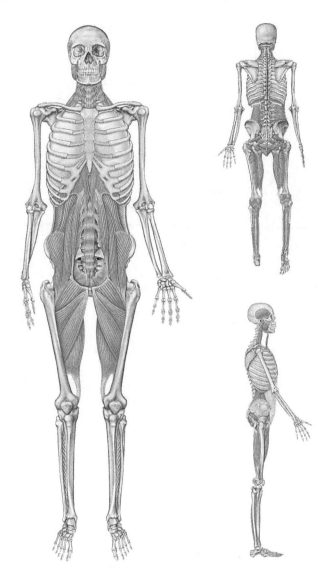

FIGURE 12.5 (Continued)   (g) the deep front line (DFL). (Courtesy of Elsevier.)

strongly anterior to the hip joint into the psoas complex, which contains two one-joint flexors frequently implicated in LBP—the iliacus and pectineus—which unlike the hamstrings or quadriceps are monoarticular to the hip and can thus maintain a postural set without restricting other joints (Figure 12.6).

The DFL continues its path anterior to the spine via the anterior longitudinal ligament and the diaphragm and mediastinum to include the anterior neck and jaw muscles in a complexity of connections that need not concern us here. Suffice it to say that in NSLBP, the DFL is directly involved in all the patterns we will now describe.

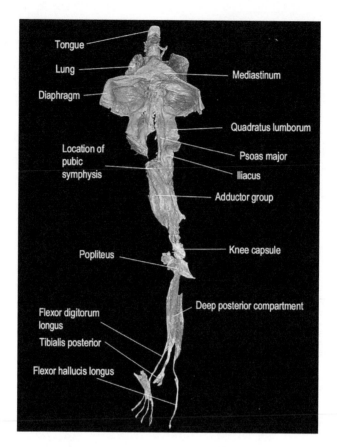

FIGURE 12.6   The deep front line runs from the inner arch to the jaw muscles in an unbroken chain of myofascial structures—many of which tie into the low back.

POSTURAL FACILITATION OF NSLBP

Although posture is not absolutely determinative of NSLBP, there are postural patterns that often accompany LBP. Here we examine three common patterns—anterior pelvic shift, pelvic tilt, and posterior rib cage shift—that outline simple assessments for those patterns and suggest corrective measures.

Heraclitus pointed out that you cannot step in the same river twice, and it is questionable whether we ever resume the exact posture we have taken before. Posture is a moving target. Still, we can recognize a friend from a few blocks away by their individual stance or gait pattern, long before we can see their face. Posture and "acture"—our characteristic way of moving—exhibits our individual, repetitive patterning. This familiar "kinesthetic set" often displays our characteristic posture. Which of these patterns might facilitate NSLBP?

ANTERIOR PELVIC SHIFT

DESCRIPTION

A very common posture in the industrialized world is to carry the pelvis / hip anterior to the ankle/feet (Figure 12.7).

ASSESSMENT

View the patient from the side. Drop a plumb line from the top of the greater trochanter. Does it fall anterior to the ankle? One can argue whether the true gravity plumb for a human should fall right through the center of the tibiotalar joint, or 1 cm in front

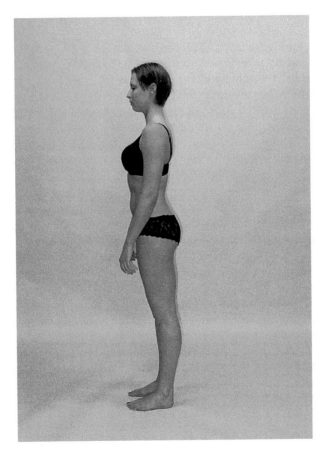

FIGURE 12.7   Although anterior pelvic shift has several variations, the consistent indicator is that the pelvis is characteristically located in front of the ankle. (Courtesy of the author.)

of it, but for many people the gravity line from the trochanter falls well in front of the ankle, in the tarsus or even through the metatarsal bases. The farther this line falls in front of the ankle, the more the pelvis is shifted anterior, and the more likely there is to be accompanying LBP.

Anatomically, the femurs and tibiae will tend to be laterally rotated, and the deep lateral rotators, notably obturator internus, will be concentrically short. The hip flexors, notably the psoas major, are eccentrically loaded, often experienced as "tight" or occasionally painful.

Myofascially, the entire SBL in the back of the leg will be eccentrically loaded and pulled up the surface of the bones. The entire SFL on the front of the leg will be pulled down. The adductor group will be turned toward the front of the thigh and working as hip flexors in gait. This arrangement tightens tissue around the sacrum (piriformis, levator ani, and sacral multifidus) and causes fixation at the sacroiliac and sacrolumbar junctions.

RESOLUTION

In terms of tissue manipulation, the entire front surface of the leg (SFL) requires freeing in an upward direction from the dorsum of the foot through the upper attachment of rectus femoris. The entire posterior myofascia (i.e., the SBL) of the leg requires freeing from the ischial tuberosity to the plantar aponeurosis. Individual deep lateral rotators will need to be identified and relaxed, usually a number of times. The psoas major is often pulled down toward the lesser trochanter and requires treatment.

In terms of movement education, the patient needs to learn the feeling of standing with the pelvis centered over the feet. Often the proprioceptive signals from muscle spindles and fascial mechanoreceptors will seem unfamiliar, and thus the patient will seek the familiar which leads to the same postural pattern and reinforce the feelings obtained (e.g., in the Golgi Tendon Organ reports from the psoas tendon and hip ligaments) when the pelvis is centered over the feet. This will involve a relaxation of the excess tension in the deep muscles under the gluteus (not the gluteus itself) and increased tonus in the psoas major to maintain the new pelvic position over the feet.

Standing behind the patient, put your forearms on their shoulders and press straight down, watching the pelvis. Does it move forward under the pressure? If so, the pelvis is still located too far forward to be mechanically efficient. Have them bring the pelvis more back over the heels, until you can feel that your downward pressure on the shoulders does not put forward pressure on the pelvis. At that point, when your pressure is taken by the skeleton and the ligamentous bed, and the pelvis no longer scoots forward under load, the pelvis is back in neutral and no longer shifted—even if it feels "unnatural" to the patient. With a bit of practice, the neutral position becomes habitual, and the predisposition to compress the lower back recedes.

ANTERIOR/POSTERIOR PELVIC TILT

DESCRIPTION

Although pelvic shift is measured relative to the feet, pelvic tilt refers to the angle at the hip joint between the hip bone proper and the femur—so it is really excessive hip flexion or hip extension in posture that we are looking for here. Because in posture the femurs are more fixed, we refer to this movement as anterior or posterior pelvic tilt. Pelvic "neutral" occurs between anterior and posterior tilt.

Pelvic "neutral" has been described in terms of goniometry, and relationships of bony landmarks. The precise coordinates of pelvic neutral are still controversial.[29] Functionally, it is a range of movement and not a precise angle.[18,30–32] A precise angle of pelvic neutral becomes more important in high level or extreme athletics, but for the common patient, neutral is not a single placement, but a range of a few degrees of arc in the middle. It is the extremes of pelvic tilt—either anterior or posterior—that seem to predispose toward NSLBP.

A strong anterior pelvic tilt (Figure 12.7a) often corresponds with what Czech physician Vladimir Janda identified as "lower crossed syndrome", where the pubic bone is down and the single joint hip flexors are concentrically loaded.[33,34] The low back, including the quadratus lumborum and lumbar erectors, will therefore be short and tight.

A strong posterior pelvic tilt (Figure 12.7b) is often associated with a flat back and an appearance of flattened buttocks. This can result in an unstable sacrum and increased concentric loading in the deep lateral rotators, the hamstrings, and the posterior adductor.

Assessment

Strong tilts can be assessed visually by viewing the patient from the side. An anterior tilt places the pubic bone and ASISs lower and the posterior iliac crest higher, often with a lumbar lordosis attached. A posterior tilt presents as a flat lumbar spine with a reduced sacral angle relative to the floor.

For the competitive athlete, or to determine less obvious tilts, a more precise test is necessary: With the patient standing comfortably on both feet, place your palm gently on the bregma at the top of their head and ask them to go slowly into an anterior pelvic tilt—"Take your pubic bone down to the floor". Notice whether the head retracts downward or "grows" into your hand as they do this. This difference is often only millimeters, so keep a sensitive hand to what happens in those first few degrees of tilt—does the head retract from or rise into your hand?

Now have them return to their normal position and try on a posterior tilt—"Tuck your tail under". Again, pay attention for those first few degrees—does the head retract from or move into your hand? Everyone will retract at the extremes of either movement—eventually either hip flexion or hip extension will pull down on the spine. The ideal position for the pelvis in this test is when the head is at its tallest, which may be a few degrees anterior or posterior to their usual normal.

Note: This test is only pertinent for those who can isolate a pelvic tilt. If the patient is compensating strongly, either in the legs or by extending or flexing the spine, the test results will be useless. In patients with such compensations, other approaches must be employed.

Resolution

Approximately 25 muscles have potential effects on pelvic tilt, so a comprehensive treatment plan is not possible here. In general, those with an anterior tilted pelvis will need myofascial release or area-specific stretching for the hip flexors and the lower

spinal extensors while simultaneously strengthening the abdominal wall and hip extensors. This includes the hamstrings, the adductor magnus, and the deep lateral rotator
group. In addition, those with an anterior tilted pelvis often have a high and tight pelvic
floor, and work with the Valsalva maneuver and generally balancing the tone of the
entire "abdominal balloon" will aid in settling the pelvis back a few more degrees.

In patients with a marked posterior tilt, the opposite strategy applies: Strengthen
the psoas, especially the inferior (L4–L5) slips, while releasing the deep lateral rotators, posterior adductor, and hamstrings as called for. The condition of the pelvic
floor varies widely from high and strongly concentrically contracted to low-toned
and spongey. Individual muscle testing is required to determine the proper corrective
for this area. Functionally those with this pattern often lack recoil, or bounce, if you
will, so work on a trampoline or rebounder can be helpful.

POSTERIOR RIB CAGE SHIFT

DESCRIPTION

The final common pattern comes from above—the tendency to shift the rib cage posteriorly relative to the pelvis (Figure 12.8), which biomechanically places increased
load on the sacrolumbar junction. This pattern also disrupts an essential "core"

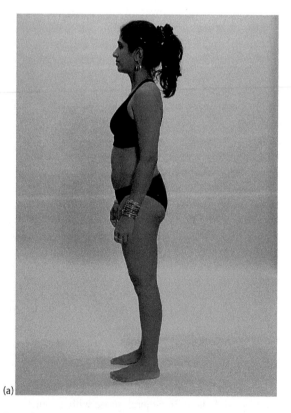

(a)

FIGURE 12.8   A strong (a) anterior or pelvic tilt.   (*Continued*)

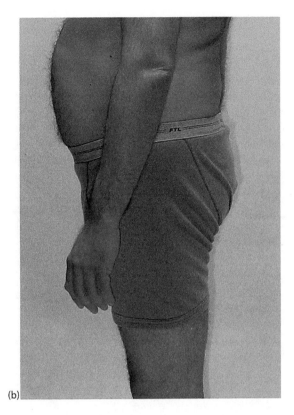

(b)

FIGURE 12.8 (Continued)   A strong (b) posterior tilt of the pelvis relative to the rib cage or femurs is a frequent contributor to nonspecific low-back pain (NSLBP). (Courtesy of the author.)

element—the reciprocity of the respiratory and pelvic diaphragm, thus robbing the client of what is called "core strength".

ASSESSMENT

The center of gravity of the pelvis is close enough to the top of the trochanter for the trochanter to be used as a measure of the center of gravity (COG) of the pelvis. A little practice will allow the assessment of the COG of the rib cage, approximately at the attachment of the serratus anterior on the fifth rib, though allowances must be made for the weight of the breasts, which, if large, affect the effective COG of the rib segment. In addition, letting the rib cage fall behind the pelvis is common to incorrect sitting, where the pelvis falls into posterior tilt and the rib cage falls back into the chair back. Think of your favorite teenager sitting in front of their phone or computer.

As with the other postural faults, the stronger the measurement, the more the predilection toward NSLBP. If it is difficult to tell whether the rib cage is behind the pelvis, then the likely effect is small. If the ribcage is significantly behind the pelvis, no matter what is happening with the head above, the increased load on the L5–S1 junction is often a predisposing factor in NSLBP (Figure 12.9).

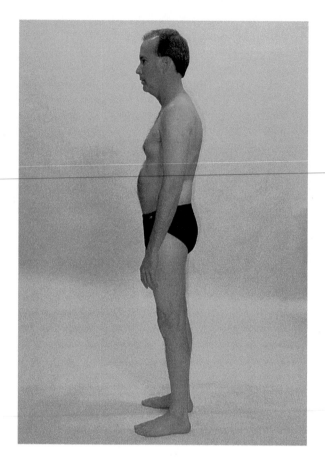

FIGURE 12.9 If rib cage, as a whole, is significantly behind the pelvis, the center of gravity is such that more weight falls on the sacrolumbar junction. This facilitates strain patterns that lead to pain patterns. (Courtesy of the author.)

This pattern routinely locks up the breathing movement of the lower floating ribs and both can inhibit and compress the area around the kidney and adrenal gland. Relieving this pattern will free up the breath in the lower posterior lobe of the lung as well as lifting a load off the sacrolumbar junction.

RESOLUTION

Think of a snowman. The goal here is to line up the balls of the snowman, with the middle ball of the chest directly over the bottom ball of the pelvis, with the head, the third ball, floating above. This involves retraining a number of muscles, and thus, it cannot be accomplished by manual therapy or stretching alone. Manual therapy can be applied to the entire erector spinae and transversospinalis group to lengthen the fascial distance from the posterior iliac crest to the lower margin of the rib cage, as far down as to include the quadratus lumborum.

The abdominal muscles must be strengthened, and the psoas major trained to hold the rib cage forward in its proper position again. Once this is accomplished, your patient will likely not only report a decrease in LBP, but also an increase in available energy as the respiratory diaphragm lines up with the pelvic diaphragm.

CONCLUSION

None of these patterns precludes the others. For example, an anterior shift of the pelvis is often accompanied by a posterior shift of the rib cage, or not. The anterior/posterior pelvic tilt is the obvious exception, as one cannot have both at the same time. Assess each piece individually but examine all the aspects.

Progressive and permanent postural correction is not without difficulties:

1. The lure of the familiar: Comfortable proprioceptive feelings will sometimes conspire to diminish progress. Therefore, specific "homework" to keep patients aware of postural correction between treatments is highly recommended.[35–38]
2. More efficient postures are often not comfortable at first: Stretching long-held tissues and/or requiring lax muscles to work can produce discomfort such as muscle soreness (DOMS) or outright pain at first, so the patient must be encouraged to persevere.
3. Fascia pulls are steady and inexorable: Although muscle stretching and training are both essential, they are often not enough on their own. Fascial sheets and structures such as the thoracolumbar fascia or the iliolumbar ligament are slower to respond, slower to heal, and thus must be reached with highly specific stretching, the hand of a manual therapist, and often both.

Aside from potentially resolving NSLBP, correcting for these patterns can have a salutary effect on health in general, so it is recommended to work with these patterns as both a corrective or a preventive for NSLBP.

REFERENCES

1. Vleeming A. 2007. *Movement, Stability and Lumbopelvic Pain.* 2nd ed. Philadelphia, PA: Elsevier.
2. Wilke J, Krause F, et al. 2016. What is evidence-based about myofascial chains? A systematic review. *Archives of Physical Medicine and Rehabilitation,* 97: 454–461. (also ref 23, 29)
3. Huijing PA. 2002. Intra-, extra-, and intermuscular myofascial force transmission of synergists and antagonists: Effects of muscle length as well as relative position. *International Journal of Mechanics in Medicine and Biology* 2: 1–15.
4. Myers T. 2020. *Anatomy Trains: Myofascial Meridians for Manual Therapists and Movement Professionals.* 4th ed. Edinburgh: Churchill Livingstone.
5. Schleip R, Findley TW, et al., eds. 2012. *Fascia: The Tensional Network of the Human Body.* Edinburgh: Churchill Livingstone.
6. Sandring S, ed. 2014. *Gray's Anatomy,* 41st ed., Edinburgh: Churchill Livingstone.

7. More terminological clarity at: https://fasciacongress.org/congress/fascia-glossary-of-terms.
8. Adstrum S, Hedley G, et al. 2017. Defining the fascial system. *Journal of Bodywork and Movement Therapies* 21(1): 173–177.
9. Langevin HM, Huijing P. 2009. Communicating about fascia: History, pitfalls, and recommendations. *International Journal of Therapeutic Massage and Bodywork* 2(4): 3–8.
10. Horwitz A. 1997. Integrins and health. *Scientific American* 276(5): 68–75.
11. Ingber D. 2006. Mechanical control of tissue morphogenesis during embryological development. *International Journal of Developmental Biology* 50: 255–66.
12. Ostuni E, Kane R. 2000. Patterning mammalian cells using elastomeric membranes. *Langmuir* 16(20): 7811–7819.
13. Moore K, Poite T. 2005. Control of basement membrane remodeling and epithelial branching morphogenesis in embryonic lung by Rho and cytoskeletal tension. *Developmental Dynamics* 232: 268–281.
14. Berry, D. Animations of unseeable biology, filmed May 2011, Sydney Australia. TedX video, 8:52, https://www.ted.com/talks/drew_berry_animations_of_unseeable_biology/transcript?language=en
15. Schuenke M, Schulte E, et al. 2006. *Thieme Atlas of Anatomy*. Stuttgart: Thieme.
16. Netter F. 2019. *Atlas of Human Anatomy*. 7th ed. Philadelphia, PA: Elsevier.
17. Muscolino J. 2002. *The Muscular System Manual*. Hartford, CT: JEM Publications.
18. Kendall F, McCreary E, et al. 2008. *Muscles: Testing and Function*. Baltimore, MD: Lippincott Williams and Wilkins.
19. Huijing PA, Baan GC, et al. 1998. Non-myotendinous force transmission in rat extensor digitorum longus muscle. *Journal of Experimental Biology* 201: 682–691.
20. Van der Waal JC. 2009. The architecture of connective tissue as parameter for proprioception – An often overlooked functional parameter as to proprioception in the locomotor apparatus. *International Journal of Therapeutic Massage & Bodywork* 2(4): 9–23.
21. Shacklock M. 1995. Neurodynamics. *Physiotherapy* 81: 9–16.
22. Schleip R. 2003. Fascial plasticity: A new neurobiological explanation. Part 1. *Journal of Bodywork and Movement Therapies* 7(1): 11–19.
23. Pollak EW. 1980. Surgical anatomy of the thoracic outlet syndrome. *Obstetrics and Gynaecology Surgery* 150: 97–103.
24. Franklyn-Miller A, Falvey E, et al. 2009. The strain patterns of the deep fascia of the lower limb. In: Schleip R & Findley T, eds., *Fascial Research II: Basic Science and Implications for Conventional and Complementary Health Care*. Munich: Elsevier GmbH.
25. Stecco C. 2015. *Functional Atlas of the Human Fascial System*. Edinburgh: Churchill Livingstone.
26. Vannabouathong C, Ayeni OR, et al. 2018. A narrative review on avulsion fractures of the upper and lower limbs. *Clinical Medicine Insights: Arthritis and Musculoskeletal Disorders* 11: 14–17.
27. Aljuraifani R, Stafford RE, et al. 2019. Task-specific differences in respiration-related activation of the deep and superficial pelvic floor muscles. *Journal of Applied Physiology* 126(5): 1343–1351.
28. Weber T, Debuse D, et al. 2017. Trunk muscle activation during movement with a new exercise device for lumbo-pelvic reconditioning. *Physiological Reports* 5(6).
29. Janda V. 1973. Muscles, central nervous motor regulation and back problems. In: Korr IM, ed. *The Neurobiologic Mechanisms in Manipulative Therapy*. Boston, MA: Springer.
30. Rolf I. 1977. *Rolfing*. Rochester, VT: Healing Arts Press.

31. Herrington L. 2011. Assessment of the degree of pelvic tilt within a normal asymptomatic population. *Manual Therapy* 16(6): 646–648.
32. Smith A, O'Sullivan P, et al. 2008. Classification of sagittal thoraco-lumbo-pelvic alignment of the adolescent spine in standing and its relationship to low back pain. *Spine* 33(19): 2101–2107.
33. Janda V. 1983. *Muscle Function Testing*. London: Butterworths.
34. Janda V. 1983. On the concept of postural muscles and posture in man. *Australian Journal of Physiotherapy* 29(3): 83–84.
35. Foster M. 2004. *Somatic Patterning*. Colorado: EMS Press.
36. Chaitow L, Bradley D, et al. 2002. *Multidisciplinary Approaches to Breathing Pattern Disorders*. Edinburgh: Churchill Livingstone.
37. Bond M. 2007. *The New Rules of Posture*. Vermont: Healing Arts Press.
38. Griffin J. 2015. *Client-Centered Exercise Prescription*, 3rd ed. Champaign, IL: Human Kinetics.

Section III

Medical Applications
Interstitial Notes on Section 3

David Lesondak

"SOMETHING IS MOVING"

According to the anecdote, someone asked Albert Einstein what he knew for sure was actually true. Einstein's answer was, "Something is moving".

In the clinical world of medical applications, what is moving would be analogous to the term "release". In this case, a fascial or myofascial release (MFR). While there is still debate over precisely what constitutes this release, physiologically speaking, in this context release is a sufficient term to describe the subjective, felt experiences on the part of both the clinician and the patient. It is the inner sensation of something "letting go", usually resulting in a net gain of greater physical ease, improved range of motion, and so forth. It turns out that there may be more to this release that meets the eye or, in this case, the hand.

An *in vitro* study sought to model repetitive motion strain (RMS) and MFR on an active, living cell culture.[1] The monofilaments, intermediate filaments, and microtubules that comprise the cytoskeleton of a living cell are mechanically active, i.e., they respond to mechanical stress. A vacuum-driven, flexible substrate, petri dish was employed to subject the cells to 8 h of RMS. The results were not pretty. The stressed cells exhibited elongated lamellopodia, decentralization, cytoplasmic condensation, reduced cell-to-cell contact areas, and an alarming 30% increase in apoptosis when compared with non-stressed control samples.

After a 3-h interval, the RMS samples were then subjected to a 60-s interval of MFR—compression, stretch, and shear (shear being a strain produced by pressure wherein the layers are laterally shifted in relation to each other). After this intervention, lamellopodia elongation and cytoplasmic condensation (a precursor to apoptosis) were reduced while intercellular distances and cell-to-cell contact areas were mostly restored. There was also a significant increase in the production of GRO, an important neutrophil in the innate immune system, in the RMS + MFR group.

This was the first, and to my knowledge the only time, that a study modeled MFR in an *in vitro* human fibroblast culture. Furthermore, it points to a deeper understanding of how manual and movement therapies may positively affect the body, right down to the cellular level.

This leads us to the following section—medical, therapeutic, applications. As with the previously highlighted research, many of these applications exist in a climate that has a relative paucity of testing and replications—not to mention robust randomized clinical trials. Our authors underscore this fact. They also point out the logic behind the various approaches and, in some instances, provide some compelling case studies.

In all cases, these modalities are thriving—both as adjuncts to more conventional treatments and as standalone procedures that get consistent results where other efforts have not. The applications covered may be more –well-known than others. Keep in mind what follows is not comprehensive.

As discussed in the preface, whenever anything "new" begins to penetrate the public sphere—especially anything that (among other benefits) purports to relieve pain—there is the inevitable "gold rush" period. During this time, therapies, approaches, and brands seem to proliferate almost overnight.

Use the same best practice principles as you would with any other medical or clinical professional when seeking out qualified individuals who practice any of these therapies.

REFERENCE

1. Meltzer KR, Cao TV, Schad JF et al. (2010) In vitro modeling of repetitive motion injury and myofascial release. J B*odyw Mov Ther.* 14 (2), 162–171.

13 Structural Integration

Michael Polon and Daniel Akins

CONTENTS

Structural integration (SI) is an interactive approach to manual and movement therapy that emphasizes embodiment education. Since SI initially gained popularity in the United States in the 1960s, people around the world have sought out structural integration for help with relieving pain and discomfort, improving posture and movement, and enhancing overall well-being. Structural integrators help their clients experience their bodies with greater ease, comfort, and efficiency. Over a series of (traditionally 10–12) sessions, SI's holistic approach is designed to address body-wide posture, movement, and pain patterns that have become habituated due to injury, stress, trauma, repetitive motion, or personality expression.

Graduates of basic programs recognized by the International Association of Structural Integrators (IASI) are trained in anatomy, physiology, kinesiology, therapeutic relationship, clinical assessment, and manual therapy application. Graduates of IASI-recognized programs are eligible to sit for an exam administered by the Certification Board for Structural Integration. Passing this exam earns the practitioner the right to refer to themselves as a Board Certified Structural Integrator (BCSI).

BACKGROUND

Ida P. Rolf, a biochemist, began developing her work of structural integration in the 1940s and founded her original school about 30 years later in Boulder, Colorado, where it still operates today.[1] There are currently 22 IASI-recognized SI training programs being offered across the United States, Australia, Europe, India, Brazil, and Japan.[2] Graduates of these programs sometimes identify with brand names associated with their respective schools, including Rolfing, Anatomy Trains, and Hellerwork Structural Integration. The term "Rolfing" was originally a nickname given to the work by Rolf's early students, but today the term is exclusively available to graduates of the Dr. Ida Rolf Institute.

Rolf synthesized concepts from the fields of osteopathy, hatha yoga, biomechanics, various posture and movement awareness therapies, the science and philosophy of consciousness, and somatic psychology.[1] She observed that the way a person carried their body was related to a wide range of factors including muscular tone, strength, balance, previous injury history, and learned patterns of movement. Furthermore, she maintained that these patterns could be related to deeply held mind-body relationships with emotionally driven factors like body image, self-concept, and personality expression. Through this awareness, Rolf developed a ten-session process of manual therapy and somatic education that paved the way for many, if not all, of the myofascial/structural bodywork modalities that evolved since her passing in 1979. The art, science, and application of SI have since been developed into a principles-driven approach that still utilizes aspects and variations of Rolf's ten-session series. Although the SI schools each present their own take on that series, the differences between their interpretations are considered relatively marginal.[3]

STRUCTURAL INTEGRATION IN THEORY

Although common use of the term *structure* tends to emphasize the physical structure of the body, modern perspectives favor more holistic definitions that are consistent with current understandings of the body as a complex biological event. Structure, when considered as any "slow pattern of long duration",[4] may include our soft tissues as well as our established neural patterns represented by our habits of posture, movement, language, and ascribed meaning.[5] Structure is both a medium and result of function[6] that might be described as "how the system predictably behaves as a response to specific conditions".[5] This definition is consistent with Rolf's view that "structure is behavior".[7]

Psychiatrist and neuroscience author Dan Siegel defines *integration* as "the linkage of differentiated components of a system, integration is viewed as the core mechanism in the cultivation of well-being... These integrated linkages enable more intricate functions to emerge".[8] Siegel describes an integrated brain as being flexible, adaptive, coherent, energized, and stable.[9] These same integrative qualities could be applied more broadly to include our physical experience. By paying attention to one's present moment, felt sense experience, the perceptive domains of interoception, exteroception, and proprioception may be integrated, resulting in an overall sense of mind-body coherence and well-being.

STRUCTURAL INTEGRATION IN PRACTICE

It is appropriate to consider SI as an *approach* to manual and movement therapy and embodiment education, as opposed to a protocol or set of techniques. A typical SI session begins with client and practitioner consulting about any changes in awareness or physical state since the previous session, and the goals and intentions for the current session. At this point, the client usually dresses down to athletic wear and the session proceeds to a physical assessment of the client, including visual and palpatory assessment of posture and movement as relevant to client concerns. The practitioner proposes a strategy for the session, and with the client's consent, the session proceeds to the therapy table where the manual and movement work will take place.

Practitioners may choose from a variety of hands-on techniques, with pressure ranging from firm to gentle in accordance with client preferences. Many SI sessions also feature movement interventions, which may include passive as well as active client movements like those seen in stretching, yoga, or coordinative movement approaches like the Feldenkrais Method. Another powerful aspect of the SI approach comes through the real-time interaction between practitioner and client. During the session, the structural integrator typically engages the client in dialogue about the client's felt sense, images, and thoughts that accompany receiving touch, performing movements, or standing or lying still. Through exploring the client's subjective experience of the session, the client can integrate and embody the work in ways that are often missed with passive modalities.

By combining these three main interventions of touch, movement, and embodiment exploration, SI addresses deeply held patterns that may show up as postural strain, movement or activity limitations, plateaued injury recovery, and persistent pain. Through a series of sessions designed to systematically address the body's habituated sensorimotor patterns, SI aims to help people with how they stand, sit, breathe, and move. These changes ultimately help clients live with a feeling of freedom in their body while having less pain, recovering lost abilities after accidents or injuries, and feeling more potential for pursuing meaningful activities. SI is commonly sought by high-level to recreational athletes, performance to casual dancers, office or desk workers, manual laborers, musicians and artists, busy parents and their children, as well as aging folks looking to feel younger and more resilient. Structural integration may be pursued as either part of an individual's wellness plan or as a component of rehabilitation and integrative medicine approaches, such as physical therapy, chiropractic, acupuncture, or fitness training.

Although there are often noticeable changes to postural alignment, muscle tone, and range of motion immediately following SI sessions, another aspect of SI's effectiveness arises from the client reorienting to their felt sense. Through touch, movement, and embodiment exploration, the work helps to introduce new possibilities of how one's body feels and functions. The goal of these interventions is to offer novel sensory input to help interrupt patterns of conditioned behavior. This helps facilitate the emergence of new options for movement, posture, and self-regulatory capacity in dealing with physical or psychological pain and stress.[10]

THE THREE MAIN INTERVENTIONS OF SI: PHYSIOLOGICAL MECHANISMS

Since its inception, the theory and practice of SI has had a strong emphasis on the manipulation and remodeling of fascial structures and behaviors. Research developments continue to point to a model where the effects of modalities like SI take place across multiple systems including the nervous, immune, and endocrine systems as well as the fasciae.[11] The changes created by SI sessions are often immediate, indicating a neuroplastic learning component, which is consistent with Rolf's original idea that SI was primarily an educational process.[12] In light of recent scientific findings in the fields of manual therapy, movement, pain, and touch-related affective neuroscience, this chapter will take a biopsychosocial view of how SI affects health outcomes.

TOUCH

In an SI setting, slow, respectful, and specific manual therapy is applied to different anatomical regions based upon client needs and mutually determined goals for the session. Using fingers, knuckles, hands, forearms, and/or elbows, a structural integrator may apply manual stretching of affected tissue layers, temporarily changing the position and forces on the related areas. These temporary positional changes communicate a cascade of information to the client's central nervous system, beginning at the nerve endings which terminate in the outer layers of the body, including skin, superficial fascia, and muscle.[13,14] While the use of manual therapy may create changes in hydration or pliability to the tissue to which it is applied,[15] changes that occur in the nervous system's feedback loops of sensitivity and response cycles are often immediate and profound.[16]

As the nervous system is provided with information from the various receptors in the addressed body tissues, there are a series of responses that may contribute toward a shift in the perception of and behavioral expression in that part of the body. Sensitive nerve endings can become less reactive, muscles can lower their tone, and the central nervous system can decrease its level of excitability, providing a local and generalized feeling of calming down.[17] These combined effects often result in lower pain sensitivity and the client becoming aware of and releasing previously unconscious patterns of tension. In this less reactive somatic climate, new options for posture, range of motion, and embodiment can emerge. These effects usually leave the client feeling taller, lighter, more spacious, balanced, stable, stronger, better coordinated, and with a sense of new possibilities.

MOVEMENT

Movement interventions can also be applied to interrupt patterns of postural, movement, and behavioral fixation. Both passive and active client movement may be standalone features of some sessions or may be done simultaneously with hands-on work. In many cases, the ways in which the various joints move are determined less by limitations of the client's anatomy and more by their habituated patterns of body use.

Guidance and support from the practitioner can help the client feel safe enough to allow their body to be taken gently through joint ranges that are difficult to achieve on their own. As joints are moved safely through new angles and dimensions, the sensory receptors around the joint tissues supply the central nervous system with novel information about what movement is safe and possible, reducing both conscious and unconscious fear-avoidant movement behaviors. With an updated movement blueprint, the body can make significant changes to complex patterns like breathing mechanics, gait, and posture that are often observed by the practitioner and perceived by the client.

Another way movement is utilized throughout SI sessions is in the form of active participation from the client while the practitioner performs hands-on techniques. For example, the client may slowly flex and extend their knee while the practitioner treats the quadriceps group. This combination of externally and internally generated forces affords the client's nervous system the opportunity to integrate their extero- ceptive, proprioceptive, and interoceptive experience. Recruiting active client move- ment concurrently with manual therapy techniques can be especially beneficial in pain-sensitive regions or where a client has become fearful, guarded, or avoidant of movement in general.[18] Beneficial outcomes of active movement performed with manual therapy may also include reduced muscle tone, increased tissue extensibil- ity, an overall sense of bodily calm, and enhanced somatosensory awareness and self-efficacy.[16,19]

EMBODIMENT

There can be clear value in changing posture or movement patterns in the presence of injury, pain, or in performance settings such as fitness or sport. Although SI tradi- tionally has focused on the alignment of the body to postural ideals, it is now under- stood that "normal" movement/posture varies tremendously across individuals.[20–22] Normal movement and posture can encompass a wide diversity due to anatomical variations; adaptations to personal illness, injury, and pain history; influences from repetitive sports or work-related motions; learned familial and cultural gestures; gen- der norms; current mood and long-term emotional tendencies; general personality expression; and any history of impactful events or trauma. Structural integration is less about teaching "proper" posture or movement patterns but more about helping clients embody safer, more capable, and more confident options for approaching the same functional tasks.

Schwartz and Maiberger define embodiment as "the combined experiences of sensations, emotions, and movement impulses in the present moment ... at its most basic level, embodiment is an integration of three sensory feedback systems: extero- ception, interoception, and proprioception".[23] The way individuals experience their emotional and physical reality is driven by interoception, the body's collection of processes that gives rise to how we feel about what is happening in our bodies.[10]

The various body tissues routinely targeted by manual therapy, including SI, have a large density of sensory nerve endings that directly inform the interoceptive parts of the central nervous system. In addition to scanning for data about depth, direc- tion, pressure, and stretch, the interoceptive aspect of the sensory nervous system is especially aware of the emotional quality of what receiving touch from this person, in this body region, in this context is like. The combination of slow, respectful touch, novel movement interventions, and interactive dialogue facilitates change in the body's interoceptive signaling.[13] This can help affect change in autonomic functions like heart rate, respiratory rate, stress-related inflammatory responses, and spinal cord-driven muscle hypertonicity.[16] Other wide-ranging nervous system responses could include changes in motivation, memory, emotion, pain, and self-awareness.

The client's engagement with the caring and thorough manual and movement work of SI can help update the lived experience of one's body in part or in whole, while facilitating global changes in somatic awareness, agency, autonomic self-regulation, and body-mind integration.

SUMMARY

The interactive nature of SI, as delivered over a series of sessions combining the therapeutic use of touch, movement, and embodiment exploration, can be highly effective for achieving various client goals. By addressing the body systematically and tailoring the pace, style, and purpose to the individual, it is an effective modality for people who are seeking help with postural improvement, movement function, recovery from accidents or injuries, or relief from stress, tension, or persistent pain. Sometimes the benefits experienced are immediate, and sometimes they emerge more slowly over time. Clients commonly report positive change in how they feel and move in both their normal activities and in the occupations most meaningful to them, enhancing feelings of self-efficacy and possibility in life. Recent research findings have shown SI to be effective as an adjunct to outpatient rehabilitation for chronic nonspecific low back pain.[24] Given the highly customizable nature of a series of SI sessions and the client's unique medical history, specific results will often vary between individuals.

REFERENCES

1. Eric Jacobson, "Structural Integration: Origins and Development," *The Journal of Alternative and Complementary Medicine* 17, no. 9 (2011): 775–80, https://doi.org/10.1089/acm.2011.0001.
2. International Association of Structural Integrators, "IASI Recognized SI Training Programs," theiasi.net, January 10, 2020, www.theiasi.net/iasi-recognized-si-training-programs.
3. Thomas W. Myers, "Structural Integration: Developments in Ida Rolf's 'Recipe'—Part 2," *Journal of Bodywork and Movement Therapies* 8, no. 3 (2004): 189–98, https://doi.org/10.1016/s1360-8592(03)00103-7.
4. L. Van Bertalanffy, *Problems of Life: An Evaluation of Modern Biological Thought* (Mansfield, CT: Martino Publishing, 1952), 134.
5. Kevin Frank and Ray McCall, "Integration: How Do We Define It? How Do We Assess It? Where Do We Place It in the Ten Series?," *Structural Integration* (2016): 5–10.
6. Daniel Akins, "Integrating the Structure of Structural Integration: A Visual Model for Professional, Conceptual, and Biopsychosocial Coherence," *IASI Yearbook of Structural Integration* 15 (2018): 25–39.
7. Ida P. Rolf, *Rolfing: The Integration of Human Structures* (New York: Harper & Row, 1997), 31.
8. Dan Siegel, "About Interpersonal Neurobiology," drdansiegel.com, 2020, www.drdansiegel.com/about/interpersonal_neurobiology/.
9. Dan Siegel, "Soul & Synapse," drdansiegel.com, April 16, 2015, www.drdansiegel.com/blog/2015/04/16/soul-synapse/.
10. Cynthia J. Price and Carole Hooven, "Interoceptive Awareness Skills for Emotion Regulation: Theory and Approach of Mindful Awareness in Body-Oriented Therapy (MABT)," *Frontiers in Psychology* 9 (2018), https://doi.org/10.3389/fpsyg.2018.00798.

11. Giandomenico D'Alessandro, Francesco Cerritelli, and Pietro Cortelli, "Sensitization and Interoception as Key Neurological Concepts in Osteopathy and Other Manual Medicines," *Frontiers in Neuroscience* 10 (2016), https://doi.org/10.3389/fnins.2016.00100.

12. Rosemary Feitis, *Rolfing and Physical Reality* (Rochester, VT: Healing Arts Press, 1990), 40.

13. Joeri Calsius et al., "Touching the Lived Body in Patients with Medically Unexplained Symptoms. How an Integration of Hands-on Bodywork and Body Awareness in Psychotherapy May Help People with Alexithymia," *Frontiers in Psychology* 7 (2016), https://doi.org/10.3389/fpsyg.2016.00253.

14. Gary Fryer, "Integrating Osteopathic Approaches Based on Biopsychosocial Therapeutic Mechanisms. Part 1: The Mechanisms," *International Journal of Osteopathic Medicine* 25 (2017): 30–41, https://doi.org/10.1016/j.ijosm.2017.05.002.

15. Carla Stecco and Julie Ann Day, "The Fascial Manipulation Technique and Its Biomedical Model: A Guide to the Human Fascial System," *International Journal of Therapeutic Massage & Bodywork: Research, Education, & Practice* 3, no. 1 (2010), https://doi.org/10.3822/ijtmb.v3i1.78.

16. Joel E. Bialosky et al., "Unraveling the Mechanisms of Manual Therapy: Modeling an Approach," *The Journal of Orthopaedic and Sports Physical Therapy* 48, no. 1 (2018): 8–18, https://doi.org/10.2519/jospt.2018.7476.

17. Robert Schleip, "Fascial Plasticity–a New Neurobiological Explanation: Part 1," *Journal of Bodywork and Movement Therapies* 7, no. 1 (2003): 11–19, https://doi.org/10.1016/s1360-8592(02)00067-0.

18. Lennard Voogt et al., "Analgesic Effects of Manual Therapy in Patients with Musculoskeletal Pain: A Systematic Review," *Manual Therapy* 20, no. 2 (2015): 250–56, https://doi.org/10.1016/j.math.2014.09.001.

19. Dan-Mikael Ellingsen et al., "The Neurobiology Shaping Affective Touch: Expectation, Motivation, and Meaning in the Multisensory Context," *Frontiers in Psychology* 6 (2016), https://doi.org/10.3389/fpsyg.2015.01986.

20. François Hug et al., "Individuals Have Unique Muscle Activation Signatures as Revealed during Gait and Pedaling," *Journal of Applied Physiology* 127, no. 4 (2019): 1165–74, https://doi.org/10.1152/japplphysiol.01101.2018.

21. Stephen J. Preece et al., "Variation in Pelvic Morphology May Prevent the Identification of Anterior Pelvic Tilt," *Journal of Manual & Manipulative Therapy* 16, no. 2 (2008): 113–17, https://doi.org/10.1179/106698108790818459.

22. Hendrik Schmidt et al., "How Do We Stand? Variations during Repeated Standing Phases of Asymptomatic Subjects and Low Back Pain Patients," *Journal of Biomechanics* 70 (2018): 67–76, https://doi.org/10.1016/j.jbiomech.2017.06.016.

23. Arielle Schwartz and Barb Maiberger, *EMDR Therapy and Somatic Psychology: Interventions to Enhance Embodiment in Trauma Treatment* (New York: W.W. Norton & Company, 2018).

24. Eric E. Jacobson et al., "Structural Integration as an Adjunct to Outpatient Rehabilitation for Chronic Nonspecific Low Back Pain: A Randomized Pilot Clinical Trial," *Evidence-Based Complementary and Alternative Medicine* 2015 (2015): 1–19, https://doi.org/10.1155/2015/813418.

14 Anatomy Trains Structural Integration

Julie Hammond

CONTENTS

WHAT IS ANATOMY TRAINS STRUCTURAL INTEGRATION?

Anatomy Trains Structural Integration (ATSI) is designed around the Anatomy Trains Myofascial Meridians concept of Thomas Myers. ATSI is a form of therapeutic bodywork that uses fascial techniques and movement education[1] to treat chronic pain, ease physical restrictions, and improve movement dysfunctions. ATSI is patient-centered. Although each session has a clear goal and anatomical territory, each treatment is modified to the individual's specific needs based on a detailed evaluation both in static posture and active function.

Overall ATSI is designed to unwind strain patterns in the body, restoring the body to its natural length and alignment, allowing the individual to move with improved efficiency and ease. To promote adaptable responsive movements, ATSI releases fascial adhesions and restores normal glide between layers of connective tissue.[2] It is also an educational/informative process, giving the patient a better understanding of their body's structure and their perceptions of it.[3]

Posttreatment, patients/clients report feeling taller and lighter, having a decrease in pain, smoother movement, having more physical/mental energy, more expressive in their communications, and overall feeling more "at home" in their body.[4]

SESSION PROTOCOL

ATSI is usually a 12-session protocol, but based on individual need this can also be adapted to a shorter series of treatments. Each session has a specific anatomical territory, based on the Anatomy Trains lines of fascial force transmission. Further specificity is developed from the client's postural evaluation and movement assessments. This includes static assessments in all anatomical planes, relevant movement assessments, and the individual's overall pattern(s). Gait assessment looks at the balance of the myofascial lines and how they act to transfer, or not transfer, force transmissions throughout the body. Gait assessment allows the whole system to be seen in a different context.[5]

SESSION GUIDELINES/PRINCIPLES

- During a treatment visual postural assessment, i.e. "Body Reading", movement assessments, and gait are used to formulate the overall strategy. The general aim is to give support to the body from the ground up and an awareness of the support from that ground. For example, we would not try to horizontalize a tilted pelvis without making sure there is adequate support from the feet and legs, which is necessary to sustain this change.
- Manual therapy is applied to match the individual's needs and tolerances. This is not a "no-pain, no-gain" treatment. It's a refined skill, some would say art, of matching the tissue response with the person's overall response in order to find that fine line of just the right amount of pressure. When there is too much pressure, the person will usually resist or guard against that pressure. This often results in a breakdown of the therapeutic connection with the patient. In ATSI, the goal is to have the person fully engaged during the process even, and especially, during moments where restrictions and adhesions make movement difficult or uncomfortable (but never painful).
- Nonjudgmental language is used to help the individual understand their patterns and restrictions as a way to invite curiosity and acceptance, rather than imply blame or shame and thereby induce avoidance.
- Developing therapeutic trust is vital. This ensures patients feel safe and in control of their treatments. People, in general, are more welcoming to touch and manipulation when in a state of safety.[6]

THE 12 SESSION PROTOCOL

Each treatment is usually of a 60-min or 90-min duration, conducted on a weekly basis. Although, as we will see in the case study that follows, this can also be modified. Treatment consists of anatomically specific fascial and myofascial manual therapy, applied in concert with slow, often stretch-like, movements and micro-movements on the part of the patient. Patients routinely get off the treatment table to better reassess gait, movement, and other physical parameters. This better informs their proprioception, allowing them to feel the specific changes that are happening during the treatment. It also serves to further inform the therapist.

ATSI is a therapy with a distinct beginning, a middle, and an end. The 12 sessions are organized progressively, working from superficial to deep. Although the order can be reorganized to better suit individual needs (e.g., the clinician might decide to first treat the superficial rotations along the spiral line on someone with a scoliosis), they often follow the following order:

SUPERFICIAL SESSIONS

Session 1: Superficial Front Line
The session starts on the dorsal surface of the foot and ends up at the mastoid process with the sternocleidomastoid. This session is about opening the superficial front line and the proximal portions of the front arm lines and serving to give "lift" to the front of the body.

Session 2: Superficial Back Line
The territory of this session is from the plantar surface of the feet to the supra-orbital ridge. This session serves to both balance the lift from the first session and increase the client's proprioceptive awareness of contact with the ground.

Session 3: The Lateral Line
The lateral line myofascia stabilizes the body with every step taken. The territory is up the sides of the body, from the foot to the occiput. Posttreatment individuals often report having more support and stability in gait, and more space to breathe as well.

Session 4: The Spiral Line
The spiral line session looks at easing restrictions in superficial rotations, balancing the scapula in the rhombo/serratus sling and the foot in the sling of tibialis anterior and fibularis longus. Working with the spiral line helps with upper body rotations, shoulder imbalances, and knee and foot arch problems.

CORE SESSIONS

Session 5: Lower Deep Front Line
The goal of this session is to support the pelvis from below by recruiting additional support from the adductor group and the deep posterior compartment of the calf. This includes the front and back of the pelvis and into the pelvic floor.

Session 6: Upper Deep Front Line
The goal of this session is to find a balance between the respiratory and pelvic diaphragm, which often involves normalizations of any remaining pelvic tilts/imbalances. The results improve lumbar support and shoulder girdle support and facilitates deeper breathing.

Session 7: The "Deep Back" Line

This session aims to further align the structural support to the back of the body, calcaneus, ischial tuberosities, sacrum, and mid-dorsal hinge—freeing the pelvis from behind and allowing the sacrum more ease in movement. It also focuses on any paraspinals, deeper spinal bends and/or rotations and also the often-strained deep lateral rotators.

Session 8: Deep Front Line, Head, Neck, and Jaw

This session looks at balancing the head on the shoulder girdle and trunk, working from superficial to deep around the fascial layers of the neck. It includes intra-oral work on the jaw and, often, intranasal procedures.

INTEGRATION SESSIONS

The final four sessions are the *integration sessions*. The integration sessions further integrate and harmonize the deeper core with the more superficial layers. They are an opportunity to improve coordination, and bring better balance to the body. After releasing remaining structural holding patterns, the changes are further supported by reeducating functional movement patterns.[7] The integration sessions, combined with the additional movement assessment/awareness, helps ensure that individuals maintain the changes they have experienced during the previous sessions.

Session 9: Integration of Lower Body

This session focuses on balance and movement in the lower body, looking at the seven lines that run through the pelvis and legs. Gait and pelvic movement are essential pieces to this session.

Session 10: Integration of Upper Body

This session promotes tonal balance and integration in the 11 lines that run through and around the ribcage. The important piece in this session is breath and functional movement of the trunk, establishing a supported core for the shoulders and arms to move freely.

Session 11: Arm Lines

While the origins of the arm lines, as they relate to the trunk, have been treated in previous sessions, here we give the arms and shoulder girdle full attention.

Session 12: Final Integration

The final session looks to promote tonal balance across the entire body. This session is about resolution and completion of the goals, and not taking on any new challenges.

BODYREADING

The BodyReading[8] assessment is initially carried out statically, examining the body in all planes. The postural assessment is not to judge a posture, or impose "perfect posture" on the client; it is a window into better understanding their patterns and how they might be contributing to their symptoms.

ATSI uses four terms to describe the skeletal geometry: *Tilt, Shift, Bend*, and *Rotate*. These terms are used to describe the displacement or distortion in the relationship of one bony portion of the body to another. It is also important when describing the skeletal geometry to clarify with what structure it is being compared. For example, an anterior tilt of the pelvis is often used to describe the pelvis in relation to the ground, but in ATSI we would first compare the tilt of the pelvis to the femur. Then the femur to the knee, the knee to the tibia, and so on. This gives better relational specificity for which structures are under tension and contributing to the pattern.

> **Tilt**—describes a deviation from the vertical or horizontal, describing a body part that is higher on one side than the other. The tilt is named for the top of the structure. If the pelvis is higher on the right than the left, it would be a left tilt of the pelvis as it is named for the direction the top of the structure is going. Anterior and posterior can also be used to describe a tilt.
>
> **Shift**—is the term used for displacement of the center of gravity of one structure of the body in relation to another. This can be right, left, anterior, posterior, superior, or inferior. For example, an anterior shift of the pelvis relative to the feet describes a common pattern of the pelvis being more forward than the feet, but the pelvis could still be neutral in the sagittal plane.
>
> **Bend**—is a series of tilts resulting in a curve and usually applied to the spine. Left, right, anterior or posterior can be used when describing a bend. An excess lordosis in the lumbars would be described as a posterior bend, named again for where the top of the bend is pointing relative to the bottom.
>
> **Rotation**—is named for the direction in which the front of the rotated structure is pointing. It usually occurs around a vertical axis in the horizontal plane, and applies to the femur, tibia, pelvis, spine, head, humerus, or ribcage.

MOVEMENT ASSESSMENTS

Movement assessments look at the body globally in motion. Static posture often serves to raise further questions. Movement helps us to be more specific. For example, a lateral tilt of the midfoot could be a shortened tibialis anterior, it could also be elsewhere along the myofascial continuity that is creating the lateral tilt, or it could be their habitual, unconscious posture. The goal in this case would be to improve the ability of the foot to better adapt to load bearing in gait. By looking at different movements, an assessment can be made to see if the tissue is already adaptable enough to allow this movement or if a myofascial meridian is helping restrict the movement.

CASE STUDY

What follows is a shortened version of an Anatomy Trains Structural Integration case study.

Initial Assessment

Patient profile: The client is a 45-year-old female bodyworker/manual therapist. She developed problems after the birth of her son in October 2014 and was diagnosed with a fourth degree perineal tear and a prolapsed bladder and bowel. Her symptoms included feelings of pain and pressure on her bowel and bladder and an inability to walk very far without feeling like she needed a bowel movement.

After seeking out a number of health care professionals including general practitioners, gynaecologists, four pelvic floor physiotherapists, and a bowel specialist, six months after diagnosis she found a physiotherapist from whom she received positive benefit. In particular, her pelvic floor symptoms improved but still didn't feel "normal". After working all day she had heaviness and pressure on her bowel. Running increased the sensation of pressure on the bowel and a sense of not being able to hold its contents. Restrictions in her breathing created an additional feeling of uncomfortable pressure on her bowel. She felt tension and heaviness in her left leg and left heel pain. This was in contrast to the ease she felt in the right leg and foot. She had three previous whiplash injuries, the first one in 2007 and the last one in 2011. She was also assaulted in 2000, that caused compression and bruising in her neck and often experienced neck pain and tension around the throat.

Her primary goal in seeking treatment was to feel more at ease in her body and to return to exercise without experiencing pelvic discomfort. Long walks, running, walking up hill, and trying to stand up on a surf board all aggravated her symptoms. She wanted to be able to return to running, surfing, and simply being able to chase after her son and play with him. Furthermore, she had travelled from Sydney to Perth (a 5-h flight) with her young son and parents in tow so she could have these treatments. Because of the distance and expense involved, the sessions were carried out on a daily basis, as opposed to the more common protocol of weekly treatments.

I asked the client why she had chosen to fly to Perth to see me. She stated that after attending several of my workshops, she immediately felt positive changes in her body that she typified as a sense of freedom and ease in her movements. She appreciated my anatomical knowledge, specifically my passion for pelvic floor anatomy. Most importantly she trusted me, and felt heard.

Postural Assessment: Anterior View

- Lateral tilt of left forefoot (Figure 14.1).
- Lateral rotation of femur and tibia.
- Left pelvic rotation relative to the feet.
- Ribcage rotated to the left relative to the feet/neutral relative to the pelvis, with a counter-rotation, upper thoracic, to the right.
- Left tilt of the ribcage relative to the pelvis.
- Forward bend of upper thoracic relative to the pelvis.
- Left shift of the head relative to the shoulder girdle.
- Right bend of upper cervical.

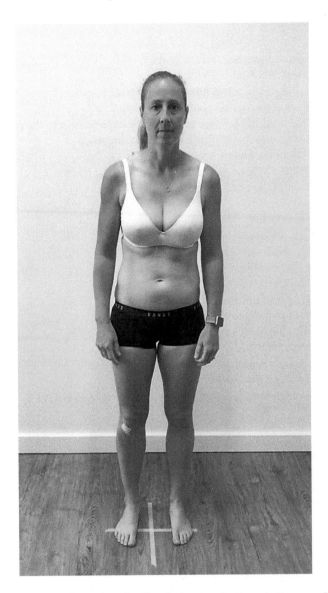

FIGURE 14.1   From the front view, the client is showing shortness in the upper SFL creating compression in the abdominals. This is a major feature of her pattern along with an anterior bend of her upper thoracic and a left tilt of the ribcage relative to the pelvis.

Right View

- Anterior tilt of lower leg relative to the feet (See Figure 14.2).
- Right knee flexed relative to the left.
- Anterior shift of the pelvis relative to the feet.
- Posterior tilt of the pelvis relative to the femur.
- Anterior shift of the shoulder girdle and ribcage relative to the pelvis.
- Forward bend of upper thoracic relative to the pelvis.
- Anterior tilt of the right scapula.
- Anterior shift of the head and neck relative to the ribcage.
- Posterior tilt of the head relative to upper cervical.

Back View

- Medial tilt of left calcaneus (Figure 14.3).
- Posterior tilt of the pelvis relative to the femurs.
- Right knee flexed relative to the left.
- Slight right tilt of pelvis relative to the feet.
- Left spinal bend and left rotation T7–L1.
- Left tilt of the ribcage relative to the pelvis.
- Right upper thoracic rotation.
- Medial rotation/anterior tilt of the left scapula relative to the ribcage.
- Anterior tilt/superior shift of the right scapula.
- Right tilt of upper cervicals relative to the shoulder girdle.

Left View

- Posterior tilt of lower leg relative to the feet (Figure 14.4).
- Anterior tilt of the femur relative to the lower leg.
- Anterior shift/posterior tilt of the pelvis.
- Anterior shift/tilt of the ribcage relative to the pelvis.
- Anterior shift of the shoulder girdle relative to the pelvis.
- Anterior tilt/medial rotation of the scapula.
- Anterior shift of the head and neck relative to the shoulder girdle.
- Posterior tilt of the head relative to upper cervical.

Summary of Initial Assessment

The client was experiencing restriction in her breathing and tightness in her throat. She felt pressure on her bowel/pelvic floor as well as general heaviness and tension in her body. This made the misalignment of her pelvic and respiratory diaphragm and the compression in her abdominals of particular symptomatic interest. She had a posterior tilt of the pelvis with an anterior bend in the thoracic spine. The anterior head position and anterior tilt of the shoulders also created more weight and compression through the pelvis and legs.

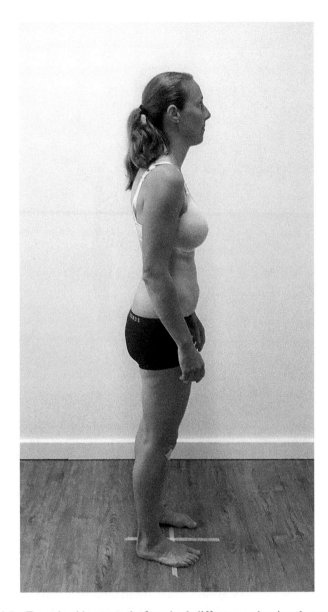

FIGURE 14.2   From the side we see the front-back differences, showing shortness and compression in the abdominals and sternal fascia going up into the front of the neck. We also see how the pelvis is held in a posterior tilt relative to the femur.

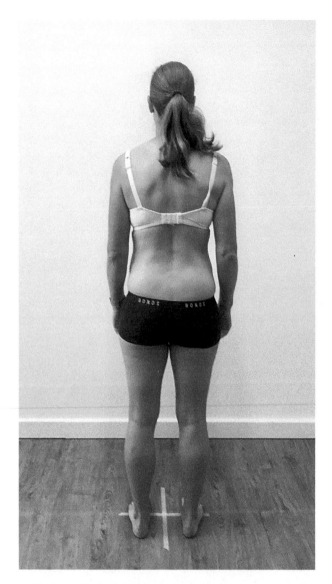

FIGURE 14.3   The back view shows more of the shoulder pattern; the left scapula has a medial rotation with an anterior tilt and the right scapula is held higher in a superior shift and anterior tilt. There is a left spinal bend from T7–L1.

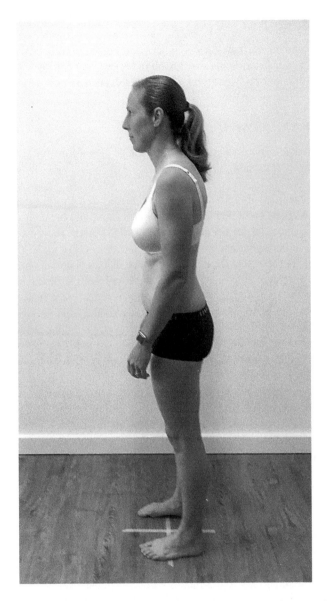

FIGURE 14.4   The left view shows a strong holding pattern on the left knee with the lower leg in a posterior tilt, along with a posterior tilt of the pelvis. If you were to draw a vertical line down the side of the body in front of the ankle, you can see how far anterior her upper body and head is in relation to the feet.

GAIT ASSESSMENT

The client initiated her walk by dropping her chest and head and walked with a short stride. There was a restriction in dorsiflexion in her left foot and she fell heavier onto her left side with upper body compression in the left ribcage.

MOVEMENT ASSESSMENTS

All assessments were performed before Session 1. Not all movement assessments were relevant to each session.

1. Overhead reach with/without arms—this test looked for the gliding ability of the superficial front line and the front arm lines, and the ability to go into extension, correlating if the arms helped or hindered the movement. She was restricted in her upper abdominals in this movement, just under the bra line. The arms contributed to the restriction, due to the medial rotation of the scapula indicating pectoralis major Superficial Front Arm Line (SFAL) and pec minor Deep Front Arm Line (DFAL). The shoulders were held tight to the ribcage and on extension with the arms pec major and latissimus (SFAL) compressed the ribcage, moving it as a block and creating hinging in the thoracics.
2. Side bend—looked at the ability of the spine to side bend as well as the obliques and intercostals to lengthen. There was restriction to side bending to the right.
3. Lunge—checked hip extension, knee extension, and ankle dorsiflexion. Her heel lifted on the left foot. The right knee held in flexion. She was already in hip extension, so this test wasn't relevant for extension but provided information on her global movement. The lunge assessment showed a lack of lengthening in the upper superficial front line, in particular the rectus abdominis. The client was unable to maintain thoracic extension while performing the lunge.
4. Hip drop—looked at the ability for the pelvis to drop/differentiate from the ribcage. The left side was restricted, showing no movement between the pelvis and the ribcage; this usually indicates restriction in the quadratus lumborum/obliques/thoracolumbar fascia.
5. Weight transfer—looked at the reciprocal relationship between the abductors of the stance leg and adductors of the opposite leg in gait. She was restricted during weight transfer to the right.
6. Quarter squat—looked at the ability of the ankle to dorsiflex and how the knees track forward. This can show a restriction in any of the plantar flexors. The client's left heel lifted.
7. Supination/pronation test—looked for adaptability in the foot as it tracked through heel strike and loading response into swing phase. The client was restricted in pronation of the left foot.
8. External/internal obliques—looked for the ability of the obliques to lengthen. When reaching forward on both sides, the distance between the ribcage and pelvis stayed the same with no lengthening of the internal or external obliques.

SESSIONS 1–4: SLEEVE SESSIONS

Summary of the treatment focus and aims: The goal of the first four sessions was to lift the upper body and unwind the superficial rotation, getting the client more upright and positioning the upper body over her pelvis.

- Superficial Front Line—The tissue on the lower right leg was lifted cephalad to bring the lower leg posterior out of its anterior tilt, easing the eccentrically loaded quads on the left leg. Lifted both sides of the abdominal and sternal fascia, more specific on left semilunar line and around the lower ribs for the Schultz[9] band around the chest. Worked into the origins of the front arm lines (pectoralis major/minor) to start to ease shoulder position and allow a deeper breath.
- Superficial Back Line—Eased the heads of the gastrocnemius and short and long heads of the biceps femoris behind the left knee for the hyperextension. The hamstrings were lifted on both sides cephalad for the posterior pelvis tilt. The fascia of the upper superficial back line was taken in a caudal direction to bring the client back over her pelvis.
- Lateral Line—Both sides of the upper lateral line were shortened and compressed. The focus was on lengthening the left for the tilt and left spinal bend. Considerable time was spent on the intercostals and working to improve the client's breathing.
- Spiral Line—Working with the lower sling of tibialis anterior and fibularii longus for the lateral tilt of the left foot. Both upper spiral lines were treated, from the hip across to opposite costal arch on the abdominals because the client had an anterior shift of the ribcage/strong forward bend of upper thoracics.

Results: She responded well to the increased frequency of the treatment. Session 3 became an emotional session, as working to improve her breathing gave her the understanding that by holding her body tense and still she was able to suppress her own emotions. There was more length in her upper body, with the most significant changes happening in the legs, abdomen, and pelvis. After four sessions, her legs looked balanced and pelvis looked even.

Client feedback, subjective: Both legs felt equal with more fluidity to their walk. She felt more open in the chest and that she could take a deeper breath. Her left foot felt balanced with no pain.

SESSIONS 5–8: CORE SESSIONS

Treatment focus and aims: The goal of these sessions was to balance the pelvic and respiratory diaphragms, give more length and lift to the abdominals along with decreasing the forward head position.

- Lower deep front line—lifted adductor magnus cephalad to ease posterior pelvic tilt and relieve tension on the posterior pelvic floor. Obturator internus to soften and relax the pelvic floor holding. Left psoas to pick up the left side of abdominals and ribcage.

- Upper deep front line—the diaphragm and costal arch were a strong focus in this session for breath and lift to the upper body. Pec minor was worked on to ease the anterior tilt of the shoulders.
- Deep back line—balance and encourage sacral ease and movement—treated both piriformii and sacral fascia. Lifted the left side erector spinae muscles for the left spinal bend and seated work on transversospinalis for the left spinal rotation.
- Head, neck, and jaw—sternocleidomastoid, anterior scalenes for the forward head posture. Tension was eased in the infra and super hyoids with gentle pin and stretch movements for the feeling of restriction in the front of the throat.

Client feedback, subjective: The biggest change was that her pelvis felt normal, with no pressure on the bowels. She could feel her gluteus maximus firing and had more hip movement. She felt taller and lifted in her abdominals and felt she could finally take a full breath. She reported she felt like her "old self" again (Figure 14.5).

Sessions 9–12: Integration

Treatment focus and aims: The main areas still under tension were the shoulders, with an anterior tilt/superior shift. The head was held in a right tilt and the thoracic spine in an anterior bend.

- Sessions 9 and 10—worked with retesting assessments. Increased adaptability in the left foot and maintained spinal length and thoracic extension in gait.
- Arm lines—medial rotation of left scapula, and anterior tilt on both scapulas; pec minor, subscapularis, and serratus anterior were all treated.
- Obliquus capitis superior for the right tilt of the occiput relative to C1/C2.

CASE STUDY RESULTS

The patient came into the sessions with pelvic problems that were made worse after either exercise or a long day at work. This was affecting her confidence in all activities. At the end of her 12 sessions, she reported feeling more confident in herself. She felt lighter and taller. There was no pressure on her bowel or pelvis. In her words, her pelvis "felt normal". The initial focus of the sessions had been to ease the pelvic imbalances, but as the treatments progressed, the focus shifted to become more about balancing the respiratory diaphragm and the jaw above to allow a full breath (compare Figures 14.2 and 14.6, and Figures 14.4 and 14.7).

One month after treatment—she reported feeling "great" and sleeping better than she ever had. She also told me her son had his birthday party, and so she had blown up lots of balloons. This was significant because before her treatments she hadn't been able to blow up balloons at all because it placed too much pressure on her bowel. This was obviously no longer the case.

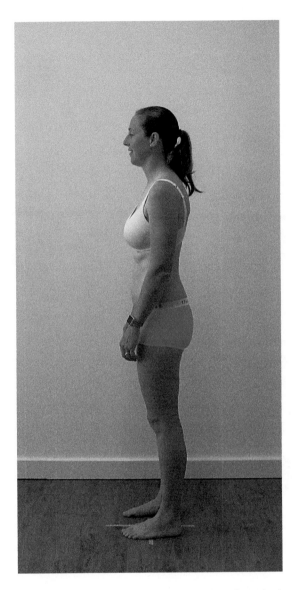

FIGURE 14.5   The diaphragm and costal arch were a strong focus in the core sessions to bring the respiratory diaphragm and pelvic floor in alignment and take away the compression on the abdominals to ease the pelvic floor.

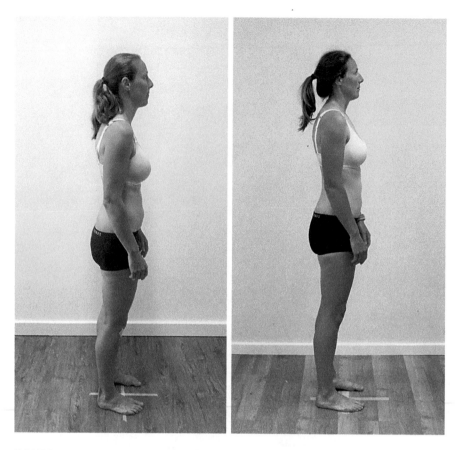

FIGURE 14.6   (Figures 14.2 and 14.6) The two right side images show before session 1 and after session 12. The client has more length in the upper body and is more aligned in the respiratory and pelvic diaphragms.

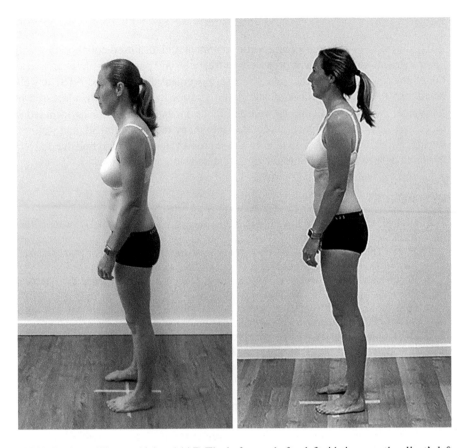

FIGURE 14.7   (Figures 14.4 and 14.7) The before and after left side images; the client's left knee is more at ease and the lower leg isn't locking back. The pelvis is lifted and balanced giving support and lift to the upper body as well as allowing the head to come back into an easier alignment.

IN SUMMARY

ATSI can be both a primary therapeutic treatment and also used collaboration with other medical and movement protocols to treat chronic pain, ease physical restrictions, unwind strain patterns, and improve movement dysfunctions. ATSI is well-positioned to address common postural and strain patterns not fully addressed by traditional western medicine, as well as unique medical conditions as included in this case study. ATSI can be incorporated into many medical, clinical, and wellness settings, working in tandem to deliver a more robust, inclusive, and holistic delivery of health care to address the needs of current and future generations.

REFERENCES

1. Maupin, Edward. *A Dynamic Relation to Gravity*. San Diego, CA: Dawn Eve Press, 2005.
2. Myers, Thomas W. *Anatomy Trains: Myofascial Meridians for Manual and Movement Therapists*. Edinburgh: Churchill Livingstone/Elsevier, 2017.
3. Bond, Mary, and Thomas W. Myers. *Your Body Mandala: Posture as a Path to Presence*. Maitland, FL: MCP Books, 2018.
4. IASI 2020, "The Benefits of Structural Integration." International Association of Structural Integrators, www.theiasi.net/the-benefits-of-structural-integration.
5. Earls, James. *Born to Walk: Myofascial Efficiency and the Body in Movement*. Chichester, UK: Lotus Publishing; Berkeley, CA: North Atlantic Books.
6. Rosenberg, Stanley. *Accessing the Healing Power of the Vagus Nerve: Self-Help Exercises for Anxiety, Depression, Trauma, and Autism*. Berkeley, CA: North Atlantic Books, 2016.
7. Aston, Judith, Ross, Kimberly and Bridgeman, Kimberly Ruess, *Moving beyond Posture: In Your Body on the Earth*. Kindle Edition, 2014.
8. Myers, Thomas W. *Anatomy Trains: Myofascial Meridians for Manual and Movement Therapists*, 249–273. Edinburgh: Churchill Livingstone/Elsevier, 2017.
9. Schultz, R. Louis, and Feitis, Rosemary. *The Endless Web: Fascial Anatomy and Physical Reality*. Berkeley, CA: North Atlantic Books, 2013.

15 Myofascial Trigger Point Therapy
History, Perspectives, and Treatment

Richard Finn

CONTENTS

INTRODUCTION

Myofascial trigger point therapy has developed significantly from the last century up to the present time. This article begins by presenting its initial development in the last century, specifically in the United States. Trigger points (TrPs)—tender contraction knots beneath dysfunctional motor endplates—are further defined and then a number of theoretical objections to their existence are counter-argued. The final section deals with how trigger points can be treated from various perspectives and approaches.

HISTORICAL DEVELOPMENT IN THE UNITED STATES

Myofascial trigger point therapy has a rich multidisciplinary history in America. The earliest written manual of this author as seen was written from a chiropractic perspective in the 1960s.[1] Ray Nimmo was a DC who discovered TrPs independent of knowledge of the work of others and initially called them "Noxious Generative Points". He described them to chiropractors as "peripheral subluxations". The next publication was from national exercise guru Bonnie Prudden, was aimed at the general public.[2] Her genius was melding her exercise program with TrP compression to create the discipline of what was then called myotherapy. Paul St John developed neuromuscular therapy, a massage therapy-style approach, from the work of Nimmo and Dr. Janet Travell. A further development in the massage field was the publication of a two-volume text by Judith DeLany and Leon Chaitow.[3,4] The first *Trigger Point Manual*, authored by Drs. Travell and David Simons, was published in 1983[5] followed by a second volume covering the lower body in 1992.[6] Additional volumes have been published for or by other disciplines including physical therapy,[7,8] massage therapy,[3,4] and acupuncture.[9] There are numerous books written for the public[10–13] and a plethora of self-treatment devices, beginning with the original Backnobber.

The earliest professional group began as the National Association of Myotherapists and now exists as the National Association of Myofascial Trigger Point Therapists. This is specifically a bodywork organization that supports trigger point therapy as a discipline as opposed to a modality. A second multidisciplinary group is the International Myopain Society.

WHAT IS A TRIGGER POINT—CLINICALLY?

> A trigger point is a hyperirritable spot in a taut band of a skeletal muscle that is painful on compression, stretch, overload or contraction of the tissue which usually responds with a referred pain that is perceived distant from the spot.[14]

According to the most recent textbook on the subject,[15] this is the most agreed upon definition of a trigger point. A recent Delphi study[16] would suggest that "referred pain that is perceived distant from the spot" be replaced by "referred sensation". That is an important distinction, as well as a departure from the previous definition.

It is not an etiological definition. It does not describe the pathology. There are frequent claims by TrP skeptics that there is no definition for a TrP. Unfortunately, this is also frequently affirmed by those who research TrPs. The second edition of the *Myofascial Pain and Dysfunction* text includes both a clinical and an etiological definition. The etiology is not currently understood in an exhaustive manner that answers all of the questions on either side of the debate, but we do have a clinical definition. Even the article by Tough et al.[17] admits in the abstract that

> the review identified 19 different diagnostic criteria. The four most commonly applied criteria were: 'tender spot in a taut band' of skeletal muscle, 'patient pain recognition', 'predicted pain referral pattern', and 'local twitch response'. There was no consistent pattern to the choice of specific diagnostic criteria or their combinations. However, one pair of criteria 'tender point in a taut band' and 'predicted or recognized pain referral' were used by over half the studies. The great majority of studies cited publications by Travell and more recently Simons as a principal authoritative source for myofascial pain syndrome (MPS) diagnosis, yet most of these studies failed to apply the diagnostic criteria as described by these authorities.

The studies cited consistently referenced the criteria developed by Travell and Simons and the recent Delphi study, referenced above, substantially agreed with the previous criteria with the exception of using the terminology of sensation instead of pain. We certainly have enough research to admit to having at least a clinical definition as well as studies that show good-to-excellent inter- and intra-rater reliability.[18–23]

In a clinical setting, it is not particularly difficult to identify the essential criteria developed in the Travell/Simons second edition [taut band, tender nodule in the taut band, patient pain recognition, painful limit to full stretch range of motion (ROM)]. That is true also of the criteria in the Delphi Study (taut band, hypersensitive spot, and referred pain/sensation). They overlap significantly. The primary differences being

1. Simons et al. use patient pain recognition, whereas the Delphi study uses sensation that may or may not be painful and
2. Simons et al. have ROM restriction as *essential* criteria, whereas the Delphi study lists it as confirmatory.

The etiological definition from the second edition of the *Trigger Point Manual* by Simons et al. gives several pages to the "integrated trigger point hypothesis". They begin with electrodiagnostic characteristics emphasizing Electromyography (EMG) findings of noise at the site of the motor endplate area and move on to an ultrasound picture demonstrating the shortened sarcomeres called for in the hypotheses. This was followed up by other ultrasound studies.[24–26] Additional input has contributed to an understanding of the biochemical milieu of the trigger point in a series of studies by Jay Shah and colleagues.[27–30]

Fernández-de-las-Peñas opined in a systematic review in 2003[31] that, "the hypothesis that manual therapies have specific efficacy, beyond placebo, in the management of MPS is neither supported nor refuted by research to date". He then went on to contribute to a number of studies that filled that research gap.[32–35]

SKEPTICAL OBJECTIONS TO TRIGGER POINTS AND THEIR TREATMENT

The preceding section gives evidence that an unbiased look at the evidence gives strong reason to think that the trigger point concept is valid. Clinical experience certainly demonstrates its utility. In spite of this, there have been a number of specific objections raised regarding the existence of trigger points, the explanatory model, and the efficacy of treating them. We will look at a few of these arguments.

1. Pain is an output of the brain, therefore, there can be no such thing as myofascial pain. Philosophically, this appears to be a formidable objection. Pain is not pain until the brain says that it is. This is true. It is also true that the brain *receives* that input from the periphery, and its response to that input is often the sensation of pain. Without that peripheral input, there would be no output, thus we can have "myofascial pain".
2. What we call myofascial pain can be explained by Neurogenic Inflammation. This is the point made by John Quintner in 2015 as an alternative to the trigger point construct.[36] Jay Shah said essentially the same thing in 2007 without denying the clinical diagnostic signs of a trigger point: "Subjects with active MTPs in the trapezius muscle have a biochemical milieu of selected inflammatory mediators, neuropeptides, cytokines, and catecholamines

different from subjects with latent or absent MTPs in their trapezius".[37] It seems logical that both conditions could coexist.

3. Occam's Razor—Occam's Razor says that the simplest explanation is most likely the right one. While it's a good principle, it's not the law, as things are often more complex than they appear. The earth is not flat, flies do not come from manure, and so on. Occam's Razor is often used to dismiss data from consideration by claiming it to be irrelevant (Occam was a theologian himself and used it in this way). When applied to trigger points, it assumes that neurology can explain the data in an alternative manner. It dismisses the research done on trigger points because it assumes trigger points do not exist. It is an argument based on deciding that the data of the opponent is not valid because of the opponent's inherent bias, usually confirmation bias. I don't think trigger points exist—therefore the data can't be relevant.

4. The *ad hominem* argument. This is rarely realized itself to be *ad hominem*. It goes like this: The arguments against the existence of trigger points are so intellectually compelling that to disagree with them is to rely upon feelings rather that thought. Those who argue this often refer to and advocate the neuromatrix model of pain, and it's worth noting that the author of that concept specifically mentions TrPs.[38] The flaw here is that they assume that their own emotions are not involved in their position. As fellow humans, they are not immune to having "affections" just like their opponents. Those who "believe" in trigger points actually do so on the basis of much of the previously cited research. They, too, are capable of thought—just as are their critics. This argument often boils down to mere name calling [a less than fancy way of saying *ad hominem*].

5. Palpatory Pareidolia is a recent common argument/explanation given to explain why practitioners "feel" that they have located a trigger point. The idea is that because we are expecting to find them, we do. They are thought to exist, so the mind creates a palpatory experience that validates the belief of the person who is palpating. It's an attempt to explain what is going on in the mind of a person who refuses to accept the argument of the skeptic.

    If we put the best possible interpretation on this argument, it may be an attempt to be charitable. Yet, it is actually another *ad hominem* argument. It is an attack on the individual making the assertion that they can indeed palpate a dysfunction of physiology with their fingers—much like a person who reads braille uses fingers. It also exists in the absence of a single study that would lend support to that specific hypothesis.

6. Muscles lie beneath thick skin and can't be palpated. This is an important objection. The question that needs to be asked is—does the scientific practice of medicine ever involve palpation through skin? Every major medical discipline has a textbook on palpation that is specific to their discipline. We have the practice in probably every emergency room and medical school of "appreciating" the organs through the skin. We have textbooks in manual therapy that discuss how to palpate nerves—through skin.[39] It is important

to acknowledge that palpation of muscles is done through the skin and that the effects of that palpation can have an effect on the nervous system. While true, it in no way demonstrates that it is not possible to palpate muscle and other tissues through the skin. It remains to be demonstrated that palpation through skin is *not* possible.

PERSPECTIVES USED IN TRIGGER POINT THERAPY

It is helpful to think in various terms or "boxes" when creating treatment protocols. I use a number of these. Rather than thinking "outside the box", I prefer to consciously place myself in a particular box or perspective. This lends a particular structure to the treatment. Although it is potentially beneficial to treat a patient according to more than one perspective at a time, for the sake of speeding up and simplifying the learning curve, it is usually better to develop skills in a particular way of thinking before utilizing another. This keeps you, and your patient, from getting lost in a less-than-therapeutic maze.

Once a couple of perspectives have been practiced, it becomes easier to move between them in a particular treatment. This provides both structure and a multidimensional picture to the treatment plan. It acknowledges and looks for a variety of approaches to an issue. Here are a few perspectives to consider.

1. A *neurological approach* considers how the nervous system might be utilized in treating the presenting complaint. A basic neurological exam should be performed with dermatomal sensitivity of particular concern. Dr. Fischer[40] demonstrates this approach. He located the dermatome in which the pain pattern manifested and the affected spinal process was palpated for tenderness. He then injected the interspinous ligament to function as a nerve block. This was followed by treating the particular muscles which contained trigger points.

   A bodyworker using this approach would also determine the affected dermatome. This would be followed by:
   - Evaluating suspected muscles for trigger points via palpation and ROM testing.
   - Treatment of the paraspinal muscles at the affected dermatome level.
   - Reassessment of the ROM of the muscles where TrPs were previously detected for change in muscle length and TrP sensitivity.
   - Treatment of TrPs.

2. A *biomechanical approach* emphasizes an assessment of posture and of the relationship of the tissues crossing the joints. It has the obvious advantage of being easily explained to the patient who is often aware of how they appear, i.e., they *know* what is wrong with their body. It is also possible that the adopted posture is part of a pattern of compensation for issues upstream or downstream from the symptomatic areas. Refocusing how the patient considers their biomechanics greatly enhances the treatment and can certainly boost their self-image. It is easy to utilize an anatomy trains approach in this model.

3. A *functional approach* has been developed by Gabriel Sella and Richard Finn.[41] Sella states, "Agonism-Antagonism-Stabilizer relationships are functional and physiological rather than anatomical". He makes this statement on the basis of his work that included 5,940 S-EMG readings on 138 muscles over ten joints. The emphasis is on treating the muscles based on the relationships found in his data as opposed to "the classic but unclear definition of muscular relationships as given in textbooks without actual proof of such relationships". Treatment is directed toward the muscles doing the first 50% of the work in cases of constant pain unaffected by motion. When motion causes pain, those muscles doing the first 50% of the activity in that particular motion are treated.

4. A *referred pain pattern approach* will identify the muscle containing the trigger point by knowledge of the referred pain patterns of the affected muscles. This may be the most common approach to treatment. Knowledge of the pain patterns can be gained in the pain and muscle guides in each version of the *Trigger Point Manual*.[5,6,15] It is advocated in these manuals that the perpetuating factors must be identified and dealt with in order for this approach to be effective.

5. The *biomechanics of injury approach*, primarily used in a physical therapy setting, has been developed by Kostopoulos and Rizopoulos.[8] If the injury was of traumatic onset, the patient is inquired of to determine how it occurred. What was their position during and after the trauma? The muscles that would have been injured during this sequence are identified and evaluated for trigger points.

6. A *yoga-based approach* is very much appreciated by those who practice it. The patient can demonstrate the issues they have in a particular pose. Areas of tightness can be evaluated for trigger points and treated. There is a reference book for which muscles are shortened and which are lengthened in particular poses[42] that was written by a yoga teacher who is also a physical therapist.

7. A *meridian-based approach* works well with those who appreciate Eastern medicine. In Japanese acupuncture, the meridians are said to be on the surface and can be made to twitch with needle insertion.[9] This may correlate with the local twitch response. Other authors have discussed how "muscle meridians" parallel the Chinese meridians.[43] There is a good deal of overlap with traditional meridians with the anatomy trains system.[44]

METHODS OF TREATMENT

1. *Compression* is a very common treatment technique utilized by massage therapists, myofascial trigger point therapists, physical therapists, and chiropractors. Simple pressure on the trigger point appears to work via Ruffini and Merkel nerve ending receptors in the skin, lengthening of actin and myosin filaments, and Diffuse noxious inhibitory control (DNIC) (brain modulating input from the cord).

2. *Contract/relax techniques* appears to lengthen shortened sarcomeres and physiological response via the Golgi tendon organs.[45]

3. *Spray and Stretch* is a technique in which a vapocoolant is sprayed over the length of the muscle and its referred pain pattern as the patient exhales. This is followed by three to five reps of full ROM and the patient is sent home with a home care stretching program.

4. *Dry needling* is becoming a popular method of treatment by physicians and practitioners of stripes, with many certification programs available. Although it utilizes the same tools as acupuncture, dry needling should not to be conflated with acupuncture. It is employed with different reasoning and intent, with trigger points identified prior to insertion.

5. *02 Derm ™Relief Topical Healing Gel* is an oxygenated gel that appears, in this author's experience, to have an effect on the irritability of the trigger point. It is useful when palpation is difficult and is best applied utilizing the above neurological perspective. It makes a good self-treatment when combined with self-compression and movement/stretching programs.

6. *Frequency-specific microcurrent*[46] (FSM) seems very effective in the treatment of trigger points.[47] Practitioners often find that trigger points resolve after treating the nervous system and other structures such as discs and facets.

7. The *Avazzia* is a hand-held microcurrent device that this author has found to be highly effective in the treatment of trigger points. There are, however, no studies to corroborate this finding. Unlike FSM, which is barely detectable, the Avazzia current is felt due to its use of a higher voltage.

CONCLUSION

Trigger point therapy works well as a specific discipline and as an adjunctive therapy in other disciplines. It can be performed with or without tools. It is best utilized when applied according to a particular perspective. Multiple methods exist that can be used to treat myofascial trigger points.

REFERENCES

1. Nimmo, R.L. 1966. *A Description of Receptor Tonus Technique.* Republished in 2001: Schneider, M., Cohen, J., Laws S. *Pioneers of Chiropractic Trigger Point Therapy: The Collected Writings.* Pittsburgh, PA: Schnieder, Cohen, & Laws.

2. Prudden, B. 1980. *Pain Erasure: The Bonnie Prudden Way.* New York: Ballantine Books.

3. Chaitow, L., and DeLany, J. 2000. *Clinical Applications of Neuromuscular Techniques Vol. 1 The Upper Body.* Edinburgh: Churchill Livingstone.

4. Chaitow, L., and DeLany, J. 2002. *Clinical Applications of Neuromuscular Techniques Vol. 2 The Lower Body.* Edinburgh: Churchill Livingstone.

5. Travell, J., and Simons, D. 1983. *Myofascial Pain and Dysfunction: The Trigger Point Manual—The Upper Extremities.* 1st ed. Baltimore, MD: Williams and Wilkins.

6. Travell, J., and Simons, D. 1992. *Myofascial Pain and Dysfunction: The Trigger Point Manual—The Lower Extremities Vol. 2.* 1st ed. Baltimore, MD: Williams and Wilkins.

7. Dommerholt, J., and Huijbregts, P. 2011. *Myofascial Trigger Points: Pathophysiology and Evidence Informed Diagnosis and Management.* Boston, MA: Jones and Bartlett Publishers.

8. Kostopoulos, D., and Rizopoulos, K. 2001. *Manual of Trigger Point and Myofascial Therapy.* Thorofare, NJ: Slack Incorporated.

9. Seem, M. 1993. *A New American Acupuncture.* Boulder, CO: Blue Poppy Press.

10. Blatman, H., and Ekvall, B. 2002. *The Art of Body Maintenance: Winner's Guide to Pain Relief.* Cincinnati, OH: Danua Press.

11. Starlanyl, D., and Sharkey, J. 2013. *Healing Through Trigger Point Therapy: A Guide to Fibromyalgia, Myofascial Pain and Dysfunction.* Berkley, CA: North Atlantic Books.

12. Davies, C., and Davies, A. 2013. *The Trigger Point Therapy Workbook.* 3rd ed. Oakland, CA: New Harbinger Publications.

13. Sauer, S., and Biancalana, M. 2010. *Trigger Point Therapy for Low Back Pain.* Oakland, CA: New Harbinger Publications.

14. Simons, D.G., Travell, J., and Simons, L. 1999. *Travell & Simon's Myofascial Pain and Dysfunction: The Trigger Point Manual. Vol 1.* 2nd ed. Baltimore, MD: Williams & Wilkins.

15. Donnelly, J., et al. 2018. *Travell, Simons & Simon's Myofascial Pain and Dysfunction: The Trigger Point Manual.* 3rd ed. Philadelphia, PA: Walters Kluwer.

16. Fernandez-de-las-Peñas, C., and Dommerholt, J. 2017. International consensus on diagnostic criteria and clinical considerations of myofascial trigger points: A Delphi study. *Pain Med* 19(1):142–150.

17. Tough, E.A., White, A.R., Richards, S., and Campbell, J. 2007. Variability of criteria used to diagnose myofascial trigger point pain syndrome—Evidence from a review of the literature. *Clin J Pain* 23(3):278–86.

18. Mayoral Del Moral, O., Torres Lacomba, M., Russell, I.J., Sanchez Mendez, O., and Sanchez Sanchez, B. 2018. Validity and reliability of clinical examination in the diagnosis of myofascial pain syndrome and myofascial trigger points in upper quarter muscles. *Pain Med* 19:2039–2050.

19. Zuil-Escobar, J.C., Martinez-Cepa, C.B., Martin-Urrialde, J.A., and Gomez-Conesa, A. 2015. Prevalence of myofascial trigger points and diagnostic criteria of different muscles in function of the medial longitudinal arch. *Arch Phys Med Rehabil* 96:1123–1130.

20. Barbero, M., Bertoli, P., Cescon, C., et al. 2012. Intra-rater reliability of an experienced physiotherapist in locating myofascial trigger points in upper trapezius muscle. *J Manual Manipul Ther* 20:171–177.

21. Bron, C., Franssen, J., Wensing, M., and Oostendorp, R.A. 2007. Interrater reliability of palpation of myofascial trigger points in three shoulder muscles. *J Man Manipul Ther* 15:203–215.

22. De Groef, A., Van Kampen, M., Dieltjens, E., et al. 2018. Identification of myofascial trigger points in breast cancer survivors with upper limb pain: Interrater reliability. *Pain Med* 19:1650–1656.

23. Donnelly, J.M., and Palubinskas, L. 2007. Prevalence and inter-rater reliability of trigger points. *J Musculoskel Pain* 15(Suppl. 13):16.

24. Sikdar, S., Shaw, J.P., Gebreab, T., et al. 2009. Novel applications of ultrasound technology to visualize and characterize myofascial trigger points and surrounding soft tissue. *Arch Phys Med Rehabil* 90(11):1829–1838.

25. Sikdar, S., Ortiz, R., Gebreab, T., et al. 2010. Understanding the vascular environment of myofascial trigger points using ultrasonic imaging and computational modeling. *Conf Proc IEEE Eng Med Biol Soc* 2010:5302–5305.

26. Ballyns, J.J., Shah, J.P., Hammond, J., et al. 2011. Objective sonographic measures for characterizing myofascial trigger points associated with cervical pain. *J Ultrasound Med* 30:1331–1340.

27. Shah, J.P., Phillips, T.M., Danoff, J.V., et al. 2005. An in vivo microanylatical technique for measuring the local biochemical milieu of human skeletal muscle. *J Appl Physiol* 99: 1977–1984.

28. Shah, J.P., Danoff, J.V., Desai, M.J., et al. 2008. Biochemicals associated with pain and inflammation are elevated in sites near to and remote from active myofascial trigger points. *Arch Phys Med Rehabil* 89:16–23.
29. Shah, J.P., and Gilliams, E.A. Uncovering the biochemical milieu of myofascial trigger points using in vivo microdialysis: An application of muscle pain concepts to myofascial pain syndrome. *J Bodyw Mov Ther* 12:371–384.
30. Hsieh, Y.-L., Yang, S.-A., Yang, C.-C., and Chou, L.-W. 2012. Dry needling at myofascial trigger spots of rabbit skeletal muscles modulates the biochemicals associated with pain, inflammation, and hypoxia. *Evid Based Complementary Alternat Med* v.2012; 2012PMC3544533. https://www.ncbi.nlm.nih.gov/pmc/articles/PMC3544533/
31. de las Penas, C.F., Sohrbeck Campo, M., Fernandez Carnero J., et al. 2005. Manual therapies in myofascial trigger point treatment: A systematic review. *J Bodyw Mov Ther* 9(1):27–34.
32. de las Peñas, C. F., del Cerro, L.P., Carneroa, J.F. 2005. Manual treatment of post-whiplash injury. *J Bodyw Mov Ther* 9(2):109–119.
33. Rodríguez Blanco, C., de las Peñas, F., Xumet, J.E. et al. 2006. Changes in active mouth opening following a single treatment of latent myofascial trigger points in the masseter muscle involving post-isometric relaxation or strain/counterstrain. *J Bodyw Mov Ther* 10(3):197–205.
34. Salom-Moreno, J., Ayuso-Casado, B., and Tamaral-Costa, B. 2015. Trigger point dry needling and proprioceptive exercises for the management of chronic ankle instability: A randomized clinical trial. *Evid Based Complement Alternat Med* Volume 2015, Article ID 790209.
35. Emilio, J., Puentedura, E.J., Buckingham, et al. 2017. Immediate changes in resting and contracted thickness of transversus abdominis after dry needling of lumbar multifidus in healthy participants: A randomized controlled crossover trial. *J Manipulative Physiol Ther* 40(8):615–623.
36. Quintner, J.L., Bove, G.M., and Cohen, M.L. 2015. A critical evaluation of the trigger point phenomenon. *Rheumatology* 54:392–399.
37. Shah, J.P. et al. 2008. Biochemicals associated with pain and inflammation are elevated in sites near to and remote from active myofascial trigger points. *APMR* 89(1):16–23.
38. Melzack, R., and Katz, J. 2013. Pain WIREs. *Cogn Sci* 4:1–15.
39. Butler, D. 2000. *The Sensitive Nervous System.* Adelaide, SA: Noigroup Publications.
40. Fischer, A. 2002. Functional diagnosis of musculoskeletal pain and evaluation of treatment results by quantitative an objective techniques, in Rachlin, R. et al. 2002. *Myofascial Pain and fibromyalgia: Trigger Point Management.* St. Louis, MO: Mosby.
41. Sella, G., and Finn, R. 2001. *Myofascial Pain Syndrome: Manual Trigger Point & S-EMG Biofeedback Therapy Methods.* Martins Ferry, OH: Genmed Publishing.
42. Stiles, M. 2000. *Structural Yoga Therapy.* Boston, MA: Weiser Books.
43. Mann, F. 1987. *Textbook of Acupuncture.* London: William Heinemann Medical Books.
44. Myers, T. 2009. *Anatomy Trains: Myofascial Meridians for Manual and Movement Therapists.* 2nd ed. Edinburgh: Churchill Livingstone.
45. Chaitow, L. 2006. *Muscle Energy Techniques.* Edinburgh: Churchill Livingstone.
46. McMakin, C. 2011. *Frequency Specific Microcurrent in Pain Management.* Edinburgh: Churchill Livingstone.
47. McMakin, C. 1998. Microcurrent Treatment in Myofascial Pain of the Head, Neck, and Face. *Topics in Clinical Chiropractic* 5(1):29–35.

16 Fascial Manipulation®

Antonio Stecco

Physiotherapist Luigi Stecco devoted his career to developing and teaching others to develop "knowing hands" in their treatment of pain and dysfunctions. *Manus sapiens, potens est*—A knowledgeable hand is a powerful one. Increased knowledge and practice will enhance your manual therapy skills, and Fascial Manipulation (FM) can be a map to deeper understanding of the fascia. What follows is the overall schema, and some of the development, of the FM approach.

Luigi understood that specific points formed the center of a vector caused by muscular contractions that operated within a particular plane of fascia. This reasoning resulted in what is defined as a myofascial unit (MFU), is a key component in FM. The MFUs are composed of a group of motor units that activate monoarticular and biarticularmuscle fibers that move a body part in a particular direction. For example, antemotion or antepulsion (forward movement in the sagittal direction). The MFU is also composed of nerves (both efferent and afferent as relating to mechanoreceptors), along with skeletal components. All of these elements are connected within the muscle spindles and are responsible for normal movement of the joint. Because the brain is responsible for a motor direction, rather than movement of specific muscles, it must depend upon the MFUs to provide the necessary information to allow our body to function in a unified and coordinated manner. The brain only interprets the movement patterns and changes in the direction. This point is critical for the understanding of motor function. The muscles function by way of MFUs as the body moves in different directions and in various ways.

MFU names are based on anatomical planes of movements and the body's ability to produce and control movements in specific directions. Every segment includes six myofascial units, i.e., two for each of the three planes of movement. Movement of the segment can be identified in three planes and each segment in six directions, forward and backward (sagittal plane), lateral and medial (frontal plane), and internal or external rotation (horizontal plane). Latin names (e.g., coxa/hip, genu/knee) are used for the segments to allow ease of understanding by practitioners worldwide.

By this sort of identifier (motion/location), points are named in every segment of the body, for example, AN-CX would indicate the point controlling the forward (anterior) movement in the hip area. For instance, HU means humerus or shoulder joint area. In FM, AN-HU means forward motion (agonist) and RE-HU means backward motion (antagonist). The same logic applies to lateral motion, LA-HU; medial motion, ME-HU; external rotation, ER-HU; and internal rotation, IR-HU. These pairs are working as agonist–antagonist, and this information is an important part of the treatment protocol with respect to creating balance in the segments. Consequently, for each joint, the abnormal vectors of movements in space for each joint can be recognized based on movement testing and palpation of MFU. Proper treatment and balancing of the involving MFU allows the joint to move in its designated direction.

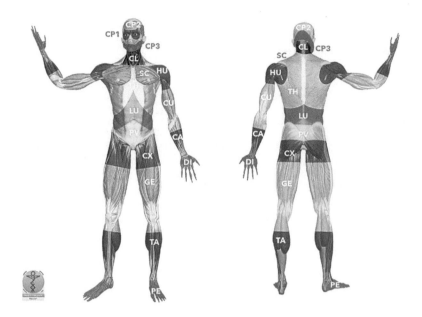

FIGURE 16.1   Fascial manipulation body segments.

Fascial manipulation (FM) divides the body into 14 body segments (Figure 16.1) that represent the functional anatomy of the major joints. Each segment is composed of six MFUs representing the six directions of motion along three anatomical planes. Segments and their MFUs can be thought of by visualizing a cake. Each piece of cake can be imagined as one direction of movement. The foot, ankle, knee, and thigh can be considered as segmental layers of the cake. In the limbs, our cake has six layers per cake, and in the trunk, we have still more layers to the "torso cake". By using terms like antemotion and retromotion it is easier to understand which way our body parts are moving or which part of the cake is missing.

In FM, specific areas within the fascia of the MFU are identified and referred to as Centers of Coordination (CCs). The CC is the site where unidirectional forces or muscular vectors converge. It's located between the deep fascia layers and it coordinates the action of unidirectional mono-articular and biarticular muscle fibers. It is the point where the vector forces act within each MFU. These are the points where FM treatment is performed. The CC points are specified by the six movement directions ante (an), retro (re), lateral (la), medial (me), external rotation (er), internal rotation (ir), and by the segment. For example, RE-CL refers to the point that functions in backward motion of the neck (CL = collum).

In each MFU described in FM, we find two specific areas: The first is on the fascia covering the muscle belly, which can be considered as the active component of the MFU. The second is around the joint. Together, these are the passive components moved by muscle contraction. The first area indicates the CC situated on the deep fascia. According to the fascial manipulation hypothesis, the forces of the muscle fibers converge on such points, as the forces of the horses converge to the coachman.

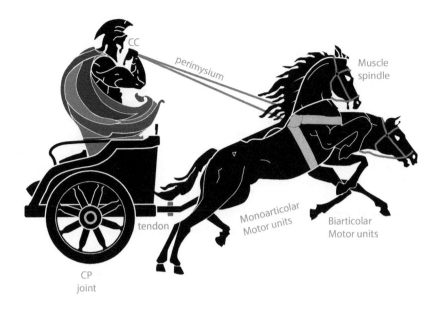

FIGURE 16.2 A myofascial unit (MFU).

The coordination of these tensile forces in the MFU is determined by the continuity of the fascia containing the important proprioceptors like muscle spindle cells. The MFU acts like a roman chariot. If one of the horses is not pulling enough the driver has a difficult time handling the chariot and the direction of the movement will be altered (Figure 16.2).

The CC can be seen as the driver of the chariot and the tensional lines are represented by the horses. If the driver (CC) is not able to handle the horses, the whole chariot will suffer from that situation, and it will lead to dysfunction. Every Chariot (MFU) has their own role and they have to be in line and move in a specific direction. This allows the body to perform coordinated and efficient movement patterns resulting in pain free movement.

When two MFUs perform a movement in one direction between two segments, a *sequence* is formed. The precise organization of the aponeurotic fasciae provides the anatomical substrate for the sequences. The biarticular muscle fibers contained in each MFU connect unidirectional with other MFUs. Also, part of the biarticular fibers found in each MFU insert onto the deep fascia via myotendineous expansions that link one segment (joint) to the next one. This tensioning between MFUs informs other segments, creating what are known as kinetic chains.[1,2] This myofascial continuity synchronizes the single MFUs in order to develop precise and forceful movements. One myofascial sequence (MFS) synchronizes the movement of several segments in a single direction on one plane. The MFSs on the same spatial plane (sagittal, frontal, or horizontal) are reciprocal antagonists. This means that if we find altered areas along the fascia of one MFS, the whole spatial plane related to that MFS can be compromised. Due to the fascia's rich innervation, the sequences also have a role of monitoring upright posture in the three spatial planes.

Direction of movement occurs along vectors within the fascial net. Normally, the fascia may be free to move, depending on the area. In some areas, it is tightly adhered to the underlying or surrounding tissue, and in others, it is attached to bone. The closer you get to the joint, the less movement of the fascial layers. In the joint area, there is more need for proprioception and stabilization. In broad elongated areas where muscles and fascia meet, for example, the upper and lower extremities, more movement is required. These areas are mostly designed for force transmission and movement. Here the layers of fascia can glide like two pieces of silk fabric if the loose connective tissue between these layers is working properly. Proper fascial tension is created by fascial expansions of muscles and direct muscle fiber attachments. All of these characteristics are responsible for creating vectored forces that reach the distal joint.

Dysfunctions and compensations in the myofascial system can alter the vectors inside the fascia and thus generate symptoms. Distal to the CC is found, usually, the center of perception (CP). The CP is the site where movement occurring at the joint is perceived. Due to densification (an increase in viscosity of the loose connective tissue inside the fascia) of the CC, the CP can become painful. This is often because of poor synchronization of the unidirectional forces of the MFU caused by inappropriate or excessive traction to the receptors located in the CP area. Functional, passive, resisted, or active testing of the CP area usually elicits pain. Also, pain from the CC could be referred to the CP area.

Functionally, it is also necessary to account for complex and intermediate movements. In 1996 Luigi Stecco began to explore another set of points he called the centers of fusion (CFs). The CFs are identified as junctions of the forces of three MFUs. For example, a CF such as ante-lateral (AN-LA) would synchronize the two MFUs and their respective CCs, AN, and LA. Associated with the CFs is always a rotational MFU consisting of either external rotation or internal rotation.

CFs are located over retinacula, over periarticular structures (near joint tendons), and in the trunk along the lines of union of some muscles. They synchronize MFU activity by way of Golgi tendon organs and muscle spindles. For example, when we flex our shoulder joint, we are moving in one anatomical sagittal plane. But, as we know, movements do not occur only along a single plane. We do not move our arm only in an anterior or lateral direction. The CF, therefore, is located in the aponeurotic fascia in the crossing of different fascial planes. This guarantees gradualism, modulation, and harmony during the change between two movement directions. Where CCs act more with muscle spindles, CFs can be related more to the Golgi tendon organs.

CFs are formed along lines similar to CCs. The CC lines are called sequences, whereas CF lines are called diagonals. There are four diagonal lines: two anterior (AN-ME and AN-LA) and two posterior (RE-ME and RE-LA). These diagonals are the result of two adjacent CC sequences. Diagonals unite unidirectional CFs. The diagonal line corresponds to movement occurring between CC sequences.

For the regulation of complex motor activities such as walking, spirals, which are the sum of the helicoidal tensions that the CFs create on the fascia, become necessary.[3] Spirals unite CFs in particular formations to account for complex movements such as swimming, running, or any athletic movements involving bilateral use of the body. Spirals synchronize CFs in opposite directions. They are involved in the coordination of complex motor patterns or opposite actions between two or more adjacent segments.

Fascial manipulation (FM) is one of the few methods that evaluate the patient from a global point of view. There are direct connections along fascial planes responsible for "connecting" the whole body. The location of the pain is often not the causation of the pain. The main goal of FM is to balance the body in a way that allows painless function.

The case history of old traumas, or even an injury dating back to childhood, usually becomes relevant during treatment. FM attempts to create homeostasis to allow the body to heal itself. This is a method that combines mental work with the physical sensitivity. In the FM method, every treatment is different, and as such, there are no specific protocols. Everything is based on patient interview and history, movement and palpatory verifications, and solid, clinical reasoning.

After the initial intake interview and movement and palpatory verification, a hypothesis is decided upon to determine which segments and fascial sequences require treatment. Treatment is then performed with fingers, knuckles, or elbows on predetermined points of the sequence. In each treatment, it is imperative that the points treated result in a balancing of the agonists and antagonists of the sequence. The impaired function is them reassessed to evaluate the immediate effects of the treatment and to ensure treating the correct sequence. Specific FM assessment charts (Figure 16.3) are used to collect data and record results. The abbreviations are in Latin so as to allow FM practitioners to communicate with other FM practitioners worldwide, regardless of language.

Every patient is unique unto themselves. Just because they might have similar symptoms does not at all indicate that they require a similar treatment. The FM is a patient-focused method based on particular guidelines that lead to individualized treatment protocols. The initial visit consists of a patient history, use of an assessment chart, and an examination.

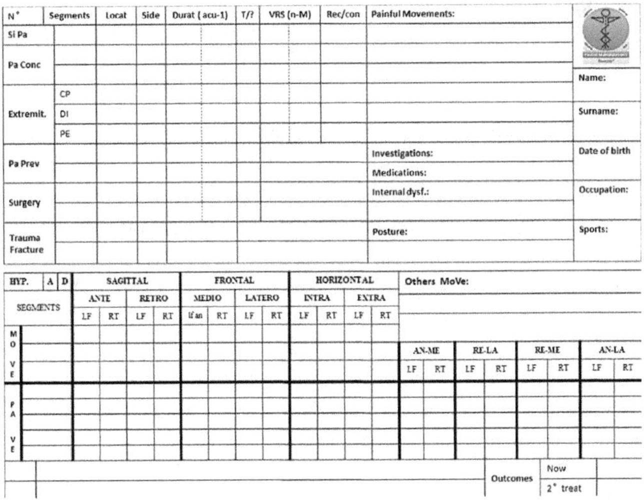

FIGURE 16.3 Sample of a Fascial Manipulation chart.

The history of the present pain should include questions such as: Is this the first time that this pain ever appeared? How long have they had the pain? Does the pain appear on weight bearing or at rest? Are past injuries or operations related to a current complaint? Is there is some sort of traumatic reason for the local pain, or did the pain appear for no apparent reason?

The therapist must determine if the painful site is compensating for a previous problem elsewhere or if it is a local issue. From the history and questions, the therapist forms a hypothesis that will lead to the particular related segments that require examination, always emphasizing the relevant fascial kinetic chain. After forming a hypothesis, movement and palpatory verifications are performed on the chosen segments relating to the patient's complaint.

In Movement Verification (MoVe), every movement in all the planes are tested. It is helpful to ask the patient what movement bothers them the most in order to check on the progress of treatment. Palptory Verification (PaVe) will be the last and most important aspect of an FM examination. Palpation determines which of the ten pathways should be treated. Is it a sequence, diagonal, or spiral or a combination of all three? In cases where the palpation disagrees with a painful movement direction, the palpation determines the line of treatment.

Treatment is guided by the "knowing hands" and the points are chosen with care according to palpatory verification findings. Treatment is performed with fingers, knuckles, or elbows. The FM method is done until the release is felt by both therapist and patient. For most musculoskeletal conditions, six to eight points are treated per session, and the results should be immediately apparent post treatment. Assessment of the progress of a patient is done both during treatment and posttreatment.

In the first session, the most densified and painful plane will be treated. It is not recommended to treat more than one plane per visit because the protocol for the second visit will be determined by the patient's response to the first. How can we know which plane was most responsible until we, and the patient, see the results? In the second treatment session, depending on the results, the same plane might be treated again or, if there is absolutely no change in movement of the pain, another plane might be decided upon. Decisions are always based on improvement in motion and palpation.

At present, Fascial Manipulation is taught in three levels. The first level is for the basic understanding of the anatomy and physiology of fascia, the CC and its sequences. The second level promotes the understanding of the centers of fusions via diagonals and spirals. The third level is intended to solve internal dysfunction by combining CCs and CFs in different settings, and superficial fascia with a specific manuality.

REFERENCES

1. Stecco C, Gagey O, Macchi V, et al. Tendinous muscular insertions onto the deep fascia of the upper limb. First part: Anatomical study. *Morphologie* 2007;91(292):29–37. PubMed PMID: 17574470.
2. Stecco A, Macchi V, Stecco C, et al. Anatomical study of myofascial continuity in the anterior region of the upper limb. *J Bodyw Mov Ther* 2009;13(1):53–62. doi:10.1016/j.jbmt.2007.04.009.
3. Stecco L. (2004) *Fascial Manipulation for Musculoskeletal Pain*. Padova, Italy. Piccin.

17 Fascial Stretch Therapy™

Chris Frederick

CONTENTS

INTRODUCTION

As a very early adopter (1998) of practitioner-assisted stretching (offered as a specific and complete whole-body therapy to patients), the author has observed this specific service category grow over the last 5 years into what is now a veritable industry. It has been reported that the number of stretch boutiques and studios has expanded dramatically, both in the United States and in other countries.[1] The fastest and largest growth has been fueled by the growth of the many different franchises now offering assisted stretching services either alone or as one of several other services that may be bundled with the stretching. Unfortunately, as was told to this author by a student who went through one franchise training, some of those companies provide only minimal instruction on how to stretch a person (a total of 4 h in that one case).

Assisted stretching in the hands of those with little training in the best case scenario may help some people with simple complaints of myofascial tightness. In the worst case scenario, as in when a specific evaluation is not conducted before getting stretched, a person may suffer any number of possible negative scenarios, from musculoskeletal injury to a sciatic flare up to an anxiety attack, all of which may necessitate the client having to go to the emergency room. The point being obvious, assisting a person to stretch is serious "business", requiring in-depth training from a reputable source in order to determine when stretching is contraindicated. When it is indicated, an experienced and highly trained practitioner must determine what specific techniques of stretching is appropriate to be implemented and then how to adjust parameters of intensity, duration, and frequency as dynamic conditions change over time and circumstance.

Rather than merely providing a conglomeration of fascial stretching techniques, Fascial Stretch Therapy (FST) was developed and has evolved for over two decades into a complete system of care. It is complete in that FST incorporates its own evaluations, assessments and corrective patterns peculiar to FST movement vocabulary and individual function. Yet, it is also recognized that integration with other effective therapies is often indicated, as well as when it is time to refer to other practitioners when a condition is not responding to FST or out of scope of the practitioner's training and experience. In the practice of FST, the treatment of the whole person—body, mind and spirit—is also acknowledged and addressed in that process.

Initially developed for dancers, then for collegiate athletes, to optimize recovery and preparation in sports, Ann Frederick (creator of FST), soon discovered its potential in helping people of all ages in eliminating common musculoskeletal and joint pain and concomitantly improving functional movement in as little as one session. She also had a number of successes with improving function and restoring hope in many clients who had reached a plateau in their progress. This included clients who had previously tried conventional and alternative care for varied diagnoses from post traumatic stress disorder (PTSD), neurological (strokes, multiple sclerosis, others), orthopedic, and various other examples of incomplete or unsatisfactory recovery from surgery.

OVERVIEW OF FST

The model upon which FST is based is called tensegrity, or alternatively biotensegrity. Described in detail elsewhere in this book, tensegrity (a neologism of tension-integrity) depends on a state of balanced tensile prestress for its mechanical stability in biological structures and the physiological systems they drive. As Ingber states, "tensional prestress is a critical governor of cell mechanics and function, and how use of tensegrity by cells contributes to mechanotransduction".[2]

Given that the human tensional network has been described by Ingber, research scientists, and other thought leaders in the science and function of fascia as being "prestressed" at rest or at "steady-state" phase in homeokinesis (or homeostasis), the author believes that it is accurate to describe this model also as a "stretch-dependent" network and system. A multitude of research studies starting from nanoscale[3] certainly seem to support this model. Therefore, as cofounder of FST, this author along with founder Ann Frederick base the principles and techniques of FST on the model that a person's structural form can be fundamentally described as being a neuro-myofascial tensional network attuned to any and all forces that then drive most of the physiological processes of life (i.e., via mechanotransduction). This model then underpins an FST evaluation, assessment, and treatment along with movement therapy prescription to return a person back to a premorbid state or to an optimal level of function or performance.

ASSESSMENT AND TREATMENT USING FST

Being primarily an orthopedic and sports medicine physical therapist, the author will use differential diagnosis methods to medically screen and evaluate patients to determine whether a person is appropriate for physical therapy (PT) management. When the patient is accepted for PT, the author will integrate an FST assessment of the neuromyofascial tensional network, which will henceforth be called the "fascial system".[4]

A functional leg length discrepancy (LLD) will be used as an example of using the FST method. After various functional tests in weight bearing as well as in non-weight bearing positions are performed to confirm suspicion of a LLD, the following additional evaluations will be conducted in supine to determine where in the fascial net, the source of the discrepancy is sourced:

- Hip capsule: Longitudinal traction in the resting joint position is performed to determine if the joint capsule is hypomobile.
- Lower lateral net: Tension testing of the lower lateral fascial net (up to about T12–L1) is performed to determine when resistance to passive range of motion (ROM) is first felt as compared with the contralateral side.
- Upper lateral net: Tension testing of the torso above T12–L1, then with addition of overhead arm and lateral head–neck ROM.

From a basic assessment of just the above three movements, one is able to determine the amount of contribution to restriction of movement. For example, restriction of active and passive movement in the lateral net may come 100% from any one of the three regions assessed; it may have an even distribution of about 33% in each region; it may have 50% restriction in one region and 25% restriction in each of the remaining regions. Naturally there are many possible combinations of restriction contributions from each or some of the regions. The point being that this evaluation helps one refine the accuracy of where the focus of treatment can occur, rather than the typical "working" assumption that it is likely one muscle (e.g., the quadratus lumborum) that is the cause of the LLD and any associated symptoms if present.

The following are instructions as to how to perform the above technique in order for the reader to try on clients/patients with a suspected LLD. Full corrective results are often seen in as little as one treatment:

Goal: To assess the hip joint capsule by performing moderate traction until slight elastic give is felt in the tissue. To find their specific "sweet spot" which is the optimal open (or "loose pack") joint position for traction. To decompress joint and create more space if indicated.

Client position: Supine and relaxed with arms at their sides.

Practitioner: Standing at the foot of the table.

Position client's leg approximately 20° flexion and abduction; with a slight external rotation of the femur.

Hold their heel with outside hand and wrap your other hand around the inside of their mid-foot, moving the foot into dorsiflexion. If this hand position does not feel secure to you, or the client's ankle is hypermobile and/or

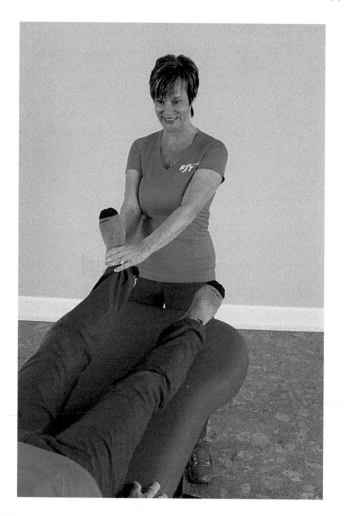

FIGURE 17.1   Hip joint capsule traction.

painful, try another variation by wrapping both hands around the malleoli and above the ankle joint (Figure 17.1).

Traction: Relax your own body. Lean back with your body to achieve the traction. Do not pull with your arms; rather, let your body do the work.

Repeat traction three times with a bit more force each time, as indicated. Reassess joint mobility for any changes after treatment is completed.

The above movements are tested in the coronal plane, then moving out of the coronal plane into the sagittal and transverse to determine specific directions that the fascial system may be inhibited or restricted in movement.

Check lateral movement (moving to the practitioner's left side)

Goal: To assess the client's ROM on the lateral side of their body and to ascertain where they may be restricted as you move them laterally.

Client position: Supine with arms at their side.

Practitioner:
- Lift both of the client's extended legs with traction at 10°–20° again.
- Hold both of their heels in the palms of your hands and gently wrap your fingers around their heels.
- Engage your core and bend your knees slightly.
- Move slowly to the left until the client's movement stops.
- If their hip begins to roll up off the table you have reached the end of their ROM.

Traction: Lean back with your body, stay relaxed (Figure 17.2).

Goal: To increase ROM in lateral lumbopelvic hip region, especially lateral quadratus lumborum(QL), tensor fasciae latae/iliotibial (TFL/IT) band and all tissue along lateral net.

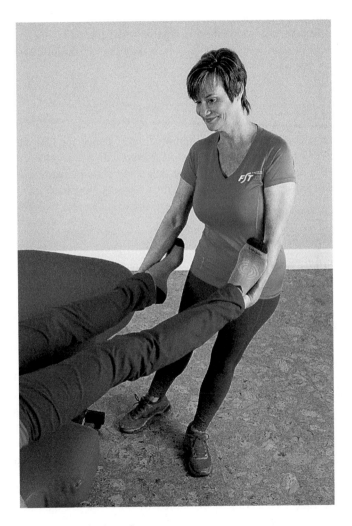

FIGURE 17.2 Assessing the lateral net.

Client position: Supine with arms at their side.

Practitioner:

- Place the client's left leg (the bottom one) on your hip or quad as you move to your left.
- Lift their top leg higher, holding at their heel.
- Place your inside hand on their medial malleolus and anchor it to your thigh on your inside leg.
- Increase ROM by increasing lateral flexion of their opposite side.
- Use your body to lean way from the table and not your arms to feel the tissue response and end feel.

Traction: Keep tractioning out as you move. Think of the traction as if you are moving together in an arc away from the table, then up toward the top of the table.

Repeat: On the other side.

Caution: Return to start position if anything like the following occurs: any sensation of pain or paresthesias which may come from unidentified disc or nerve issues.

RESEARCH ON FST

Although there is also currently no high-quality evidence for FST in the science literature, a 2017 pilot cohort study was conducted with participation of the author and Ann Frederick, founder of FST. The two study authors examined the clinical intervention of using FST in treating chronic nonspecific low back pain.[5]

STUDY ABSTRACT

Background: Numerous fascia-focused therapies are used to treat pain, most relying on direct manipulation and/or tool-mediated techniques. FST, on the other hand, uses distally applied techniques to yield both local and global desired tissue outcomes and subjective pain improvement, including those related to low back pain (LBP). We hypothesize that subjects receiving FST will have reduced nonspecific LBP and enhanced activities of daily living (ADL) scores.

Methods: Eleven subjects who met study criteria (7 females, 4 males; Age 22–32 years) underwent 1 ($n = 11$), 2 ($n = 7$), or 3 ($n = 5$) successive FST treatments (Tx in table below), which consisted of 30 min of three-strap stabilization-mediated body stretch (eight per side). Subjects had pain and ADL scores (Bathing: BAT; Car egress/ingress: CEI; Toilet use: TOI; Forward bending: FOB; Dressing: DRE) measured pre- and 1- and 3-day post-FST. We used a linear mixed-effects model to ascertain the relative percentage change in scores over time using the pretreatment time point as the reference group. All p-values were two-sided and $p < 0.05$ was considered statistically significant.

Results: Statistically significant improvements in pain and ADL scores (*) were found at the time points shown in the table:

SCORE	1 Tx; 1 Day Post	1 Tx; 3 Day Post	2 Tx; 1 Day Post	2 Tx; 3 Day Post	3 Tx; 1 Day Post	3 Tx; 3 Day Post
PAIN	*	*		*	*	
BAT				*		
CEI	*	*	*	*	*	*
TOI						
FOB	*	*	*	*	*	*
DRE	*		*		*	*

Score improvements noted in the table ranged between 31% and 57% compared with pretreatment time point.

Case study by Stephanie LeTourneau, Level 3 FST practitioner

CLIENT INFORMATION:

NICKNAME: A-Dawg

GENDER: Female

AGE: 10 (now)

LEVEL OF FST ADMINISTERED: Level 1 at time of first session

REASON FOR TREATMENT: Improve Range of Motion, flexibility, body control

LIFE GOALS: Play for the Toronto Raptors, meet the Nashville Predators, and changing occupations daily

MEDICAL INFORMATION:

- Sotos Syndrome
- Attention Deficit Hyperactivity Disorder (ADHD) and Attention Deficit Disorder (ADD)
- Anxiety Disorder (unlabeled)
- Microseizures (two seizures every minute when regulated with medication, and temperament regulation)
- Dietary regulations secondary to multiple food allergies
- On the Spectrum (Autistic)

Sotos Syndrome

Sotos Syndrome is a genetic disorder which can occur from the mutation of the *NSD1* gene, or the absence of a gene. Primarily, the mutation is most common, and it is passed down from the carrier parent(s). People that are carriers of Sotos Syndrome are 50% likely to pass it on to their offspring.

The disorder is visible at infancy and early childhood because it affects the physical development of the child, primarily, overgrowth. Their facial structure will be long and narrow, with an enlarged forehead, as well as a small pointed chin. Sotos Syndrome causes hypotonia of the upper body, where motor control and muscle development are lax. They have little control over their upper limbs, whereas the lower body has hypertonia. The legs and hips do not stretch, and children tend to be toe walkers, and lack of separation when observing their gate. Children with Sotos are much larger than their counterparts due to the accelerated growth, but as adults, are of "normal" size.

Another main factor due to the improper development is the lack of pain reception. People with Sotos Syndrome feel very little pain, and usually none at all; they tend to be quite accident prone and have many underlying injuries that go unnoticed.

Although separate, those diagnosed with Sotos Syndrome will typically also have mental development issues, disorders, and emotional difficulties. These can be observed as tantrums, lack of ability to express oneself, ADHD, and underdeveloped cognitive abilities. Learning and speech patterns are often altered and can present in lack of verbal communication skills. Seizures are common with those diagnosed but are not necessarily codependent; someone with Sotos Syndrome do not always suffer from seizures, just as someone who suffers from seizures does not necessarily have Sotos Syndrome.

A-DAWG SPECIFICS

Although symptoms and development presented itself right at infancy, A-Dawg was not confirmed with the diagnosis until nearly 18 months old. Being a premature birth, there were several other precautions, tests, and critical issues that were addressed first. There is also no testing in Canada done for Sotos Syndrome, which delayed the confirmation of the disorder.

A-Dawg feels next to no pain. She has broken several bones without knowledge of the pain. She is extremely accident prone.

We describe her as being "Tinman" from the waist down and "Scarecrow" from the waist up. As an infant, she needed two nurses to change her diaper: one to pry open her legs, and the other to change the diaper itself. Whereas, when picking up an arm, it would flop to the side like a spaghetti noodle.

Her gait is shallow, with one foot (it changes) turned medially for stability. Her knees barely extend, and she walks on her toes. She has never been able to straighten her legs, nor touch her toes due to the hypertonia.

She displays all of the facial features that are to be expected, but is considered "small" for a child with Sotos Syndrome due to having been a premature baby, despite be much taller than children her own age, with much larger feet.

A-Dawg has been to over 450 medical appointments to treat her disorders, test new medications, and help with her psychotherapy and behavior, and for counseling as well as treatments for her mobility including chiropractic, massage therapy, electroshock therapy, reflexology, acupuncture, osteotherapy, and others with minimal to no success or change in her posture, gait, or overall range of motion.

A-Dawg and Microseizures

When properly medicated, for not only the seizures, but for her behavioral issues, she suffers from a microseizure twice every minute. When she is agitated, having a fit, feels stress, or medication needs to be regulated, her seizures can occur every 7 s.

A-Dawg and Behavioral Issues

A-Dawg has both ADD, as well as AD/HD. She will throw fits and tantrums that can last for days without any regulation, which can also manifest physically, and shows in her gait, as well as increased lack of control to her upper body.

She is on the spectrum for autism, and even though she has no personal boundaries (does not understand personal space, or someone's bubble) she is quite intelligent and has a mind like a steel trap. She remembers everything she is told and will try to manipulate to get what she wants, leading to fits when not given what she demands, causing physical issues, and increased seizure activity.

Although learning disabilities are common in patients with Sotos Syndrome, it is possible that hers are also caused by her PTSD, which has been confirmed to have developed *in utero*. Her mother was physically abused throughout, which *may* have also caused the premature labor. The labor itself was traumatizing, also resulting in PTSD. Recently, A-Dawg has also been assaulted, which has heightened the PTSD and caused a plethora of behavioral issues, as well as an increased tightness rate in her lower quadrants.

A-Dawg also presents with lack of bladder control, both voluntary, and involuntary. If overexcited, or overstimulated, she can lose bladder control. She also will intentionally wet herself to be defiant, or to get attention, which is a result of her behavioral disorders and expression of her suffering.

Primary Observations Prior to First Stretch

A-Dawg's mother approached to set up a session to see if fascial stretch therapy would be beneficial for her. She had explained how there hadn't been any success with anything else, and that given other results that she had seen, as well as her own, she felt confident that there could be a chance at minimal improvements (Figure 17.3).

A-Dawg Primary Session: Attempting to Keep Legs as Straight as Possible

- Does not stand up straight, knees bent, tilted forward, slight lean to one side (changes)
- Bent over position, unable to touch toes, knees bent
- Limited flexion/extension in hips
- Limited dorsiflexion in ankles
- Toes curled
- Upper body loose, limited control/strength
- Uneven hips, right side lower than left with slight anterior tilt
- Slight pigeon toed
- Rounding of the spine when bent forward

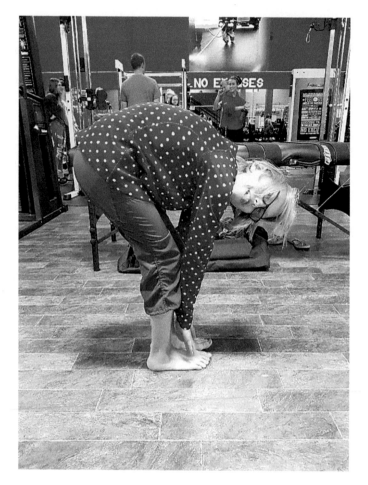

FIGURE 17.3   A-Dawg before FST.

- Immediately comfortable and wanted to be "best friends" as she is eager to please
- Wants to impress me, and not disappoint, attentive.

Given the list of conditions and limitations, there were a number of modifications that were taken to accommodate, as well as maximize her sessions. In this circumstance, the primary session is the one that is going to be discussed.

TREATMENT MODIFICATIONS MADE

- TIME: 20 min, as opposed to 60 min
- Storytime: School talk, interests, etc. to keep her distracted
- Changing verbal queues: "go limp like a spaghetti noodle" as opposed to "relax" or "let go"

- Primary focus on circumduction, and traction, lots and lots of traction of the hips
- Encouraged proprioceptive neuromuscular facilitation (PNF) to allow for her participation—easier for her to relax with engagement
- Having no pain tolerance, or body awareness, crucial to try to hear the tissue, and determine where and if there is an initial barrier to stretch (R1) via multiple passes in a nonrhythmic pattern.

RESULTS (FIGURE 17.4)

- She was able to straighten her legs.
- Able to stand with her heels on the ground.
- Hip flexion able to go deeper, and hips moving further back.
- Back able to extend further/less rounding bending forward.

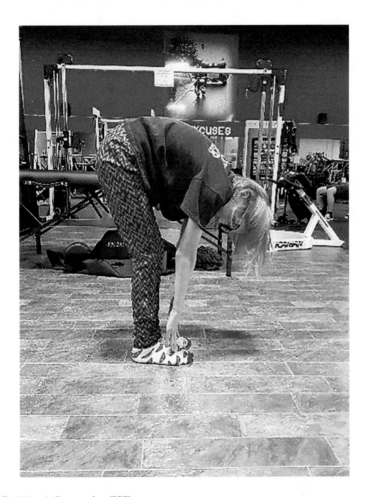

FIGURE 17.4   A-Dawg after FST.

- Gait pattern significant change:
  - Stride much longer.
  - Heel-to-toe strike as opposed to walking on her toes.
  - Standing straighter, spinal column elongated.
  - Arm swing/foot strike opposite and more evenly spaced as opposed to arms swinging in all directions.
  - Forward lean with stride decreased.
  - Knees straightening and bending evenly, able to go to a 90° angle and extend straight out.
- Running strides more evenly spaced and less lateral movement to accommodate balance discrepancies.
- Too comfortable on the table; easily distracted/not as willing to listen—trying to test boundaries.
- Wants to "show off" her toe touch, and feels better with her steps.
- Increase in confidence, and feeling safe on the table (protected).

LOOKING AHEAD

Due to her sensory reception and her lack of ability to feel pain, we want to continue to encourage better gait and movement. Being able to develop and learn deeper and more specific techniques will allow for even more successful results. Hopefully, it will also keep her motivated and welcome new things and experiences. Providing a sense of relief to her mother, as well as her younger sister (who says she is nicer after stretching), and her sense of ability for more efficient movements and confidence in sports, FST is now considered an essential element in improving the quality of life for A-Dawg and her family. Being able to find greater range, and relaxation in her lower extremities, is the goal, and maintaining what has been accomplished thus far.

Every case is unique, and every individual is different, which allows for a multitude of options and opportunities for development; it could never have been anticipated to find so many in one client. It helps me as a therapist to stay alert and continuously look for modifications and growth, which in turn, benefits my ability to adapt, and continue to grow as well. Although she does not have an ailment that can be "cured", being able to continue to make her life a little easier, and calming her nervous system is a reward in itself, with a push to keep going forward in the future.

SUMMARY

This case study was chosen as one example among many of how FST has been used where multiple and varied types of treatment have been attempted with little lasting effect while FST made a significant and long-lasting impact. It was all the more poignant because of the multifactorial nature of a particular genetic disorder in a child with many biopsychosocial challenges.

Although no claims are being made here about FST being a superior treatment over any other, there is something of undeniable benefit going on here that warrants further research. Unfortunately, because it is far more difficult to find high-quality studies of individuals with genetic disorders, we chose the much more prevalent symptom of chronic nonspecific low back pain to do our first cohort research study owing to the multitude of unfortunate people who suffer from this affliction. In the near future, the author would like to move to randomized control studies (RCTs) to get higher quality research going in this area.

When FST was first utilized, it was with collegiate and then Olympic and professional athletes. Even during the very first years of developing FST, athletes reported significant improvement in their athletic performance, faster recovery, reduced injuries, and extended careers. We would like to see RCTs that address and study those claims.

Until that happens, however, a cumulative body of a few hundred case studies such as this is currently being made available to certified FST practitioners so that help and hope may be offered to those suffering where hope has been lost. The author plans to offer these case studies to both researchers and clinical professionals practicing other fascial therapies in the near future in order to expand the possibilities of hope to even more people.

REFERENCES

1. Kaufman, J. Stretching exercises are in as the next fitness fad. www.nytimes com/2017/02/01/business/smallbusiness/stretching-muscles-in-as-the-next-fitness-fad. html.
2. Ingber, D.E., Wang, N., Stamenović, D. 2014. Tensegrity, cellular biophysics, and the mechanics of living systems. *Reports on Progress in Physics*, 77(4):1–42. https://doi. org/10.1088/0034-4885/77/4/046603.
3. Standley, P.R. Meltzer, K. 2008. In vitro modeling of repetitive motion strain and manual medicine treatments: Potential roles for pro- and anti-inflammatory cytokines. *Journal of Bodywork & Movement Therapies*, 12(3):201–203.
4. Adstrum, S., Hedley, G., Schleip, R., et al. 2017. Fascia Nomenclature Subcommittee Report: Defining the fascial system. *Journal of Bodywork & Movement Therapies*, 21:173–177.
5. Ayotunde, O., Standley, P.R., Frederick, C., Kang, P., Frederick, A. 2019. Effects of Fascial Stretch Therapy (FST) on pain index and Activities of Daily Living (ADL) in patients with chronic non-specific Low Back Pain (LBP). *Journal of Investigative Medicine*, 67:1. http://dx.doi.org/10.1136/jim-2018-000939.224

18 Scar Tissue Management

Catherine Ryan and Nancy Keeney-Smith

CONTENTS

INTRODUCTION

The information in this chapter is directed at pathological scarring within the fascial system and the subsequent impact on movement, posture, and visceral function.

The prevalence of occurrence and sequelae associated with pathological scars of varying etiology present important clinical, social, and economic considerations. Postsurgical scar/adhesion complications can occur as a result of even minimally invasive "keyhole" incisions, cauterizing, suturing, or fusing together of segments that are normally meant to be separate from one another.[1,2] It is estimated that 93% of abdominal surgeries result in abdominal adhesions.[1]

Given the impact on the patient and cost burden, improved preventative measures warrant important consideration. Reoperating to lyse problematic scar tissue may not always be necessary to restore function and improve patient quality of life.

FASCIA INTERRUPTED

Regardless of etiology (surgery, burns, accidental injury, overuse/repetitive strain) fascia, like other tissues, will reconcile trauma via the wound healing process, culminating in the repair/restoration of tissue integrity. Fibroblasts, myofibroblasts (MFBs), and transforming growth factor beta 1 (TGF-β1) play fundamental roles in fascial healing.[3–5] Fibroblasts mediate several key processes. MFBs play a primary role in wound closure and signaling TGF-β1 activity—a potent stimulator of collagen deposition. Collagen fibers constitute the physical *fabric* of scars. Along with collagen deposition, angio-, lympho-, and neurogenesis ensure that pre-injury form and function are achieved, as much as possible.

WHEN THINGS GO SIDEWAYS

Regulatory mechanisms ensure that remodeling terminates once tissue homeostasis is reestablished. If these mechanisms fail, unchecked/anomalous collagen proliferation, or fibrosis, ensues, typified by chaotic organization, pathological cross-links, abnormal crimp, and stiffness.

Fibrotic collagen constitutes the common physical presentation shared by all types of pathological scars/adhesions.[6–8] Once established, fibrosis can be a challenging issue to reconcile; therefore, inhibiting profibrotic activity is an important clinical consideration.[9]

Two primary drivers of profibrotic activity have been identified:

- *Excessive/prolonged inflammation*[6,10–12]
- *Anomalous extracellular matrix (ECM)/tissue mechanical tension*[6,9,10,13] (Figure 18.1).

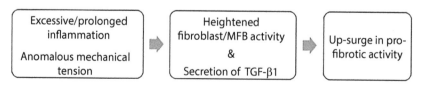

FIGURE 18.1   Primary drivers of fibrogenesis.

MANAGEMENT STRATEGIES

Two general classes of receptors are sensitive/responsive to mechanical forces:

- Integrins
- Neural/fascial Mechanoreceptors.

Mechanoreceptors can be targeted by Massage/Manual Therapy (MMT) to facilitate a positive impact on wound healing, modulating pain, and improving function.[14–17]

EARLY STAGES OF WOUND HEALING

Attenuating dysregulated inflammatory responses and anomalous ECM/tissue tension are key to preventing/tempering profibrotic activity.[10,18] Other important factors to consider are neural hyperactivity/sensitivity, immobilization, and the patient's psychological state.

EXCESSIVE/PROLONGED INFLAMMATION

Normal inflammatory response activates wound healing. Several factors can instigate deviation from natural resolution, potentiating the risk of excessive/prolonged inflammation.

Edema

Following tissue damage, the lymphatic system is tasked with managing consequent edema/swelling and clean-up of debris. Several factors can impact the lymphatic system's ability to uptake fluid and its constituents from the interstitium. Transport inadequacy occurs when local lymphatic load exceeds lymphatic system capacity. Mechanical inadequacy occurs when lymphatic transport capacity slows due to functional or organic causes such as surgery, radiation, and trauma. Following tissue rupture, the volume of local edema coupled with factors that may impede lymphatic flow (e.g., patient immobility or decreased movement, disruption of lymphatic vessels/nodes and compression of lymphatic vessels) may lead to a state of temporary transport inadequacy contributing to stasis and/or impaired drainage. Lymph stasis potentiates prolonged/excessive tissue distention, heightened cytokine/pain mediator concentration, compromised diffusion of cellular waste, nutrients and oxygen—delaying or impairing healing and contributing to fibrogenesis. For example; axillary web syndrome or cording is thought to be fibrosis of the fascial sheath surrounding lymph vessels and/or small veins that occurs as a result of disruption of lymphatic flow due to node dissection or surgical procedure.

Swartz et al.[19] assert that the pre-lymph is information-rich, supplying important details about the state of the tissue from which it drained. Facilitating the movement of, information-rich, fluid from the interstitium into the lymphatic system may prove vitally important in healing and other aspects of patient care (e.g., oncology).

Further, post-trauma edema causes a rapid expansion of local connective tissue (CT) microvacuoles, resulting in mechanical distension of fibrillar structures. The swollen, distended fibers are unable to perform their role in the distribution of tension, and the impact on the microvacuoles can also compromise the sliding mechanism.[20] Prolonged, unchecked edema can also increase the risk of irreversible tissue creep (i.e., plastic deformation), resulting in laxity/instability.

Superficial Fascia; Fibrosis, Lymphedema, and Thermoregulation

A clinical hallmark in lymphedema patients is a predisposition for progressive fibrosis in regional tissues.[21,22] Larger vessels (blood and lymphatic) and nerves track through the superficial fascia (SF). Stecco et al.[23] suggest that if the SF is altered (e.g., fibrotic), lymphatic flow can be compromised. Further, blood flow to the skin plays a role in controlling body temperature, and similarly, the impact of fibrotic SF on resident arteries can impair thermoregulation.[23]

Neurogenic Inflammation and Hyperactivity/Sensitivity

Noxious stimuli triggers the release of neuropeptides such as substance P and calcitonin gene-related peptide (CGRP). Altered neuropeptide levels are implicated in excessive inflammation, pruritus, complex pain, and pathological scar formation.[13,24,25] In addition to acute pain signaling, substance P is implicated in mediating certain complex pain related symptoms, such as hyperalgesia and allodynia, seen with mature hypertrophic scars.[23,26]

Keloids and Pruritus

With burn scars, antihistamines have been shown to be largely ineffective for reducing itch, suggesting that factors other than histamine release, play a role in pruritogenesis. Fourteen days post-injury, a rebound increase in substance P–responsive nerve fibers is observed in pathological/pruritic scars, implicating prolonged/excessive inflammation with subsequent pathological neurogenesis.[25,27,28]

MMT, Inflammation Regulation, and Immune Modulation

MMT methods that facilitate the uptake of exudate laden fluid by the lymphatic system can temper prolonged/excessive inflammation, concentration of pro-inflammatory and pain mediators, and edema-mediated tissue distension.[29–31]

Following soft-tissue injury, MMT is capable of evoking immunomodulatory and wound healing responses such as inducing phenotype change (M1 macrophage to M2), stimulating anti-inflammatory/resolving agents, and suppressing pro-inflammatory agents.[30,32,33]

In addition to diluting the concentration of inflammatory and sensitizing agents, the MMT-mediated influence on interstitial osmotic pressure and lymphatic flow may promote a healthy nerve environment by improving axonal blood flow and reducing intraneural edema.[29] MMT-mediated influence on nerve sensitization and collateral sprouting may reduce the risk of pain translation and, if implemented early, may attenuate intraneural fibrogenesis, preserving peripheral nerve motility.[7,33–35]

Undue Tissue Tension

Appropriate intrinsic wound tension, mediated by MFBs, is necessary for closure and subsequent remodeling. Remodeling is also highly influenced by extrinsic tensional forces (e.g., edema distension and neural-mediated tension).[6] In addition to driving collagen proliferation, undue tension/strain potentiates fibrotic changes that can impact tissue slide capacity.[36] Compressional-tension can also compromise the patency of the SF, with subsequent impact on the vessels/structures tracking throughout.[23]

Mechanical Tension, Nerve Growth Factor, and Pathological Scars

Undue mechanical tension stimulates mechanosensitive receptors. A subsequent hyper-release of neuropeptides and nerve growth factor (NGF) can occur even in the absence of mechanical tension once the malignant cycle has begun. Excessive neuropeptides and NGF are implicated in pathologically innervated scars and may contribute to fibrogenesis.[27,37]

MMT and Tension

MMT-mediated normalizing of mechanical forces in/around the wound environment can play an important role in mitigating fibrogenesis via impact on fibroblast/MFB activity, downregulation of TGFβ1, and upregulation of collagenase.[7,17,38] Restoring tensional homeostasis may also mitigate consequences associated with neural, hematic, and lymphatic compression.

Tension and Keloids

The margins of keloid scars tend to pull outward (i.e., they exhibit considerable peripheral tension), whereas the center of the scar is subjected to milder tension.[6,39] Therefore, tension normalization methods applied along the margins of the scar may result in better outcomes.

Immobilization

The seriousness of injury, pain avoidance, medications, and casting can all impact the patient's movement capacity. The lack of regular movement or total immobility can alter fibroblast activity, leading to fibrotic changes such as anomalous fiber organization and diminished crimp.[40–42] Stiffness, related to fibrosed intramuscular fascia, can occur as quickly as within 2 days of immobilization. Disruption of the structure and organization intramuscular collagen and subsequent impairment of biomechanical properties contributes to functional declines.[43,44] Further, over time, lack of movement/sensory stimulus results in correlating gray matter plasticity changes, with subsequent diminished or lost ability for movement stimulus and/or coordination.[45] Consequently, each of these factors; fibrosed/stuck (can't move) and impact on neural network governing movement (can't generate, control, or coordinate movement) potentiates the other—perpetuating a vicious cycle (Figure 18.2).

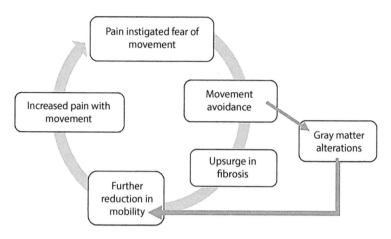

FIGURE 18.2   Immobilization/movement avoidance—fibrosis cycle.

Postoperative Peritoneal Adhesions

Postoperative abdominopelvic adhesions[35] (anomalous/fibrotic anatomical attachments between articulating structures) can lead to detrimental consequences such as bowel obstructions, infertility, pain, and potential reoperations to lyse adhered structures. Bove et al. hypothesize that adhesions develop from a lack of movement of the abdominopelvic organs in the immediate postoperative period while the patient is rendered immobile by surgery and opiates.

MMT and Immobilization

When patient active movement would be unsafe, harmful, or unattainable, non-nocicepting/non-threatening manual mobilization of skin and fascia provides a safe alternative. Bove et al.[35] found that immediate postoperative MMT of abdominopelvic structures resulted in reduced frequency and size of adhesions. It is important to note that treatment did not inhibit healing or induce undesirable complications following strictureplasty. According to Wasserman et al.,[1] there is preliminary strong evidence that MMT applied to acute surgical abdominal adhesions has a positive outcome on pain and function and preliminary weak evidence in treating pain, function, and mobility in the chronic postsurgical abdomen.

Gentle methods that facilitate cellular stimulation are desirable when more profuse tissue deformation would be considered unfavorable, for example, following surgery as a means to avoid tissue dehiscence. Because fascia is a biotensegrity system, it is not always necessary to apply methods directly to the wound-site in order to facilitate productive outcomes.

Bouffard et al.[44] demonstrated that brief tissue stretch, beyond the habitual range of motion, reduces TGF-β1 concentrations—resulting in downregulation of fibrogenesis and subsequent reduction in adhesions in mouse subcutaneous connective tissue (CT).

Active and passive movement and mechanical loading are essential for optimal healing of joints and adaptation of fascia.[46–48] Manual manipulation and movement can influence collagen organization during healing, reducing the risk of restrictions that may impair tissue slide capacity.[36]

PROLONGED STRESS RESPONSE, PAIN, AND WOUND HEALING

The effects of prolonged pain and stress response on healing are moderate to large, resulting in poor surgical outcomes and poor wound healing.[49–51] Elevated levels of cortisol and other glucocorticoids during prolonged stress are associated with sympathetic nervous system (SNS) hyperarousal. According to Christian et al.,[52] dysregulation of both glucocorticoid and cytokine function are key biological links between stress and healing.

MMT and Prolonged Stress Response and Pain

Interventions designed to reduce stress and its concomitants warrant worthwhile consideration in the prevention of pathological scars. Research supporting MMTs impact on pain, stress, anxiety, and SNS hyperarousal and immune function, affirm its utility.[30,48,53] For example, according to Schleip,[54,55] manual manipulation of fascia can impact the nervous system in ways that lead to a global decrease in SNS tone. SNS hyperarousal is implicated in increased fascial tension, mediated by MFB contraction.[43,56,57] Conversely, SNS sedation may normalize fascial tension, theoretically—reducing the risk of profibrotic activity.

MMT has been shown to have a positive impact on inflammation, tissue tension, immobilization, neural distress and patient mood, augmenting the early wound healing process and reducing the risk of fibrogenesis and associated sequelae.[58–60] The biological and psychological mechanisms by which various MMT methods modulate the wound healing process involve interrelated responses within multiple systems.[17,29,61]

MATURE SCARS

In addition to fibrotic changes, mature scars/adhesions can present with anomalous ingrowths of capillaries, adipose tissue, smooth muscle, and nerves.[62]

Tendon Sliding and Restrictions

In his exploration of the tendon sliding system, Guimberteau noted, at the FRC III 2012, that when tendons move, the movement is barely discernible in neighboring tissues if no restrictions are present (e.g., adhesions, fibrosis, densification). According to Guimberteau, variances in non-injured tissue and in tissue during and after scar formation can be seen endoscopically. Notably, with irregular or abnormal healing (even though the surface tissue looks normal), below the surface, undifferentiated tissue can be present for several months (e.g., thick/dense and devoid of loose sliding tissue)[20]. Additionally, the hypervasculization typically seen in the early stages of normal healing will persist far longer with abnormal or irregular healing. When orthopedic/reconstructive hardware is used, normal scar formation does not occur. In addition to biomechanical implications, reduced sliding appears to limit the functionality of the endocannabinoid system, which is of concern as endocannabinoids are believed to better manage inflammation and pain information originating in the fascial system.[63]

Distressed (e.g., fibrosed) somatic tissues adjacent to nerve structures release inflammatory substances that can chemically irritate neural elements. This suggests that neural function can be impacted by not only by the direct influence of scarring on neural components but also by pathological scarring in neighboring tissue. Higher than normal concentrations of MFBs are found in injured fascia, constituting a potential source of ongoing undue tissue tension, collagen proliferation, and subsequent contracture.

Although fibrotic tissue is often considered an inactive scaffold, precluding potential for change, fibrosis is neither static nor irreversible but, rather, a continuous remodeling process—susceptible to intervention.[64–66] Given the extraordinary tensile strength of collagen, it is evident that it is physiologically implausible to *break down* (i.e., lyse) profuse/dense mature scar tissue/adhesions by application of manual methods. Nor would it be considered patient-considerate to try.

Like steel, collagen is highly ductile, meaning that when subjected to *extreme* forces, it will slowly deform, rather than break like porcelain or glass.[41] The operative word being *extreme*—therefore, it seems physiologically implausible to facilitate functionally meaningful deformation of dense fascia by application of manual methods.[67]

What then are physiologically plausible changes that constitute the rationale for the clinical outcomes commonly seen in MMT practice when addressing mature scars/adhesions?

MMT and Mature Scars

When treating any type of mature scar/adhesion within the fascial system, MMT methods are directed at facilitating collagen (fiber) and ground substance (fluid) changes. Fiber and fluid environment alterations in fascia can impact force transmission, slide capacity, elasticity, pliability and muscular, neural, visceral, circulatory and lymphatic function. Desirable fiber changes include improved hydration and organization, disruption of pathological cross-links, and promoting favorable features such as crimp, suppleness, and smoothness. Fluid environment changes include shifts in volume and/or viscosity. The mechanisms by which various methods facilitate fiber and fluid changes involve interrelated responses within multiple systems.[17,68,69]

Fascial collagen is capable of slowly remodeling itself over time, influenced by the mechanical forces to which it is subjected.[41] If mature (fibrotic) collagen (including intraneural loose connective tissue) is in an ongoing state of flux (remodeling), it then seems plausible to intervene in order to temper any ongoing proliferation and facilitate changes in certain fiber features (e.g., crimp, smoothness, pliability, and organization). Experimental (animal model) evidence provides rationale for how MMT may promote better healing outcomes—where remodeling is still in process.[7,36,70]

Injury, immobilization, and inflammation have been shown to impact fluid environment viscosity (densification) and volume (fluid gap)—leading to mal-sliding.[71–73] Injury and posttreatment densification changes can be visualized via ultrasonography.[74,75] It is suggested that alterations in hyaluronan amount and organization may play a role in the MMT-mediated posttreatment changes (e.g., tissue softening, improved pliability, and slide capacity).[64,76] Some of the clinical outcomes commonly seen may be due to changes in the intra- and interfibrillar fluid environment (volume and viscosity) and within the loose CT serving a sliding function[77]; for example see "Clinical Consideration", Pohl.[78]

CLINICAL CONSIDERATION

Summary: Afflicted areas were determined by patient report of pain, other discomfort, and impaired function—further supported by therapist assessment of concomitant tissue changes. Thirty patients were measured with high-frequency ultrasound (22 MHz) immediately before and after initial treatment in the afflicted area. A specialized form of skin rolling was administered. Non-afflicted regions were also measured as a comparison.

Results: In the afflicted areas, highly significant posttreatment differences are visible in the structure of the collagen matrix within the dermis: There appears to be more fluid within the collagen fibers and the fibers are better distributed in the surrounding interstitial fluid (Figures 18.3 and 18.4). The visualized changes also reflect what was felt by the therapists—differences in

- Tension
- Softness/pliability
- Regularity/texture (smoothness).

It is important to note that in non-afflicted areas, treatment did not elicit any collagen changes.

(Continued)

CLINICAL CONSIDERATION (Continued)

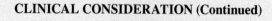

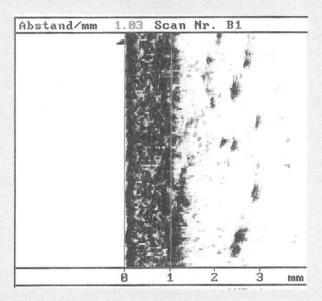

FIGURE 18.3   Pretreatment image of the afflicted area. (Used with Kind Permission from Dr. Helga Pohl – Pohl, H., *J. Bodyw. Mov. Ther.*, 14, 27–34, 2010.)

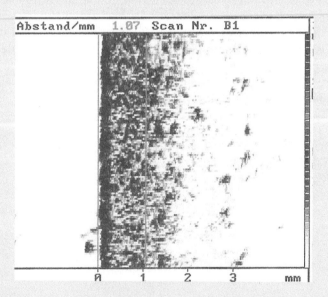

FIGURE 18.4   Posttreatment image of the afflicted area showing a reduction in density and a more homogenous fiber structure. (Used with Kind Permission from Dr. Helga Pohl – Pohl, H., *J. Bodyw. Mov. Ther.*, 14, 27–34, 2010.)

In some circumstances, MMT may effectively address the patient's, scar-related, pain and dysfunction while offsetting the impact of subsequent surgery, including the burden of cost and risk of more scar tissue[79] In both developing and mature scars, changes in certain scar characteristics may be attainable. With post-burn hypertrophic scars, MMT appears to be a viable modality for attenuating pain, pruritus, and scar characteristics such as thickness, melanin deposition, erythema, transdermal water loss, and tissue elasticity/mobility.[28]

Although the effects of MMT on remodeling are not fully known, it may shorten the time needed to form a healthy, mature scar.[28] An important aspect of care is addressing functional declines associated with compensations or adaptations within the fascial system and the associated multisystem consequences related to mal-sliding and restrictions. MMT shows solid utility for addressing fibrosis-related functional declines within the fascial system.[17,29]

Drain Sites

Surgical drain site scarring is commonly problematic. Any, midstream interruption in the healing process increases the risk of fibrosis. For example, following mastectomy, restricted shoulder range of motion can be related to fibrotic tethering/restriction around the surgical drain site, well below the glenohumeral joint. If standard protocols of care (e.g., joint mobilizations and range of motion exercises) are not achieving expected outcomes—look beyond the local area of complaint.

A biotensegrity (myokinetic chain or myofascial meridian) approach is considered key when addressing dysfunctional adaptations/compensations. Various methods (e.g., Structural Integration/Rolfing® and Fascial Manipulation®) are influenced by the biotensegrity model. Other important sequalae requiring consideration include impact on proprioception and interoception.

CONCLUSION—THE IMPORTANCE OF EARLY INTERVENTION AND COLLABORATION

An Ounce of Prevention

It appears that MMT tempers inflammation and consequent changes in function and tissue pathology, possibly by reducing collagenous tethers between tissues and maintaining mobility between structures. It is hypothesized that fibrotic collagen around and between structures likely impedes normal sliding, instigating ongoing inflammation and nociception as tethered tissues begin to tear during excursion while performing normal tasks. Because the methods used in this study were translated from the MMT clinic to the laboratory, translating this data back to the MMT clinical population is likely to have substantial preventive effects in people performing repetitive tasks. In repetitive motion/strain injuries, Bove et al.[7,70] identified that fibrotic and fluid changes in/around neural interfaces (i.e., loose CT serving a sliding function) are a potential source of peripheral axon compression, agitation of mechanoreceptors, leading to subsequent pain and sensory dysfunction.[70] They demonstrated that MMT intervention before severe problems developed rescues most if not all metrics of deleterious changes in sensory function, task performance, and tissue integrity.

This research supports that early treatment, before pathological changes progress, may mitigate undue pain, functional declines, and prolonged medical expenses. Because stages of healing are largely the same across etiologies, it is reasonable that adhering to early standardized treatment protocols may improve patient outcomes across fascial-trauma etiologies.

INTERPROFESSIONAL COLLABORATION

Although postsurgical patient self-care instructions commonly include a recommendation to self-massage the scar, there is a paucity in patients receiving direction to seek out early treatment administered by an MMT professional, constituting an important missed opportunity in preventative care.[80–82]

Generally considered minimally invasive and safe, MMT is not without risk entirely. More assertive methods pose some risk in the early stage of wound healing and therefore patients are often advised to not receive "massage" for several weeks post-surgery. It is unfortunate that the word *massage* is used as an umbrella term to describe a wide variety of MMT methods. When treatment is provided by an MMT professional, the risk of adverse events is low and outcomes are enhanced.[1,83]

Fascially skilled MMT professionals can assist the medical management team with augmenting wound healing, mitigating fibrogenesis, early detection of nascent issues, and evaluating existing issues.

Surgeons and manual therapists share similarities—we are both in direct contact with tissues. Patients would be better served by surgeons and manual therapists working together

Jean-Claude Guimberteau MD & Thomas Hausner MD,
Surgery and Fasciatherapy,
4th International Fascia Research Congress 2015

REFERENCES

1. Wasserman, J. B., Copeland, M., Upp, M., et al. (2019). Effect of soft tissue mobilization techniques on adhesion-related pain and function in the abdomen: A systematic review. *Journal of Bodywork and Movement Therapies*, 23(2), 262–269.
2. Fourie, W. (2014). Management of scars and adhesions. In: Chaitow, L., (ed.), *Fascial Dysfunction: Manual Therapy Approaches*. Ch. 18. Handspring Publishing, Pencaitland, UK.
3. Tomasek, J. J., Gabbiani, G., Hinz, B., et al. (2002). Myofibroblasts and mechano-regulation of connective tissue remodelling. *Nature Reviews Molecular Cell Biology*, 3(5), 349.
4. Hinz, B. (2007). Formation and function of the myofibroblast during tissue repair. *Journal of Investigative Dermatology*, 127(3), 526–537.

5. Darby, I. A., Laverdet, B., Bonté, F., et al. (2014). Fibroblasts and myofibroblasts in wound healing. *Clinical, Cosmetic and Investigational Dermatology*, 7, 301.

6. Ogawa, R. (2011). Mechanobiology of scarring. *Wound Repair and Regeneration*, 19, s2–s9.

7. Bove, G. M., Harris, M. Y., Zhao, H., et al. (2016). Manual therapy as an effective treatment for fibrosis in a rat model of upper extremity overuse injury. *Journal of the Neurological Sciences*, 361, 168–180.

8. Citrin, D. E., Prasanna, P. G., Walker, A. J., et al. (2017). Radiation-Induced Fibrosis: Mechanisms and Opportunities to Mitigate. Report of an NCI Workshop, September 19, 2016. *Radiation Research*, 188(1), 1–20.

9. Barnes, L. A., Marshall, C. D., Leavitt, T., et al. (2018). Mechanical forces in cutaneous wound healing: Emerging therapies to minimize scar formation. *Advances in Wound Care*, 7(2), 47–56.

10. Ogawa, R. (2017). Keloid and hypertrophic scars are the result of chronic inflammation in the reticular dermis. *International Journal of Molecular Sciences*, 18(3), 606.

11. Ogawa, R., Okai, K., Tokumura, F., et al. (2012). The relationship between skin stretching/contraction and pathologic scarring: The important role of mechanical forces in keloid generation. *Wound Repair and Regeneration*, 20(2), 149–157.

12. Wong, V. W., Rustad, K. C., Akaishi, S., et al. (2012). Focal adhesion kinase links mechanical force to skin fibrosis via inflammatory signaling. *Nature Medicine*, 18(1), 148.

13. Widgerow, A. D. (2013). Hypertrophic burn scar evolution and management. *Wound Healing Southern Africa*, 6(2), 79–86.

14. Huang, C., Holfeld, J., Schaden, W., et al. (2013). Mechanotherapy: Revisiting physical therapy and recruiting mechanobiology for a new era in medicine. *Trends in Molecular Medicine*, 19(9), 555–564.

15. Ng, J. L., Kersh, M. E., Kilbreath, S., et al. (2017). Establishing the basis for mechanobiology-based physical therapy protocols to potentiate cellular healing and tissue regeneration. *Frontiers in Physiology*, 8, 303.

16. Bialosky, J. E., Beneciuk, J. M., Bishop, M. D., et al. (2018). Unraveling the mechanisms of manual therapy: Modeling an approach. *Journal of Orthopaedic & Sports Physical Therapy*, 48(1), 8–18.

17. Chaitow, L. (Ed.). (2018). *Fascial Dysfunction—Manual Therapy Approaches*. 2nd ed. Handspring Publishing.

18. Hinz, B. (2015). The extracellular matrix and transforming growth factor-β1: Tale of a strained relationship. *Matrix Biology*, 47, 54–65.

19. Swartz, M. A. (2014). Immunomodulatory roles of lymphatic vessels in cancer progression. *Cancer Immunology Research*, 2(8), 701–707.

20. Guimberteau, J. C., and Armstrong, C. (2015). *Architecture of Human Living Fascia: The Extracellular Matrix and Cells Revealed Through Endoscopy*. Handspring Publishing.

21. Rockson, S. G. (2013). The lymphatics and the inflammatory response: Lessons learned from human lymphedema. *Lymphatic Research and Biology*, 11(3), 117–120.

22. Mukherji, A. (2018). *Managing Complications: Lymphoedema and Fibrosis. In Basics of Planning and Management of Patients during Radiation Therapy* (pp. 357–366). Springer, Singapore.

23. Stecco, A., Stern, R., Fantoni, I., et al. (2016). Fascial disorders: Implications for treatment. *PM&R*, 8(2), 161–168.

24. Henderson, J., Terenghi, G., McGrouther, D. A., et al. (2006). The reinnervation pattern of wounds and scars may explain their sensory symptoms. *Journal of Plastic, Reconstructive & Aesthetic Surgery*, 59(9), 942–950.

25. Scott, J. R., Muangman, P., and Gibran, N. S. (2007). Making sense of hypertrophic scar: A role for nerves. *Wound Repair and Regeneration*, 15, S27–S31.

26. Henderson, J., Ferguson, M. W., and Terenghi, G. (2012). The feeling of healing. *Plastic and Reconstructive Surgery*, 129(1), 223e–224e.

27. Xiao, H., Wang, D., Huo, R., et al. (2013). Mechanical tension promotes skin nerve regeneration by upregulating nerve growth factor expression. *Neural Regeneration Research*, 8(17), 1576.

28. Cho, Y. S., Jeon, J. H., Hong, A., et al. (2014). The effect of burn rehabilitation massage therapy on hypertrophic scar after burn: A randomized controlled trial. *Burns*, 40(8), 1513–1520.

29. Fryer, G., and Fossum, C. (2009). Therapeutic mechanisms underlying muscle energy approaches. In: Fernandez-de-las-Peñas, C., Arendt-Nielsen, L., Gerwin, R.D. (eds.), *Physical Therapy for Tension Type and Cervicogenic Headache*. Jones & Bartlett, Boston, MA.

30. Crane, J. D., Ogborn, D. I., Cupido, C., et al. (2012). Massage therapy attenuates inflammatory signaling after exercise-induced muscle damage. *Science Translational Medicine*, 4(119), 119ra13.

31. Rasmussen, J., Fife, C., and Sevick-Muraca, E. (2019). Imaging the lymphatic response to manual lymphatic drainage and pneumatic compression devices. *Journal of Vascular Surgery: Venous and Lymphatic Disorders*, 7(2), 285.

32. Fadok, V. A., Bratton, D. L., Guthrie, L., et al. (2001). Differential effects of apoptotic versus lysed cells on macrophage production of cytokines: Role of proteases. *The Journal of Immunology*, 166(11), 6847–6854.

33. Waters-Banker, C., Dupont-Versteegden, E. E., Kitzman, P. H., et al. (2014). Investigating the mechanisms of massage efficacy: The role of mechanical immunomodulation. *Journal of Athletic Training*, 49(2), 266–273.

34. Gilbert, K. K., Smith, M. P., Sobczak, S., et al. (2015). Effects of lower limb neurodynamic mobilization on intraneural fluid dispersion of the fourth lumbar nerve root: An unembalmed cadaveric investigation. *Journal of Manual & Manipulative Therapy*, 23(5), 239–245.

35. Bove, G. M., Chapelle, S. L., Hanlon, K. E., et al. (2017). Attenuation of postoperative adhesions using a modeled manual therapy. *PloS One*, 12(6), e0178407.

36. Franchi, M., Ottani, V., Stagni, R., et al. (2010). Tendon and ligament fibrillar crimps give rise to left-handed helices of collagen fibrils in both planar and helical crimps. *Journal of Anatomy*, 216(3), 301–309.

37. Gabriel, V. (2011). Hypertrophic scar. *Physical Medicine and Rehabilitation Clinics*, 22(2), 301–310.

38. Langevin, H. M. (2013). The science of stretch. *The Scientist*, 27(5), 32.

39. Akaishi, S., Akimoto, M., Ogawa, R., et al. (2008). The relationship between keloid growth pattern and stretching tension: Visual analysis using the finite element method. *Annals of Plastic Surgery*, 60(4), 445–451.

40. Schleip, R., and Müller, D. G. (2013) Training principles for fascial connective tissues: Scientific foundation and suggested practical application. *Journal of Bodywork and Movement Therapies*, 17(1), 103–111.

41. Lesondak, D. (2018). Fascial syndromes: Emerging, treatable contributors to musculoskeletal pain. In *Metabolic Therapies in Orthopedics*, 2nd ed. (pp. 357–368). CRC Press.

42. Jarvinen, T. A., Jozsa, L., Kannus, P., et al. (2002). Organization and distribution of intramuscular connective tissue in normal and immobilized skeletal muscles. An immunohistochemical, polarization and scanning electron microscopic study. *Journal of Muscle Research and Cell Motility*, 23(3), 245–254.

43. Schleip, R., Naylor, I. L., Ursu, D., et al. (2006). Passive muscle stiffness may be influenced by active contractility of intramuscular connective tissue. *Medical Hypotheses*, 66(1), 66–71.

44. Bouffard, N. A., Cutroneo, K. R., Badger, G. J., et al. (2008). Tissue stretch decreases soluble TGF-β1 and type-1 procollagen in mouse subcutaneous connective tissue: Evidence from ex vivo and in vivo models. *Journal of Cellular Physiology*, 214(2), 389–395.

45. Granert, O., Peller, M., Gaser, C., et al. (2011). Manual activity shapes structure and function in contralateral human motor hand area. *Neuroimage*, 54(1), 32–41.

46. Grinnell, F. (2000). Fibroblast–collagen-matrix contraction: Growth-factor signalling and mechanical loading. *Trends in Cell Biology*, 10(9), 362–365.

47. Ingram, K. R., Wann, A. K. T., Angel, C. K., et al. (2008). Cyclic movement stimulates hyaluronan secretion into the synovial cavity of rabbit joints. *The Journal of Physiology*, 586(6), 1715–1729.

48. Fryer, G. (2017). Integrating osteopathic approaches based on biopsychosocial therapeutic mechanisms. Part 1: The mechanisms. *International Journal of Osteopathic Medicine*, 25, 30–41.

49. Broadbent, E., Kahokehr, A., Booth, R. J., et al. (2012). A brief relaxation intervention reduces stress and improves surgical wound healing response: A randomised trial. *Brain, Behavior, and Immunity*, 26(2), 212–217.

50. Padgett, D. A., and Glaser, R. (2003). How stress influences the immune response. *Trends in Immunology*, 24(8), 444–448.

51. Lucas, V. S. (2011). Psychological stress and wound healing in humans: What we know. *Wounds: A Compendium of Clinical Research and Practice*, 23(4), 76–83.

52. Christian, L. M., Graham, J. E., Padgett, D. A., et al. (2006). Stress and wound healing. *Neuroimmunomodulation*, 13(5–6), 337–346.

53. Tejero-Fernández, V., Membrilla-Mesa, M., Galiano-Castillo, N., et al. (2015). Immunological effects of massage after exercise: A systematic review. *Physical Therapy in Sport*, 16(2), 187–192.

54. Schleip, R. (2003). Fascial plasticity–a new neurobiological explanation: Part 1. *Journal of Bodywork and Movement Therapies*, 7(1), 11–19.

55. Schleip, R. (2003). Fascial plasticity–a new neurobiological explanation: Part 2. *Journal of Bodywork and Movement Therapies*, 7(2), 104–116.

56. Staubesand, J., and Li, Y. (1996). Zum Feinbau der Fascia cruris mit besonderer Berücksichtigung epi-und intrafaszialer Nerven. *Manuelle Medizin*, 34(34), 196–200.

57. Bhowmick, S., Singh, A., Flavell, R. A., Clark, R. B., O'Rourke, J., and Cone, R. E. (2009). The sympathetic nervous system modulates CD4+ FoxP3+ regulatory T cells via a TGF-β-dependent mechanism. *Journal of Leukocyte Biology*, 86(6), 1275–1283.

58. Cho, Y. S., Jeon, J. H., Hong, A., et al. (2014). The effect of burn rehabilitation massage therapy on hypertrophic scar after burn: A randomized controlled trial. *Burns*, 40(8), 1513–1520.

59. Anthonissen, M., Daly, D., Janssens, T., et al. (2016). The effects of conservative treatments on burn scars: A systematic review. *Burns*, 42(3), 508–518.

60. Ault, P., Plaza, A., and Paratz, J. (2018). Scar massage for hypertrophic burns scarring—A systematic review. *Burns*, 44(1), 24–38.

61. Rodríguez, R. M., and del Río, F. G. (2013). Mechanistic basis of manual therapy in myofascial injuries. Sonoelastographic evolution control. *Journal of Bodywork and Movement Therapies*, 17(2), 221–234.

62. Herrick, S. E., Mutsaers, S. E., Ozua, P., et al. (2000). Human peritoneal adhesions are highly cellular, innervated, and vascularized. *Journal of Pathology*, 192(1), 67–72.

63. Bordoni, B., and Zanier, E. (2014). Skin, fascias, and scars: Symptoms and systemic connections. *Journal of Multidisciplinary Healthcare*, 7, 11.

64. Wynn, T. A. (2007). Common and unique mechanisms regulate fibrosis in various fibroproliferative diseases. *The Journal of Clinical Investigation*, 117(3), 524–529.

65. Kisseleva, T., Cong, M., Paik, Y., et al. (2012). Myofibroblasts revert to an inactive phenotype during regression of liver fibrosis. *Proceedings of the National Academy of Sciences*, 109(24), 9448–9453.

66. Troeger, J. S., Mederacke, I., Gwak, G. Y., et al. (2012). Deactivation of hepatic stellate cells during liver fibrosis resolution in mice. *Gastroenterology*, 143(4), 1073–1083.

67. Chaudhry, H., Schleip, R., Ji, Z., et al. (2008). Three-dimensional mathematical model for deformation of human fasciae in manual therapy. *The Journal of the American Osteopathic Association*, 108(8), 379–390.

68. Stecco, L., Basmanjian, J. V., and Day, J. A. (2004). Fascial manipulation for musculo-skeletal pain.

69. Schleip, R., Findley, T. W., Chaitow, L., et al. (2012). *Fascia: The Tensional Network of the Human Body*. Churchill Livingstone, London, UK.

70. Bove, G. M., Delany, S. P., Hobson, L., et al. (2019). Manual therapy prevents onset of nociceptor activity, sensorimotor dysfunction, and neural fibrosis induced by a volitional repetitive task. *Pain*, 160(3), 632–644.

71. Stecco, C. et al. (2011). Hyaluronan within fascia in the etiology of myofascial pain. *Surgical and Radiologic Anatomy*, 33(10), 891–896.

72. Roman, M., Chaudhry, H., Bukiet, B., et al. (2013). Mathematical analysis of the flow of hyaluronic acid around fascia during manual therapy motions. *The Journal of the American Osteopathic Association*, 113(8), 600–610.

73. Guimberteau, J. C., and Delage, J. P. (2012). The multifibrillar network of the tendon sliding system. *Annales de chirurgie plastique et esthetique*, 57(5), 467–481.

74. Pavan, P. G., Stecco, A., Stern, R., et al. (2014). Painful connections: Densification versus fibrosis of fascia. *Current Pain and Headache Reports*, 18(8), 441.

75. Stecco, A., Meneghini, A., Stern, R., et al. (2014). Ultrasonography in myofascial neck pain: Randomized clinical trial for diagnosis and follow-up. *Surgical and Radiologic Anatomy*, 36(3), 243–253.

76. Evanko, S. P., and Wight, T. N. (1999). Intracellular localization of hyaluronan in proliferating cells. *Journal of Histochemistry and Cytochemistry*, 47, 1331–1342.

77. Stecco, C., Fede, C., Macchi, V., et al. (2018). The fasciacytes: A new cell devoted to fascial gliding regulation. *Clinical Anatomy*, 31(5), 667–676.

78. Pohl, H. (2010). Changes in the structure of collagen distribution in the skin caused by a manual technique. *Journal of Bodywork and Movement Therapies*, 14(1), 27–34.

79. Diamond, M. P. (2012). Scars and Adhesion Panel. Lecture notes from The 3rd International Fascia Research Congress, Vancouver, March 28–30.

80. Jette, A. M., and Delitto, A. (1997). Physical therapy treatment choices for musculoskeletal impairments. *Physical Therapy*, 77(2), 145–154.

81. Bishop, P. B., and Wing, P. C. (2003). Compliance with clinical practice guidelines in family physicians managing worker's compensation board patients with acute lower back pain. *The Spine Journal*, 3(6), 442–450.

82. Li, L. C., and Bombardier, C. (2001). Physical therapy management of low back pain: An exploratory survey of therapist approaches. *Physical Therapy*, 81(4), 1018–1028.

83. NIH. (2015). Massage therapy for health purposes: What the science says. Available: https://nccih.nih.gov/health/providers/digest/massage-science [Accessed February 21, 2015].

19 Exercise and Fascial Movement Therapy for Cancer Survivors
Potential Benefits and Recommendations

P. J. O'Clair

CONTENTS

INTRODUCTION

Cancer is one of the world's most common major diseases, with over 18 million people diagnosed each year. The four most common cancers reported globally are lung, female breast, bowel, and prostate cancer. It is estimated that by the year 2040 there will be 27.5 million new cases of cancer worldwide.[1] Fortunately, due to early detection, advancements in screening, and improvements in treatment, many patients diagnosed will survive and go on to live out their normal life expectancy. Cancer deaths have declined by 27% over the past decade and, according to the American Cancer Society, there were 16.9 million cancer survivors in the United States in 2019—with a projected 22.1 million survivors in 2030.[2] Despite this good news, cancer treatments still take an enormous toll on the body. Survivors are often left to face lasting and unique health issues from both the disease and treatment-associated side effects.

TREATMENT AND SIDE EFFECTS

Cancer treatments aim both to rid the body of disease and to minimize the possibility of the cancer returning. They are either local or systemic, with patients receiving one form or a combination based on individual needs. Local treatments are used to remove or destroy damaged tissue at and around the cancer site. Systemic treatments are used to destroy or control cancer cells throughout the entire body rather than at a specific site; these methods include chemotherapy, hormonal therapy, targeted therapy, and immunotherapy. Both local and systemic treatments substantially impact the life a cancer patient.

Side effects include:

- *Anxiety*
- *Reduced bone health*
- *Cardiotoxicity*
- *Chemotherapy-induced peripheral neuropathy*
- *Cognitive function*
- *Depressive symptoms*
- *Falls*
- *Cancer-Related Fatigue*
- *Lymphedema*
- *Nausea*
- *Pain*
- *Physical function*
- *Sexual function*
- *Sleep*
- *Treatment tolerance.*

Treatments can cause collateral damage to the heart and weaken many of the body's operating systems: cardiorespiratory, circulatory, lymphatic, hormonal, nervous, and musculoskeletal.[1] The most common toxicities reported from cancer treatments include

- Increased risk for fractures and cardiovascular events with hormonal therapies
- Neuropathies related to certain types of chemotherapy
- Musculoskeletal morbidities secondary to treatment
- Treatment-related cardiotoxicity.

The decline in cardiorespiratory fitness during chemotherapy has been well documented,[3] along with the loss of muscular strength due to the inability of the patient to be physically active during treatment. Unfortunately, even after treatment ends many cancer patients struggle to rebuild their pre-diagnosis physical fitness. This is especially true in the case of advanced or metastatic cancers. The standard care for advanced or metastatic prostate cancer is a hormone therapy, androgen deprivation therapy (ADT). ADT is designed to either stop the production of testosterone or to block it from acting on prostate cancer cells. The block of testosterone from ADT results in an abrupt loss of lean body mass and a rapid reduction in muscular strength and endurance. Men on ADT may not be able to build lean tissue mass even when participating in a resistance training program.[4,5]

CASE STUDY 1—CLIENT WITH METASTATIC PROSTATE CANCER

One of my clients, diagnosed with stage four metastatic prostate cancer, struggles with his inability to build lean tissue and regain his pre-diagnosis fitness level. He went into the disease a very fit endurance athlete at 59 years of age. His oncology team told him that due to his physical and mental strength they would be able to administer an aggressive treatment protocol, which, by all measures, did him well. Within just 2 months of his treatment, which included surgery, oral medication, and ADT, he was cleared to resume supervised physical activity. We began him with a restorative Pilates reformer regimen. The Pilates reformer uses spring tension to rebuild strength and endurance. As soon as his nephrostomy tube with drainage bag was removed, he added in low-intensity cycling.

Within 8 months posttreatment, he resumed his pre-diagnosis exercise routine consisting of

- 2–4 h of moderate-intensity outdoor road and mountain biking 5–6 days per week
- 60 min of supervised moderate-to-high intensity resistance training two times per week
- 20 min of core and total body mobility sessions one to two times per week.

Clearly, he is highly motivated and works hard to return to his pre-diagnosis state of health. Yet, due to his ongoing ADT treatments he struggles with weight gain, fatigue, and frustration. He is unable to regain his strength and endurance despite all his efforts.

This case study brings about the importance of listening to the individual and trying to understand where they are at emotionally. It is easy for those of us who haven't had to deal with a life-threatening disease to think that the person is doing great and that they shouldn't worry about the way they look or feel. It will take time for them to rebuild. What we may not appreciate is the real day-to-day hardship caused by the traumatic side effects. These emotional setbacks can linger and cause depressive symptoms. I keep a careful watch out for signs of emotional decline. Along with the others in our fitness community, I work to encourage him and praise him for his efforts.

LIVING WITH CANCER

Throughout diagnosis, treatment, and recovery, cancer survivors struggle to maintain a positive attitude and are often plagued by several major concerns:

1. Cancer recurrence
2. Life expectancy
3. Employment issues
4. Family matters
5. Short/long term effects on the body.

The patients look to their medical teams for support, advice, and direction. Clinicians, well aware of the physical and emotional toll the disease takes on the individual, are encouraged to seek accessible, inexpensive ways to improve the lives of their cancer patients and to reduce the risk of recurrence. Based on the abundance of evidence, exercise is shown to be a beneficial solution for the cancer patient's journey through recovery and survivorship. In fact, the Physical Activity Guidelines for Adults with Chronic Conditions (including cancer) urge survivors to avoid inactivity and be as physically active as possible.[6]

Physical activity above all other possible lifestyle modifications, including weight management, diet, cessation of tobacco, reduction in alcohol consumption, may have the most robust effect on reducing breast cancer recurrence.[7] Exercise is also believed to slow down the progression of cancer, thus reducing mortality.[8] The health and function of a patient pre-diagnosis will play a role in exercise tolerance.[9] Physically active individuals, prior to diagnosis, have a greater chance of feeling recovered in as little as 3 weeks posttreatment than their deconditioned counterparts; and breast cancer patients who participated in preoperative exercise experienced enhanced shoulder range of movement and upper extremity functional recovery with a reduction in postoperative pain.[10]

Symptomology such as pain, temporary swelling, tenderness, infection, increased stiffness in joints, "hardness" due to scar tissue that forms at the surgical site,[11] weight fluctuations, and low self-esteem all factor into their lack of motivation to exercise. Survivors confess that along with lifestyle disruptions that may limit the prioritization of regular exercise, they lack energy and/or motivation. This lack of motivation to exercise may be largely due to Cancer-Related Fatigue (CRF). CRF often begins immediately upon diagnosis with studies reporting a prevalence in patients of up to 96%.[12] Compared with the fatigue experienced by healthy individuals, CRF is more severe and distressing and often not relieved with rest. For many CRF can persist for years, even after treatment has ended, drastically affecting their ability to return to the workplace, restore independent living, and resume normal activities of daily life.

CELLULAR ENVIRONMENT

For much of the twentieth century, the vast majority of scientific efforts to understand and destroy cancer have focused on the cells but not on the environment in which they live: the microenvironment. Cells in the human body, when operating under normal conditions, have specific jobs to do. They receive instructions from both their genetic material and signals from their environment. They respond by obeying these commands. Cancer researcher Helene Langevin said that, "cancer cells are cells that have gone rogue: they march to the beat of their own drum".[13] Under normal circumstances there is a dynamic yet stable interaction between cells and their surrounding extra cellular matrix (ECM). Cancer development results when there are alterations to those normal interactions. Cancer cells seem to behave as masters of division, multiplying out of control and not stopping when it is appropriate, gradually invading the body.

Cellular response to both chronically inflamed tissue and cancer-associated tissues is to become contractile, increasing stiffness in the ECM by generating sustained and continued tension on the ECM. Increased stiffness in the ECM is accompanied by greater interstitial pressure and lymphatic flow, which may predispose an individual to fibrosis, cancer invasion, and metastasis.

EXERCISE AND CANCER

In the last two decades it has become clear that regular physical exercise plays a vital role in the prevention and/or management of several chronic medical conditions, including various forms of cancer.[14] The strongest evidence exists for colon cancer, breast cancer, and cardiovascular diseases.[15] Previously, there was a lack of scientific evidence to support that exercise was safe for cancer patients or that it was a wise choice. It was typical for clinicians to advise patients to rest and recover post-treatment and avoid physical exercise. This has changed. There is a growing body of exercise-oncology research that strongly suggests exercise greatly reduces the risk of cancer recurrence as well as enhances quality of life.[16–18]

Numerous organizations provide evidence-based, physical exercise guidance for cancer patients. The American Heart Association (AHA),[19] the American College of Sports Medicine (ACSM),[20] and the U.S. Department of Health and Human Services (HHS)[6] recommend that individuals with chronic conditions such as cancer should be as physically active as their abilities and conditions allow. AHA recommends that cancer patients follow a cardio rehab plan to as some cancer treatments can weaken or damage the heart. In 2018, HHS reported that physically active cancer survivors have a lower risk of death due to cancer, improved fitness and physical function, reduced risk of heart disease, and fewer adverse treatment side effects. ACSM published recommendations and guidelines with specific Exercise Guidelines for Cancer in 2010.[21]

American College of Sports Medicine (ACSM) 2010 Exercise Guidelines for Cancer

- Exercise can lower the risk for colon, breast, endometrial, kidney, bladder, esophagus, and stomach cancers.
- Exercise is generally safe for cancer survivors.
- Exercise during and after cancer treatment can relieve fatigue, anxiety, depression, and improve physical function and quality of life and mitigate cancer-related fatigue.

- Exercise can improve common cancer-related health outcomes, including anxiety, bone health, depressive symptoms, falls, fatigue, health-related quality of life, lymphedema, nausea, pain, physical functioning, and sleep. Implications for other outcomes, such as chemotherapy-induced peripheral neuropathy and cognitive functioning, remain uncertain.
- Exercise programming should focus on a combination of aerobic, resistance, and flexibility training. Cancer survivors should aim for 150 min per week of aerobic activity, two or more days a week of resistance training for all major muscle groups, and flexibility training.

At the time the ACSM 2010 guidelines were published, there was insufficient scientific evidence to inform specific exercise prescriptions for cancer, therefore only general recommendations were given. However, that 2010 landmark publication triggered an influx of interest in research increasing the number of randomized controlled exercise trials in cancer survivors by 281% (PubMed Search completed March 2018) to over 2,500 published randomized controlled trials.

The increased availability of high-quality randomized controlled trials of exercise in cancer survivors prompted the ACSM in 2018 to convene an International Multidisciplinary Roundtable on Physical Activity and Cancer Prevention and Control, with the goal to update the 2010 recommendations. It was acknowledged that the exercise recommendations put forward in 2010 may be unachievable for cancer survivors with physical limitations and that benefits may come from less exercise. The roundtable recognized the need for more specific evidence-based exercise prescription to improve common side effects of a cancer diagnosis and treatment, namely anxiety, depressive symptoms, fatigue, health-related quality of life, and physical function, along with safety of exercise training in persons with or at risk of breast cancer-related lymphedema.

The exercise prescription recommendations are based on frequency, intensity, time, and type (FITT). These changes in recommendations are designed to better guide fitness and other health care professionals who train or care for cancer survivors. In 2019 ACSM published their consensus of the findings[9]:

- Exercise is generally safe for cancer survivors and that every survivor should "avoid inactivity".
- Specific doses of aerobic, combined aerobic plus resistance training, and/or resistance training could improve common cancer-related health outcomes, including anxiety, depressive symptoms, fatigue, physical functioning, and health-related quality of life.
- Exercise programming should be monitored and customized to suit the immediate needs of the cancer patient and programming should be designed to address specific outcomes survivors wish to tackle including anxiety, depressive symptoms, fatigue, physical functioning, and health-related quality of life.
- Supervised training programs are more effective than unsupervised or home-based interventions with outcomes such as anxiety, depressive symptoms, health-related quality of life, and physical function.

The 2019 recommendations should serve as a guide for the fitness and health care professionals working with cancer survivors. Treatment for cancer patients differ from individual to individual due to many factors: age, extent of disease, comorbid state, and current physical condition.

Practitioners should be well versed in the type of cancer, current stage of treatment, type of medication(s), and potential side effects with exercise. Appropriately directed exercise therapy is a critical component in the cancer patient's journey to recovery. More research is needed to fill remaining gaps in knowledge to better serve cancer survivors, as well as fitness and health care professionals, to improve clinical practice.

CANCER, FASCIA, AND MOVEMENT THERAPY

While the relationship between cancer and fascia has been a relatively quiet topic in the scientific and therapeutic worlds, researchers are starting to recognize the potential importance of fascia in cancer, especially when it comes to integrative medicine, not just drugs and pharmacology.[22] Therapeutic work to rebuild the body may involve rehabilitation of the fascia, which could have been damaged in treatment.

Recent findings that favor exercise over drugs and pharmacology

- Exercise helps reduce the risk of developing cancer, cancer progression, and recurrence.[8]
- Cardiovascular and intense exercise increases the circulation of immune cells, which helps fight off disease.[23]
- Intense exercise stimulates production and circulation of the Natural Killer (NK) and Killer T cells.[24] These protect against bacteria and viruses and reduce systemic inflammation. Inflammation is an extremely problematic human condition and is related to chronic musculoskeletal pain, different types of inflammatory diseases, and cancer. The reduction of inflammation is favorable for cancer patients.
- Stress reduction practices like yoga, meditation, and/or breath work could be possible solutions to increased stress levels brought on by cancer. Clinical studies of breast cancer patients, 3 years posttreatment, show that stress-induced inflammatory markers could lead to an increase in morbidity and mortality.[25] And, that chronic stress can play a role in the etiology of tumor growth, progression, and metastasis.[26]
- Mechanical factors, such as physical force or exercise, can be a potential target for therapeutic intervention. As observed in animal models, just 10 min a day of simple stretching can potentially slow down the advance of cancer.[27]
- Exercise may have an analgesic effect on the body.[28] Manual therapies and exercise may stimulate the endocannabinoid system, located deep in the fascial tissue, thus increasing significant serum levels of the "bliss molecule" anandamide.[29]
- Having strong fascial tissue may help prevent tumors from spreading. Resistance exercise mechanically loads the fascial elements strengthening the fascial membranes, which could help prevents tumorigenesis and metastasis.[30]

ALTERNATIVE MOVEMENT THERAPIES

Most all of the published exercise recommendations are specific to cardiorespiratory and resistance training. There is not as much mainstream awareness of therapies that address the psychological trauma patients experience. Dealing with a life-threatening disease and living with extended periods of stress, can often lead to an increase in sympathetic nervous system (SNS) activity.[31] Sympathetic activation may cause fascial contractions and potentially lead to an increase in fascial stiffness.[32,33]

The combination of moderate-to-low intensity movement therapy with integrative, contemplative practices such as yoga, meditation, Pilates, and tai chi has shown improvements in sleep, anxiety, depression, and quality of life for cancer patients.[34,35] Given contemplative practices help decrease sympathetic tone, it could be speculated that it may, in turn, help decrease fascial stiffness.

Throughout the past decade there has been a positive trend toward movement therapies that target the body's fascial system and fascial structures. The fascial movement programming protocols include exercises and procedures that foster proper force transmission and hydration in the myofascial continuities and joint structures, employ better elastic recoil in the tendinous structures, and improve on sensory stimulation to enhance kinesthetic awareness and proprioception. There are various props such as foam rollers, spiky mats and/or balls, vibration rollers or sticks, and elastic bands all designed to facilitate tissue hydration, enhance the elastic properties, increase parasympathetic activity, and enhance sensory function.

I've been fortunate to witness some of these programs and to work on teams to design specific fascial fitness programs for both healthy individuals and those with chronic disease including cancer. In fact, many of the cancer patients my team and I have worked with report feeling better postexercise and believe fascial movement therapy played a role in helping them tolerate the side effects and symptoms from cancer-related treatments such as chemotherapy and radiation.

PRETREATMENT

Upon diagnosis patients may undergo a continuum of defensive and protective behaviors, both emotional and physical. This pretreatment phase is the time to begin preparing the mind and body for what is to come. Teaching patients/clients meditative practices and breathing techniques can assist in the mind-body connection. Because this is pretreatment, there are not many exercise restrictions. However, there should be a significant focus on muscular strength and endurance. Daily movement is key to keeping both the mind stimulated and all systems of the body functioning.

GODARD EXPERIMENTS

For almost a decade, Hubert Godard and a team of researchers from the National Cancer Institute in Milan observed the physical and psychological damage of women with breast cancer. They conducted experiments with different groups of patients while walking and performing movements of daily life. One group was in the preoperative phase and the other in the postsurgical phase. In the preoperative group, they observed as many as 50% had already begun to lose "pendulousness", i.e., the rhythmic swinging quality of gait. This loss was observed in the affected limbs (arms), often with just the news of the diagnosis. In the postsurgical group, they found unusual postsurgical limitations of the shoulder girdle that could not be explained through traditional examinations The pendulousness would further decrease after surgery, with 65% demonstrating a loss of pendular motion during gait in the arm on the affected side. In some cases, there was a complete cessation of movement in the arm. The arm appeared almost lifeless, anchored to the trunk. Yet, when prompted to swing their arms symmetrically they did so with no difficulty.[36]

The experiments by Godard and his team have had a significant impact in my practice and programming of both preoperative and postoperative exercise programs. As witnessed in these experiments, patients diagnosed with breast cancer will begin to guard their body, subconsciously protecting the arm on the affected side. They keep it close to their side and do not allow it to hang loosely or swing naturally with gait. The early onset of this protective behavior may result in a physical manifestation, making the connective tissue more rigid and stiff, impacting the health and function of the muscles. In a rat model, immobilized limbs become rigid and lose elasticity and the connective tissue fibers become adhesive in as little as 2–3 weeks.[37]

In my experience, the patients who enter the treatment process more aware of their bodies and physically stronger have an easier time dealing with the physical limitations post-surgery. It is such a benefit when, as a movement therapist or practitioner you have the luxury to work with an individual pretreatment. You can make a significant impact on their state physically and emotionally.

POSTTREATMENT

Postoperative programming should include steps to restore the health of the damaged or compromised myofascial continuities, facilitate slide and glide of tissues between adjacent structures, decrease excessive scar tissue build, build strength of the entire kinematic chain, address postural dysfunctions, help to regain sensory awareness, teach or restore proper breathing techniques, and regain strength and endurance to improve their quality of life.

I have broken down the rehabilitation process into two segments and begin after preliminary tissue rehabilitation has occurred and/or the medical team has cleared the patient to do gentle range of motion and low-load strengthening. These phases are designed to reeducate the body-mind connection and to develop a strong physical foundation. The exercises can be used throughout the course of the patient's cancer journey to restore and rebuild their bodies.

CASE STUDY—CLIENT WITH BREAST CANCER

A female patient was looking for exercises to help with her hip pain. She was 60 years old. While completing her comprehensive health history screen, she revealed she had been diagnosed with breast cancer 9 months before. Her treatment included having a mastectomy with a Transverse Rectus Abdominus Muscle (TRAM) flap reconstruction. Her TRAM flap surgery involved making an incision along the lower abdomen and taking an oval section of skin, fat, blood vessels, and the rectus abdominis muscle from the lower half of the belly and rerouting it to the chest to form a breast. The rectus abdominis muscle mobilizes the trunk into flexion by pulling the ribs and pelvis inward, but it also serves as a facilitator in upright posture and, along with the deeper abdominal muscles, acts as a shield and protects the viscera. The absence of this muscle could result in movement compensation.

During evaluation we found she had overactive hip flexors with a resulting tightness of the ipsilateral lumbar erector spinae and quadratus lumborum. We concluded that her hip pain was likely due to her years of movement compensation post breast cancer surgery and not necessarily an isolated hip joint problem. The client also shared that when she asked her medical team what she should do for physical therapy, she was advised to walk regularly. Just weeks post-surgery, lacking in motivation but anxious to recover her pre-surgery strength, she began her daily walking regimen. Her neighborhood was up on a steep hill, which challenged her, but she didn't give up. It was then that she started to experience hip pain and hip clicking.

Upon initial examination, her entire body was weak and deconditioned. She was very stiff and lacked coordination. Also, during a static postural analysis her navel was revealed to be completely off center. It shifted to the opposite side of where the rectus had been removed, likely due to postsurgical scar tissue. I noted it in her chart and brought it to her awareness.

I asked her to give up her walking for a short while in order to reestablish proper biomechanics and gain strength. We started with two 30-min sessions per week. We used the Pilates reformer, stability chair, and various small props to help increase her proprioceptive awareness and restore the slide and glide of her connective tissue. She had significant lack of sensation in her shoulder and chest area, with minimal if any movement of the scapula on the thorax. We followed a gentle, restorative exercise protocol for her shoulders and hips, strengthened her core, and worked on balance and walking biomechanics.

In only 2 months, our 30-min supervised sessions were increased to 60 min. After 3 months, she was pain free and had begun to regain physical confidence. Also, after gentle assisted fascial stretching of the abdominal area and mobilization of the hip, the connective tissue around her abdomen began to soften. Gradually her navel moved closer to center. It has never completely re-centered, but the tissue below her skin is more pliable. Within 9 months, her audible hip clicking with basic everyday movements was gone and she was able to resume her passion for long walks and hiking without discomfort or pain. After 13 months, she was able to join a group Pilates Reformer class.

For over a decade, she has remained physically active, she does Pilates twice per week, resistance training once per week, plays tennis once or twice per week and goes on long walks three to five times per week. For her yearly vacation, she joins a group for a week-long walking trip. Four years from our first session, she was diagnosed with breast cancer of her other breast. Her treatment included a lumpectomy and radiation. Due to her high level of fitness, her recovery was, in a word, remarkable.

She is now in her early 70s, cancer free, and claims she is stronger than she has ever been in her entire life.

This case study illuminates our central points—that being physically prepared for cancer treatment helps with both the physical and emotional recovery, and physical activity posttreatment helps restore physical function and reduces pain.

CONCLUSION

Exercise and being physically active has been proven to be a powerful, inexpensive, and joyful way to prevent disease. Strengthening the body through the combination of aerobic, resistance training, and fascial movement therapy is the best prescription. Although there is still much to learn about the absolute role various exercise modalities play, we know it can make an individual feel better, potentially look better, and most certainly move better.

Cancer patients ultimately have to choose the path that is best suited for them and adheres to their lifestyle. Individuals who were not involved in an exercise program pre-diagnosis face the biggest challenge. We only need to inspire them to get moving and ensure them that it will indeed add to their quality of life long term. We find being part of a community program or working out with a buddy is always good reinforcement and yields better compliancy.

It is highly recommended for cancer patients to seek out qualified practitioners who are well versed in cancer care and recovery. A qualified, compassionate therapist will teach the cancer patient to become self reliant, help them improve their physical functional for everyday activities and empower them to live a quality life. The stronger an individual is before and during treatment, the better the results posttreatment.

REFERENCES

1. Cancer Research UK. 2020. www.cancerresearchuk.org/health-professional/cancer-statistics/worldwide-cancer#heading-Zero (accessed February 10, 2020).
2. Miller, K.D., Nogueria, L., Mariotto, A.B., et al. 2019. Cancer treatment and survivorship statistics. *Cancer Journal for Clinicians* 69:363–85.
3. Scott, J.M., Nilsen, T.S., Gupts, D., et al. 2018. Exercise therapy and cardiovascular toxicity in cancer. *Circulation* 137(11):1176–91.
4. Galvao, D.A., Newton, R.U., Taaffe, D.R., et al. 2008. Can exercise ameliorate the increased risk of cardiovascular disease and diabetes associated with ADT? *Nature Clinical Practice Urology* 5(6):306–7.
5. Galvao, D.A., Taaffe, D.R., Spry, N., et al. 2009. Reduced muscle strength and functional performance in men with prostate cancer undergoing androgen suppression: A comprehensive cross-sectional investigation. *Prostate Cancer and Prostatic Diseases* 12(2):198–203.
6. U.S. Department of Health and Human Services. 2018. Physical activity guidelines advisory committee report, 78–86. www.hhs.gov/fitness/be-active/physical-activity-guidelines-for-americans/index.html (accessed February 10, 2020).
7. Dieli-Conwright, C.M. and Orozco, B.Z. 2015. Exercise after breast cancer treatment: Current perspectives. *Breast Cancer: Targets and Therapy* 7:353–62.
8. Hoffman, P. 2018. Cancer and exercise: Warburg hypothesis, tumour metabolism and high-intensity anaerobic exercise. *Sports* 6(1):10.
9. Campbell, K.L., Winters-Stone, K.M., Wiskemann, J., et al. 2019. Exercise guidelines for cancer survivors: Consensus statement from international multidisciplinary roundtable. *Medicine & Science in Sports & Exercise* 51(11):2375–90.

10. Yang, A., Sokolof, J. and Guliati, A. 2018. The effect of preoperative exercise on upper extremity recovery following breast cancer surgery: A systematic review. *International Journal of Rehabilitation Research* 41(3):189–96.

11. Fourie, W. 2008. Considering wider myofascial involvement as a possible contributor to upper extremity dysfunction following treatment for primary breast cancer. *Journal of Bodywork and Movement Therapies* 12(4):349–55.

12. Stasi, R., Abriani, L., Beccaglia, P., et al. 2003. Cancer-related fatigue: Evolving concepts in evaluation and treatment. *Cancer* 98:1786–801.

13. Langevin, H. 2018. Connective tissue, inflammation and cancer. Lecture presented June 5, 2018 at Grand Rounds at Osher Center for Integrative Medicine, Harvard Medical School, Boston, MA.

14. Courneya, K.S. and Friedenreich, C.M. 2007. Physical activity and cancer control. *Seminars in Oncology Nursing* 23(4):242–52.

15. Kruk, J. 2007. Physical activity in the prevention of the most frequent chronic diseases: An analysis of the recent evidence. *Asian Pacific Journal of Cancer Prevention* 8(3):325–338.

16. Katlin, C.M., Coltrera F., Gardiner, J., et al. 2006. *The Breast Cancer Survivor's Fitness Plan: A Doctor-Approved Workout Plan for a Strong Body and Lifesaving Results.* New York: McGraw-Hill Education.

17. Mutrie, N., Campbell, A.M., Whyte, F., et al. 2007. Benefits of a supervised group exercise programme for women being treated for early stage breast cancer: Pragmatic, randomised, controlled trial. *BMJ* 334(7592):517. https://doi.org/10.1136/bmj.39094.648553.AE

18. Sprague, B.L., Trentham-Dietz, A., Newcomb, P.A., et al. 2007. Lifetime recreational and occupational physical activity and risk of in situ and invasive breast cancer. *Cancer Epidemiology, Biomarkers & Prevention* 16(2):236–43.

19. American Heart Association. 2019. How can therapy for heart attack patients help cancer survivors? www.heart.org/en/news/2019/04/08/how-can-therapy-for-heart-attack-patients-help-cancer-survivors (accessed February 10, 2020).

20. Haskell, W.L., Lee, I.M., Pate R.R., et al. 2007. Physical activity and public health: Updated recommendation for adults from the American College of Sports Medicine and the American Heart Association. *Medicine & Science in Sports & Exercise* 39(8):1423–34.

21. Schmitz, K.H., Corneya, K.S., Matthews, C., et al. 2010. American college of sports medicine roundtable on exercise guidelines for cancer survivors. *Medicine & Science in Sports & Exercise* 42(7):1409–26.

22. Langevin, H., Keely, P., Mao, J., et al. Connecting (tissues): How research in fascia biology can impact integrative oncology. *Cancer Research* 76(2):6159–62.

23. Kwak, S., Lee, J., Zhang, D., et al. 2018. Angiogenesis: Focusing on the effects of exercise in aging and cancer. *Journal of Exercise Nutrition & Biochemistry* 22(3):21–26.

24. Idorn, M. and Hojman, P. 2016. Exercise-dependent regulation of NK cells in cancer protection. *Trends in Molecular Medicine* 22(7):565–77.

25. Pierce, B.L., Ballard-Barbash, R., Bernstein, L., et al. 2009. Elevated biomarkers of inflammation are associated with reduced survival among breast cancer. *Journal of Clinical Oncology* 27(21):3437–44.

26. Thaker, P.H., Jan, L.Y., Kamat, A.A., et al. 2006. Chronic stress promotes tumor growth and angiogenesis in a mouse model of ovarian carcinoma. *Natural Medicine* 12:939–44.

27. Berrueta, L., Bergholz, J., Munoz, D., et al. 2018. Stretching reduces tumor growth in a mouse breast cancer model. *Scientific Reports* 8:1–7. https://doi.org/10.1038/s41598-018-26198-7

28. Zügel, M., Maganaris, C.N., Wilkey, J., et al. 2018. Fascial tissue research in sports medicine: From molecules to tissue adaptation, injury and diagnostics: Consensus statement. *British Journal of Sports Medicine* 52:1497.

29. Fede, C., Albertin, G., Petrelli, L., et al. 2016. Expression of the endocannabinoid receptors in human fascial tissue. *European Journal of Histochemistry* 60(2):2643.

30. Pozzi, A., Yurchenco, P.D. and Iozzo, R.V. 2017. The nature and biology of basement membranes. *Matrix Biology* 57–58:1–11.

31. Won, E. and Kim, Y.K. 2016. Stress, the autonomic nervous system, and the immune-kynurenine pathway in the etiology of depression. *Current Neuropharmacology* 14(7):665–73.

32. Staubesand, J. and Li, Y. 1996. On the fine structure of the crural fascia, with particular reference to the epi- and intrafascial nerves. *Manuelle Medizin* 34(5):196–200.

33. Bhowmick, S., Singh, A., Flavell, R.A., et al. 2009. The sympathetic nervous system modulates CD4(+)FoxP3(+) regulatory T cells via a TGF-beta-dependent mechanism. *Journal of Leukocyte Biology* 86(6):1275–83.

34. Stan, D.L., Collins, N.M., Olsen, M.M., et al. 2012. The evolution of mindfulness-based physical interventions in breast cancer survivors. *Evidence-based Complimentary and Alternative Medicine* 2012:758641. https://doi.org/10.1155/2012/758641

35. Buettner, C.H., Kroenke, R.S., Phillips, R.B., et al. 2006. Correlates of use of different types of complementary and alternative medicine by breast cancer survivors in the Nurses' Health Study. *Breast Cancer Research and Treatment* 100(2):219–27.

36. Godard, H. et al., 2001. Motion ed e-motion in oncologia. In *Psiconologia*, ed. M. Bellani and D. Amadori, 875–81. Paris: Elsevier-Masson.

37. Järvinen, T.A., Józsa, L., Kannus, P., et al. 2002. Organization and distribution of intramuscular connective tissue in normal and immobilized skeletal muscles. An immunohistochemical, polarization and scanning electron microscopic study. *Journal of Muscle Research and Cell Motility* 23(3):245–54.

20 Clinical Foundations and Applications for Self-Myofascial Release with Balls, Rollers, and Tools

Jill Miller

CONTENTS

INTRODUCTION

Self-myofascial release (SMFR) is a tool for prehab and rehab using an object as a stress transfer-medium (STM). This self-directed form of care is a way to manage pain, improve movement, boost recovery, improve arterial function, and stimulate parasympathetic arousal. SMFR gives the user ability to apply their own therapeutic intervention for little, if any, cost. This chapter presents the current state of SMFR research and offers a holistic view of perspectives around pain management, chronic disease, performance enhancement, stress reduction, and tool hardness.

WHAT IS SMFR?

To define SMFR, we must first define myofascial release (MFR). MFR originates from the founder of Osteopathy, A.T. Still.[1] The "release" work uses a therapist's palpation skills to engage the fascial stretch barrier of a client with appropriate sustained pressure or a variety of manual mobilizations. Conversely, release can be achieved by shifting fascial tissues away from a restriction. In SMFR, an individual performs this MFR with a tool and uses it to assist its application in a self-guided manner. (See SMFR Tools below.)

There are many studies researching how therapist-applied fascia specific manual therapy affects fascial tissues. A quick glance at PubMed on December 20, 2019 using search terms "myofascial release" tabulated 462 papers; "myofascial massage" had 229. On the other hand, when seeking self-directed treatment, "self-massage" revealed 1,050; "self-myofascial release" rendered 107 articles; and "self-myofascial massage" provided 69.

It's important to note, that the term "myofascial release" implies that fascial tissues are being released and may be undergoing morphological changes. Two recent studies question the use of the term "release" when using SMFR tools. One study found that no morphological changes are actually taking place.[2] Another states: "The current evidence indicates that the term *self-myofascial release* is misleading and a misnomer … self-myofascial release may become prevalent and ubiquitous since it was widely incorporated before the likely rolling mechanisms were determined and elucidated".[3] Thus, for accuracy, the accepted term SMFR may need to transform in the future.

SMFR BENEFITS

Many benefits of SMFR are supported by current research. The list below includes only a fraction of representative studies.

1. Improves movement coordination[4,5]
2. Improves joint range of motion (ROM)/mobility[6–11,12,13]
3. Increases torque[10,11]
4. Decreases muscle fatigue/soreness/delayed onset muscle soreness (DOMS)[14]
5. Decreases pain[15,16]
6. Reduces arterial stiffness and improves vascular endothelial function[17,18]
7. Induces physiological relaxation and increased parasympathetic features[12]
8. Helpful for lymph edema[19,20]
9. Ideal for individuals who are touch averse[21]

Many SMFR benefits run parallel with manual MFR, although some manual MFR benefits supported by research such as scar tissue attenuation[22] and mental health are not yet exclusively researched with SMFR. Although user and therapist reported SMFR benefits like scar tissue mitigation, improved sleep, and emotional self-regulation have not yet been studied, anecdotal evidence exists.[23–25]

SMFR TOOLS

Any object used to knead, compress, stroke, prod, or vibrate your body without breaking skin is considered a stress transfer medium (STM). Throughout history, people have used such objects to rub their aches and pains. The oldest device found to date, a Neolithic jade ritual blade from China, is thought to be from 2000 BCE.[23,26] STM tools can be classified as various sized balls, broad foam rollers (FR), and rolling sticks (RS). STM are crafted from a variety of rubber, foam, plastic, metal, and wood textiles of differing indentation hardness measured on a Shore scale via a durometer.[27] A durometer is the measure of hardness of a material, which can be defined as the material's resistance to permanent indentation. Three different scales using a Shore measurement are used depending on the material properties within the object. There are 12 different scales within Shore, the most common are Type A for soft rubber and plastics (rubber shoe heel, hockey puck), Type D for hard rubber and plastics (hard hat, bowling ball), and Type OO for sponge and foam rubber and plastics (racquet ball, chewing gum). Only one published paper disclosed durometer specifics.[28]

Some tools are specifically designed for STM, while others like commonly found sports balls, are used for self massage. Tool choice is vast and provides "different strokes for different folks". One person's body mass and pressure pain threshold (PPT) will favor certain tools, while another finds that same tool does not address every symptom or need. Some tools are suitable to one body part, i.e., a wand for internal pelvic floor,[29] but are nonsensical for another part, i.e., FR are more often used on large myofascial units of the thighs, not on the smaller myofascial units of the face (there were no studies with FR and face, however there were two studies with ball and foot).

TOOL HARDNESS

Is there an advantage to using hard tools vs. soft tools? Given the hardness variances of different objects, as well as personal touch sensitivity, it can be challenging to determine. Standardizing pressure is tricky for research design because each person's PPT and stretch tolerance (ST) will be different regardless of their athletic training or health. In many studies, especially with foam rollers, there is a repetitive instruction of subjects to apply "maximum tolerable pressure".[18,30] Perhaps this reveals a bias that more pressure is better, or more colloquially "no pain, no gain".

Tool hardness is likely a key factor in allowing a person's tissues to comply with STM, or conversely to brace against it (muscle spindle reactivity). Pain perception and PPT would seem to be activated by tool hardness and yet, there are few studies analyzing this.

Softer tools seem to have the 'edge' on restoring tissues. Blyum and Driscoll were the first to present on this topic; "Mechanical stress transfer—the fundamental physical basis of all manual therapy techniques" at the 2012 Fascia Congress and revealed that "using a weaker STM during manual therapy (for example soft foam or rubber vs. hard foam or wood) techniques may improve stress transfer. It is therefore advisable to adopt a STM that will facilitate and optimize stress transfer to the targeted tissues".[31]

A 2018 study on tool hardness displayed significant differences in a group of 30 subjects in their mid-60s with neck pain. The research team used a soft inflatable rubber ball with Shore A hardness of 45 and a hard massage ball with Shore A hardness of 90 (the equivalent of a Lacrosse sport ball)[27] (Figure 20.1).

While analyzing posterior neck muscles, "a soft inflatable rubber ball (SIRB) is more advantageous than a hard massage ball (HMB) for pressing the soft tissue

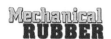 **Shore Durometer* Conversion Chart**

Approximate Hardness Value
(to be used as a guide)

Type	Extra Soft / Soft (Chewing Gum)				Medium Soft (Pencil Eraser)			Medium Hard (Windshield Wiper Blade)							Hard (Skate Wheel)			Extra Hard (Bowling Ball)		
Shore A Rubber, Soft Plastic & Polyurethane	5	10	15	20	25	30	35	40	45	50	55	60	65	70	75	80	85	90	95	100
Shore B** Rigid Rubber				6	12	17	22	27	32	37	42	47	51	56	62	66	71	76	81	85
Shore C** Rubber & Plastic						9	12	14	17	20	24	28	32	37	42	47	52	59	70	77
Shore D Hard Rubber & Plastic						6	7	8	10	12	14	16	19	22	25	29	33	39	46	58
Shore O** Soft Rubber	8	14	21	28	35	42	48	53	57	61	65	69	72	75	79	84				

Type	Soft (Slice of Bread)				Medium Soft (Seat Cushion)			Medium Firm (Mouse Pad)							Firm (Tennis Ball)	
Shore OO Sponge	45	55	62	70	76	80	83	86	88	90	91	93	94	95	97	98

Type	Very Soft (Slice of Bread)	Extra Soft (Pillow)	Soft (Mattress)	Firm (Tennis Ball)	Extra Firm (Styrofoam Cup)	Very Firm (Life Preserver)
Density (lb/ft³) Foam	0 - 2	2 - 5	5 - 9	9 - 13	13 - 16.5	16.5+

*Durometer is the standard for hardness measurement of rubber, plastic, sponge & non-metallic material.

** Not commonly used

www.mechanicalrubber.com

FIGURE 20.1   Durometer Conversion Chart illustrating hardness comparisons for rubbers, plastics, foams, and so on. A helpful guide to understanding the indentation hardness of different self-myofascial release tools. (Courtesy of Mechanical Rubber.)

deeply. This finding would be related to reduced muscle tension and discomfort in the SIRB condition when compared with the HMB condition".[28] The Korean team also found a significant increase in neck extension ROM and a decrease in tissue thickness with the SIRB. This decrease allowed the SIRB to approximate the bony prominence and presumably lengthen fascial tissues. "Our findings suggest that firm pressure by an HMB increases muscle tension, which resists pressure propagation into the deep muscles".

Although their results are favorable toward a softer tool, further studies are needed to clarify what the optimal hardness is for SMFR and how much pressure provides ideal release.

The majority of SMFR studies use FR or RS, and no durometers were disclosed. FR and RS are constructed from a variety of compressed foams, and many use the extra-hard plastic PVC pipe as a base layer that is surrounded by foam or rubber. It is possible that results in many studies would be different if hardness were factored in as a variable. A hard SMFR tool of any shape comes with potential risks. A May 2019 case report[32] in *Medicine (Baltimore)* describes a rare injury to the tibial division of the sciatic nerve in a 50-year-old woman who used a hard massage ball in her gluteals.

- Clinically, I observe that patients respond better with soft STM. It doesn't have to hurt to work. The STM is not exclusively interacting with myofascia, it is also interfacing with skin, mobilizing fluids (blood, lymph, extracellular matrix, interstitial fluids), migrant cells (especially immune cells) within tissues, and multiple neural and vascular tissues as well as approximating non-moving bony prominences. Thus, a hard tool may activate the body's innate defense system/protective mechanism to minimize risk. The user feels that as "tension" and may decide that SMFR is uncomfortable and give up their attempt to self treat, or they may suffer through their own neurological tension, which is counterproductive for therapeutic results.

Less can be way more when it comes to application.[33] According to Paul Standley the duration and rate of loading can alter fibroblast production of cytokines. In *in vitro* experiments, he "stretched cells 6% beyond their resting length at a loading rate of 3%/s. Strain was held for 60s before being released at a rate of 1.5%/s back to resting length". This low grade pressure helped damaged muscle cells to repair. "If clinically translatable, restorative strain regimens such as myofascial release applied to a fibroblast-rich tissue following injury may facilitate muscle repair".[34] Further stress does not result in more stretch but can induce non-therapeutic tissue damage.[35]

Pressure variables, time under load, and tool hardness are a blind spot in current research. These are factors that imitate the intention of skilled therapeutic human touch and merit further study. Now, let's take a closer look at some other research findings.

PERFORMANCE AND RECOVERY

Performance and mobility gains are of great interest to the athletic and rehab community. Clinicians would like to see patients return to function, and sports therapists and trainers celebrate performance enhancements that are non-drug generated. A number of studies show improvements in whole body mobility[3,9] torque, single joint ROM,[9,10,11,13,14] and attenuation of DOMS.[15]

A systematic review of SMFR papers published prior to 2015 reveals "SMFR with a foam roll or roller massager appears to have short-term effects on increasing joint ROM without negatively affecting muscle performance and may help attenuate decrements in muscle performance and DOMS after intense exercise. Short bouts of SMFR prior to exercise do not appear to effect muscle performance".[35]

A 2019 meta-analysis of 21 studies compared and contrasted FR and RS rolling pre vs. post activity (known colloquially as "Precovery vs. Recovery"). "Overall, it was determined that the effects of foam rolling on performance and recovery are rather minor and partly negligible, but can be relevant in some cases (e.g., to increase sprint performance and flexibility or to reduce muscle pain sensation). Evidence seems to justify the widespread use of foam rolling as a warm-up activity rather than a recovery tool".[16] However, this meta-analysis with heterogeneous samplings of FR and RS also states "The largest average effects of FR in general and post-rolling in particular were found for the alleviation of perceived muscle pain".[16] Minimizing DOMS is a great motivator for those who need or want to play hard in their next game tomorrow. It is interesting to note that the phenomenon of DOMS has been shown to generate the greatest sensitivity at the epimysial fascia, rather than within the muscle belly.[36]

Balls have yet to merit their own systematic review or meta-analysis, but these spherical tools provide additional insights. Capobianco's recent studies in 2018, 2019 demonstrate rolling the gastrocnemius on a soft rubber ball in a sample of both college-aged and middle-aged adults was able to offset a stretch-induced force deficit. Both cohorts displayed increases in torque and ROM[10,11] The middle-aged adults showed the strongest ROM increase: ankle dorsiflexion doubled (24.5%) compared with stretching alone (12.5%). Their average muscle force production increased by 16%. As humans age, ankle ROM and strength often decrease, this decline is a primary driver of slip and falls. In other words, these ball studies with an aging population provide a different perspective on "Precovery/Recovery" as a longevity strategy.

An even newer study evaluated rolling a hard foam ball on the plantar fascia of a sample of 168 participants with a wide range of ages, 19–85 years.[37] These participants performed a sit-and-reach test, then rolled for 2 min per foot and then re-performed their test. Hamstring extensibility increased across all age groups, but the ROM increase lessened as participants' age increased. This study could act as a template for other researchers to provide insights into the spectrum of fascial behavior throughout a life cycle.

CHRONIC PAIN/DISEASE MANAGEMENT

Chronic pain treatments using STM can potentially reduce or eliminate the need for pain medication.[15,19–21,23,29] Studies that showed improvements from disease-related injuries include functional improvements post stroke using a tennis ball protocol,[38] and pain reduction and movement improvements after a 20 week multi-tool program for fibromyalgia.[15] Vascular improvements might point to using SMFR for circulation issues.[12] Chronic pelvic pain and medication was significantly reduced using a pelvic wand tool.[29]

SMFR can also be performed with one's own hands. An 11-month study of temporomandibular pain benefited 71% of the participants who followed a self-massage protocol.[39] Another 2016 study[20] followed 1,000 women after radical mastectomy for 1 year. All 1,000 were given physical exercises, and half of these women were also taught light touch massage strokes to mobilize their scars and promote lymph flow. "Manual lymph drainage, when combined with physical exercise, effectively prevents upper limb lymphedema, alleviates scar formation, and stimulates functional recovery". These studies are notable because they illuminate questions that future research might investigate about how to utilize tools in a light pressure manner rather than maximum tolerable pressure.

ACUTE USE

The majority of studies demonstrate time-limited (AKA acute) results, with subjects in the lab rolling a single body part for 60 s–2 min. Beardsley and Skarabot published a systematic review[40] of self-myofascial release and found an abundance of studies covering acute use.

> SMFR appears to have a range of potentially valuable effects for both athletes and the general population, including increasing flexibility and enhancing recovery. Specifically, SMFR seems to lead to increased joint ROM acutely and does not impede athletic performance acutely. SMFR therefore seems suitable for use by athletes or the general population prior to exercise, training sessions or competition. SMFR seems to alleviate DOMS acutely and may therefore be suitable for use by athletes or the general population for enhancing recovery from exercise, training sessions or competition. There is also limited evidence that SMFR may lead to improved arterial function, improved vascular endothelial function, and increased parasympathetic nervous system activity acutely, which may also be useful in recovery.

In Beardsley's review, only four "long-term studies" were compared, their durations ranged from 1 to 8 weeks. The studies produced conflicting results on flexibility.[40]

LONGER DURATION STUDIES

A 2017 Spanish study is the first to provide 20 weeks of SMFR in a cohort with Fibromyalgia (FM). This study used a variety of STM's including balls and FR of different densities. Subjects were also led in twice weekly classes for 50 min and were given pressure options as their lessons progressed. "The application of a 20-week SMFR program may lead to a series of anatomical changes to myofascial tissue, correcting common pathological processes such as myofascial densification, fibrosis, adhesions and dehydration. With the improvement of myofascial viscoelasticity, these changes can enable correct gliding of the different fascial layers and therefore facilitate proper joint function".

They conclude "The continued application of a supervised program based on SMFR exercises that develop an adequate progression of pressure intensity on the muscles through the use of materials of different sizes and densities can improve the health-related quality of life of people with FM while having beneficial effects in terms of stiffness, fatigue, widespread pain intensity, and ROM".[15]

In contrast, another 4-week study compared rolling stick (RS) massage three times weekly vs. six times weekly. The participants rolled a RS from proximal to distal quadriceps for 30 s, followed by using the RS along their distal to proximal hamstrings for 30 s. They repeated this circuit four times (4 min of total rolling per session). They performed it either three times per week or six times per week for 4 weeks. The use of RS seemed to have no effect on ROM, PPT, muscle contraction, or jump performance of the young college-aged participants.[41]

It is unfair to directly compare these two studies, duration of rolling is radically different between the groups, as is the tool. But it demonstrates a gap in the research for longer duration studies and illuminates potential differences in tool hardness and application.

PARASYMPATHETIC AROUSAL

Massage is documented as inducing the relaxation response.[42] But can SMFR do the same? The interaction of an STM with skin, fascia, and myofascial tissues potentiates the relaxation response.[23,40] The shear friction on the body's tissues stimulates interstitial receptors and Ruffini endings, which dampen sympathetic tone.[43] Cardiac, vasculature, and nervous system effects are also evident.

To elaborate further, approximately 15 min of FR on different sections of the legs and back had a 30-min downregulating impact on subjects. "Our findings indicate that foam rolling decreases sympathovagal balance for 30 min postintervention, which is concurrent with an important hypotensive effect"[12] Nitric Oxide (NO), an endogenous vasodilator is also produced by FR, this decreases arterial stiffness and expands arteriole perfusion.[17] Manually massaging trigger points alters the activity of the autonomic nervous system via the prefrontal cortex to reduce subjective pain,[44] it decreases sympathetic tone and upregulates vagal tone.[45] "Because increased NO plays a major role in blood pressure (BP) regulation, and the current study showed acute decreases in BP, it is possible that the effect of FR on cardiac autonomic activity and BP can be mediated, at least in part, by this major regulator of vascular function".[12]

Another FR study targeted cortisol levels. When measuring cortisol levels 30 min after running on a treadmill, a control group who rested on the floor was compared with a group who FR'd for 30 min. Both groups had significant decreases in cortisol, but no significant differences between the two groups. The foam rolling group had slightly lower cortisol levels, but they were not significantly different.[46]

CLINICAL SUMMARY

Though limited data is published on the efficacy of SMFR, the existing studies are building a body of awareness about it. In a 2018 survey of allied health students at 12 universities in the United States, more than 50% of respondents knew about SMFR and more than 50% intended to use them in their future practices.[47] Thus, more research can help foster the benefits of this emerging intervention, especially as medical care costs rise. Performing SMFR is cost effective for users. A one-time tool purchase for on-demand treatment is more budget-friendly than paying for ongoing clinical services. This is especially advantageous for those with medical conditions who benefit from regular therapy or for populations not residing in proximity to providers. For clinicians who administer manual therapies, instructing clients to perform SMFR for home care is also a potential thumb/wrist/elbow repetitive-stress injury preventative strategy for the clinician, and could speed patient progress and positive outcomes.

Further research is needed to understand the potential mental health and wellness benefits of SMFR.[25,48] For touch-averse individuals, or those living touch-starved lives, SMFR can add a positive benefit. One 9-month study tracked caregivers of those with dementia and used ball self-massage in combination with relaxation strategies and breath work found that it improved "certain dimensions of psychological well-being".[25] With chronic insomnia a growing concern, appropriate SMFR application to boost parasympathetic physiology could potentially improve good sleep and reduce sleep-aid drug dependency given that users report sleep improvements with SMFR.[23,49]

What should researchers focus on for the future to improve accuracy and practical applications?

1. Tool hardness disclosures and/or comparisons.
2. Tool hardness interactions with different body parts and different body morphologies.
3. Tool application variations and myofascial technique variety. The majority of studies rolled their tools up and down along muscles bellies from origin to insertion The majority of these studies also looked at thigh muscles or posterior calf (the vastus lateralis and neighboring iliotibial band (IT) were very popular). What would happen if the tool were moved in a different manner, perhaps across a muscle, or by creating tissue shear rather than rolling?
4. Examine differences between self-directed SMFR, SMFR through instructor-led guidance, SMFR via prerecorded video instruction.
5. Longer duration studies.
6. What is the optimum length of time to perform SMFR? What is the optimum pressure?
7. Research on older populations and disease populations are needed. The majority of studies are performed on healthy college-aged adults.
8. Treatment based protocols for specific conditions/morbidities/populations. Researchers could use successful manual myofascial release protocols and adapt methods to replicate treatment with STM self-application. This could potentially enlarge the scope of self-treatment that enables autonomy and decreases care costs.
9. Mental health outcomes.

In summary, SMFR case reports that index morbidities and individual protocols may be useful as a cross-reference for patients who wish to make self-care health care a cost-sustainable priority. But as suggested earlier in this chapter, the term "self-myofascial release" may need to be re-languaged to a more accurate representation.[3] Terms like "self-myofascial stimulation", "self-myofascial manipulation" "self-myofascial mobilization" or simply "self-massage" would all be more accurate, but it is often difficult to change a term once it has traction in the public vernacular.

In the near future, more data is expected on vibration-based tools,[24] and we will know more about SMFR's impact on the brain. Current research in Germany (launched November 2018, concluding January 2021) is including SMFR as the placebo/control group in a large-scale study on breast cancer patients. This study focuses on cognitive impact of high-intensity interval training, the control group will have 20–35 min SMFR sessions three times weekly while undergoing chemotherapy.[50]

More than 100 patients will reveal a range of results never analyzed before, including systemic inflammation, neurotrophin, growth factor expression, brain vasculature changes, and more. It will also provide data on anxiety, depression, quality of life, sleeping disturbances fatigue, and more.

More specifically, this author encourages the reader to be their own laboratory, by doing their own SMFR self-research. Although subjective experience is uneven, there are abundant benefits to being the agent of fascial-tissue connection within oneself, whenever and wherever you need it. Soft-tissue and nervous system modulation are within everyone's grasp. It's possible that we enrich our somatosensory processing by using tools to help locate ourselves and enlarge our scope of embodiment.[51] Future generations may look forward to this form of preventative care and self-empowered rehabilitation.

DISCLOSURES

Author of a book on self-myofascial massage *The Roll Model*, Victory Belt Publishing 2014, and co-owner of Tune Up Fitness Worldwide, Inc.

REFERENCES

1. Boyajian-O'Neill, Lori A, Cardone, Dennis A. 2008. Practical Application of Osteopathic Manipulation in Sports Medicine in *The Sports Medicine Resource Manual*. Amsterdam, NL: Elsevier.
2. Yoshimura A, Inami T, Schleip R, et al. 2019. Effects of Self-myofascial Release Using a Foam Roller on Range of Motion and Morphological Changes in Muscle: A Crossover Study. *J Strength Cond Res*. 2019. doi:10.1519/JSC.0000000000003196.
3. Behm DG, Wilke. 2019. Do Self Myofascial Release Devices Release Myofascia? Rolling Mechanisms: A Narrative Review. *J Sports Med*. https://doi.org/10.1007/s40279-019-01149-y.
4. Le Gal J, Begon M, Gillet B, et al. 2018. Effects of Self-Myofascial Release on Shoulder Function and Perception in Adolescent Tennis Players. *J Sport Rehabil*. 27(6):530–535.
5. David E, Amasay T, Ludwig K, et al. 2019. The Effect of Foam Rolling of the Hamstrings on Proprioception at the Knee and Hip Joints. *Int J Exerc Sci*. 12(1):343–354.
6. Monteiro ER, Škarabot J, Vigotsky AD, et al. 2017. Acute Effects of Different Self-Massage Volumes on the FMS™ Overhead Deep Squat Performance. *Int J Sports Phys Ther*. 12(1):94–104.
7. Monteiro ER, Cavanaugh MT, Frost DM, et al. 2017. Is Self-Massage an Effective Joint Range-of-Motion Strategy? A Pilot Study. *J Bodyw Mov Ther*. 21(1):223–226.
8. Williams W, Selkow NM. 2019. Self-Myofascial Release of the Superficial Back Line Improves Sit-and-Reach Distance. *J Sport Rehabil*. 12:1–19. doi:10.1123/jsr.2018–0306.
9. Joshi DG, Balthillaya G, Prabhu A. 2018. Effect of Remote Myofascial Release on Hamstring Flexibility in Asymptomatic Individuals—A Randomized Clinical Trial. *J Bodyw Mov Ther*. 22(3):832–837. doi:10.1016/j.jbmt.2018.01.008.
10. Capobianco RA, Mazzo MM, Enoka RM. 2019. Self-Massage Prior to Stretching Improves Flexibility in Young and Middle-Aged Adults. *J Sports Sci*. 4:1–8. doi:10.1080/02640414.2019.1576253.
11. Capobianco RA, Almuklass AM, Enoka RM. 2018. Manipulation of Sensory Input Can Improve Stretching Outcomes. *Eur J Sport Sci*. 18(1):83–91. doi:10.1080/17461391.2017.1394370.

12. Lastova K, Nordvall M, Walters-Edwards, et al. 2018. Cardiac Autonomic and Blood Pressure Responses to an Acute Foam Rolling Session. *J Strength Cond Res.* 32(10):2825–2830.

13. Guillot A, Kerautret Y, Queyrel F. 2019. Foam Rolling and Joint Distraction with Elastic Band Training Performed for 5–7 Weeks Respectively Improve Lower Limb Flexibility. *J Sports Sci Med.* 18(1): 160–171.

14. Schroeder AN, Best TM. 2015. Is Self Myofascial Release an Effective Preexercise and Recovery Strategy? A Literature Review. *Curr Sports Med Rep.* 14:200–208.

15. Ceca D, Elvira L, Guzmán JF, et al. 2017. Benefits of a Self-Myofascial Release Program on Health-Related Quality of Life in People with Fibromyalgia: A Randomized Control Trial. *J Sports Med Phys Fitness.* 57(7–8):993–1002.

16. Wiewelhove T, Döweling A, Schneider C. 2019. A Meta-Analysis of the Effects of Foam Rolling on Performance and Recovery. *Front Physiol.* 10:376.

17. Okamoto T, Masuhara M, Ikuta K. 2014. Acute Effects of Self-Myofascial Release Using a Foam Roller on Arterial Function. *J Strength Cond Res.* 28(1):69–73.

18. Hotfiel T, Swoboda B, Krinner S, et al. 2017. Acute Effects of Lateral Thigh Foam Rolling on Arterial Tissue Perfusion Determined by Spectral Doppler and Power Doppler Ultrasound. *J Strength Cond Res.* 31(4):893–900.

19. Zhang L, Fan A, Yan J, et al. 2016. Combining Manual Lymph Drainage with Physical Exercise after Modified Radical Mastectomy Effectively Prevents Upper Limb Lymphedema. *Lymphat Res Biol.* 14(2):104–108.

20. Temur K, Kapucu S. 2019. The Effectiveness of Lymphedema Self-Management in the Prevention of Breast Cancer Related Lymphedema and Quality of Life. A Randomized Controlled Trial. *Eur J Oncol Nurs.* 40:22–35.

21. Miller, J. 2012. Self-Myofascia Massage Transforms Chronic Pain in Client with Charcot-Marie Tooth (CMT) Disease aka: Hereditary Sensory Motor-Neuropathy (HSMN). www.fasciacongress.org/2012/Abstracts/52_Miller.pdf.

22. Wasserman JB, Copeland M, Upp M, et al. 2019. Effect of Soft Tissue Mobilization Techniques on Adhesion-Related Pain and Function in the Abdomen: A Systematic Review. *J Bodyw Mov Ther.* 23(2):262–269.

23. Miller, J. 2014. *The Roll Model: A Step by Step Guide to Erase Pain, Improve Mobility and Live Better in Your Body.* Las Vegas, NV: Victory Belt Publishing.

24. Gordon C, Lindner S, Birbaumer N, et al. 2018. Self-Myofascial Vibro-Shearing: A Randomized Controlled Trial of Biomechanical and Related Changes in Male Breakdancers. *Sports Med Open.* 4(1):13.

25. Alonso-Cortes B, Seco-Calvo J, Gonzalez-Cabanach R. 2019. Physiotherapeutic Intervention to Promote Self-Care: Exploratory Study on Spanish Caregivers of Patients With Dementia. *Health Promot Int.* 1–12. doi:10.1093/heapro/daz045

26. Calvert, R. 2002. *The History of Massage: An Illustrated Survey from Around the World.* Rochestor, VT: Healing Arts Press.

27. Elbex Custom & Standard Rubber Extrusions. n.d. Durometer. www.elbex-us.com/sites/default/files/Durometer_0.pdf.

28. Kim Y, Hong Y, Park HS. 2019. A Soft Massage Tool Is Advantageous for Compressing Deep Soft Tissue with Low Muscle Tension: Therapeutic Evidence for Self-Myofascial Release. *Complement Ther Med.* 43:312–318.

29. Anderson, RU, Harvey RH, Wise D. 2015. Chronic Pelvic Pain Syndrome: Reduction of Medication Use after Pelvic Floor Physical Therapy with an Internal Myofascial Trigger Point Wand. *Appl Psychophysiol Biofeedback.* doi:10.1007/s10484-015-9273-1.

30. Pearcey G, Bradbury-Squires D, Kawamoto J, et al. 2015. Foam Rolling for Delayed-Onset Muscle Soreness and Recovery of Dynamic Performance Measures. *J Athl Train.* 50(1):5–13.

31. Blyum L, Driscoll M. 2012. Fascia Congress. www.fasciacongress.org/2012/Abstracts/78_Blyum.docx.

32. Cho JY, Moon H, Park S, et al. 2019. Isolated Injury to the Tibial Division of Sciatic Nerve after Self-Massage of the Gluteal Muscle with Massage Ball: A Case Report. *Medicine (Baltimore)*. 98(19):e15488.

33. Hitzmann, S. 2019. *Melt Performance: A Step-by-Step Program to Accelerate Your Fitness Goals, Improve Balance and Control, and Prevent Chronic Pain and Injuries for Life*. New York: HarperOne.

34. Hicks M, Cao T, Campbell D, Standley P. 2012. Mechanical Strain Applied to Human Fibroblasts Differentially Regulates Skeletal Myoblast Differentiation. *J Appl Physiol*. 113(3):465–472.

35. Cheatham SW, Kolber MJ, Cain M, et al. 2015. The Effects of Self-Myofascial Release Using a Foam Roller or Roller Massager on Joint Range of Motion, Muscle Recovery, and Performance: A Systematic Review. *Int J Sports Phys Ther*. 10(6):827–838.

36. Gibson W, Arendt-Nielsen L, Taguchi T, et al. 2009. Increased Pain from Muscle Fascia Following Eccentric Exercise: Animal and Human Findings. *Exper Brain Res*. 194(2): 299–308.

37. Wilke J, Kalo K, Banzer W. 2019. Gathering Hints for Myofascial Force Transmission Under In Vivo Conditions: Are Remote Exercise Effects Age Dependent? *J Sport Rehabil*. 28(7): 758–763.

38. Park DJ, Hwang YI. 2016. A Pilot Study of Balance Performance Benefit of Myofascial Release, with a Tennis Ball, in Chronic Stroke Patients. *J Bodyw Mov Ther*. 20(1):98–103.

39. Henien M, Sproat C. 2017. Interactive Group Therapy for the Management of Myofascial Temporomandibular Pain. *Br Dent J*. 223(2):90–95.

40. Beardsley C, Skarabot J. 2015. Effects of Self-Myofascial Release: A Systematic Review. *J Bodyw Mov Ther*. 19(4):747–758.

41. Hodgson DD, Lima CD, Low JL, et al. 2018. Four Weeks of Roller Massage Training Did not Impact Range of Motion, Pain Pressure Threshold, Voluntary Contractile Properties or Jump Performance. *Int J Sports Phys Ther*. 13(5):835–845.

42. Barreto DM, Batista MVA. 2017. Swedish Massage: A Systematic Review of its Physical and Psychological Benefits. *Adv Mind Body Med*. 31(2):16–20.

43. Schleip, R. 2003. Fascial Plasticity–A New Neurobiological Explanation: Part 1. *J Bodyw Mov Ther*. 7:11–19.

44. Morikawa Y, Takamoto K, Nishimaru H, et al. April 2017. Compression at Myofascial Trigger Point on Chronic Neck Pain Provides Pain Relief through the Prefrontal Cortex and Autonomic Nervous System: A Pilot Study. *Front Neurosci*. 11:186.

45. Takamoto K, Sakai S, Hori E, et al. 2009. Compression on Trigger Points in the Leg Muscle Increases Parasympathetic Nervous Activity based on Heart Rate Variability. *J Physiol Sci*. 59:191–197.

46. Kim K, Park S, Goo BO, et al. 2014. Effect of Self-Myofascial Release on Reduction of Physical Stress: A Pilot Study. *J Phys Ther Sci*. 26:1779.

47. Cheatham SW, Stull KR. 2018. Knowledge of Self-Myofascial Release among Allied Health Students in the United States: A Descriptive Survey. *J Bodyw Mov Ther*. 22(3):713–717.

48. Halvorson, R. 2016. When Myofascial release Gets Emotional. *Idea Fitness J*. 2016:70–73.

49. Hitzmann, S, Karch, D. 2013. *The Melt Method*. New York: Harper Collins.

50. Oberste M, Schaffrath N, Schmidt K, et al. 2018. Protocol for the "Chemobrain in Motion – study" (CIM – Study): A Randomized Placebo-Controlled Trial of the Impact of a High-Intensity Interval Endurance Training on Cancer Related Cognitive Impairments in Women with Breast Cancer Receiving First-line Chemotherapy. *BMC Cancer*. 18(1):1071.

51. Miller L, Montroni L, Koun E. 2018. Sensing with Tools Extends Somatosensory Processing Beyond the Body. *Nature*. 561(7722):239–242.

Index

Note: Page numbers in bold and italics refer to tables and figures, respectively.